A history of the case study

MANCHESTER
1824

Manchester University Press

A history of the case study

Sexology, psychoanalysis, literature

Birgit Lang, Joy Damousi
and Alison Lewis

Manchester University Press

Published by Manchester University Press
Altrincham Street, Manchester M1 7JA

www.manchesteruniversitypress.co.uk

British Library Cataloguing-in-Publication Data
A catalogue record for this book is available from the British Library

Library of Congress Cataloging-in-Publication Data applied for

ISBN 978 0719 09943 4 *hardback*

First published 2017

Typeset in Bodoni and Futura
by R. J. Footring Ltd, Derby
Printed in Great Britain
by TJ International Ltd, Padstow

Contents

Acknowledgements

This volume was made possible by the Australian Research Council (ARC), which funded the Discovery Project titled 'Making the Case: The Case Study Genre in Sexology, Psychoanalysis, and Literature' led by Birgit Lang and Joy Damousi. The authors acknowledge the vital importance of the ARC in providing generous support for the project.

Thank you to the unfailingly helpful staff of the following archives and libraries (in alphabetical order): Bavarian State Archives Munich; German Literary Archive (Marbach); Monacensia, Literary Archive of the City of Munich; Rare Book and Manuscript Library and the A. C. Long Health Sciences Library at Columbia University (New York); Saxon State and University Library (Dresden); Wellcome Library (London).

Warmest thanks to Katie Sutton, the former Australian Postdoctoral Fellow attached to the ARC project, for commenting on the manuscript. We acknowledge Jana Verhoeven and Mary Tomsic for their outstanding research assistance in Melbourne and New York respectively. The authors extend special thanks to Cynthia Troup, who has managed the editorial process, and prepared and polished all aspects of the manuscript with extraordinary thoroughness and diligence.

We owe much to Emma Brennan, Commissioning Editor and Editorial Director at Manchester University Press. Also at Manchester University Press we sincerely thank the anonymous reviewers and editorial board, and Paul Clarke, Assistant Editor, and Ralph Footring, freelance production editor, for their expertise, efficiency and responsiveness.

Birgit Lang, Joy Damousi, Alison Lewis

Introduction

Birgit Lang, Joy Damousi
and Alison Lewis

A History of the Case Study represents a critical intervention into contemporary debate concerning the construction of knowledge which – after Michel Foucault's elaborations on modern discourses of power – considers the medical case study in particular as an expression of new forms of disciplinary authority. This volume scrutinises the changing status of the human case study, that is, the medical, legal or literary case study that places an individual at its centre. With close reference to the dawning of 'sexual modernity' during the nineteenth and twentieth centuries, and to ideas about sexual identity in the period immediately before and after the fin de siècle, the following chapters examine the case writing practices of selected pioneers of the case study genre.[1] Alertness to the exchange of ideas between the empirical life sciences and the humanities is key to *A History of the Case Study.*

Defined by desire to unravel the mystery of human sexuality and the depths of the human condition, the case study can be linked to the modernist project itself. Indeed, the case study can be defined as one of modernity's vital narrative forms and means of explanation. *A History of the Case Study* builds on our earlier edited collection, *Case Studies and the Dissemination of Knowledge*, and outlines how case knowledge actively contributed to the construction of the sexed subject.[2] The present volume tells the story of the medical case study genre in a historically and geographically contingent manner, with a focus on Central Europe, extended also to the USA. The lives of individual brokers of case knowledge are pivotal to this book, as is the task of mapping their agency and interventions. 'Brokers of case knowledge', however, can be shown to include newly emerging sexual publics, as well as members of professional elites (psychiatrists, psychoanalysts and jurists) and creative writers.

These practitioners took up case studies as a representational practice so as to demonstrate or classify a new phenomenon or pathology; to register a deviation from existing knowledge; to raise questions concerning the meaning of a given example (and by implication its explanatory framework); and to disseminate specialist knowledge to reading publics.

In this context, case studies regularly became sites of reinterpretation and translation, sometimes of resistance. There resulted a range of case modalities. Such 'incarnations of case studies' across different social and disciplinary contexts came to encompass published psychiatric, sexological and psychoanalytic case studies of individuals, as well as case study compilations; unpublished medical notes and juridical case files; autobiographical or journalistic case studies; and fictionalised or fictional case studies ('case stories'). All of these iterations of the case study are inseparable from the history of three fields or kinds of knowledge: sexology, psychoanalysis and literature.

The case study pioneers at the centre of our investigation all participated and were actively involved in discourses connected to the disciplinary sphere of medicine, and especially to the psychiatric realm: Austrian psychiatrist Richard von Krafft-Ebing embraced patient narratives in an attempt to quantify what he could not measure – the sexual paradigm he presupposed. Psychoanalysts, the majority of whom were trained physicians, used the case study genre to reconceptualise the role of creative genius in the light of new scientific and medical insights, or to explore newly urgent socio-political questions, as did Viola Bernard in her analysis of race. State prosecutor Erich Wulffen was able to revitalise the judicial case study genre through the new field of forensics, an imbrication of legal and medical discourse. Physician-writers Oskar Panizza and Alfred Döblin developed new literary cases that incisively commented on specific case writing practices. Each of these writers exemplifies a new language and paradigm, often in competition with other case writers, through which to explore challenges that presented themselves in their time and in their respective fields. An aim of this volume is to chart the emergence and development of the case study in historical terms, and through the medium of biography.

Definitions of the case study

For the key modern theoretician of the case, André Jolles, case studies belong to the very archetypes of narration.[3] Two distinct features define the discursive possibilities of the case study genre: the intrinsic element of judgement; and the 'abductive' or 'guessing' nature of the case study, which can be used in both inductive and deductive styles of reasoning.[4]

Case studies are examples or instances that can be used either to illustrate a rule or a norm, or to signal a deviation from it.[5] In turn, readers of case studies in varying professional, cultural and historical contexts measure the examples or singular events against the norm. In what Umberto Eco would have called 'closed' case studies, clear discursive rules exist within well established fields of knowledge and power, such as the judicial system or institutional religion.[6] These fields shape the structure and wording of a case study, but also presume certain values and beliefs on the part of the readership. A case study simultaneously lends itself to reinterpretation, because the genre 'hovers about' – to cite Lauren Berlant's phrase – 'the singular, the general, and the normative'.[7] In comparison with 'closed case studies', 'open case studies' manipulate their readership in more subtle ways, and with greater insight about their readers, as seen in some psychoanalytic and literary case studies discussed herein. They exploit the genre's tendency towards undecidability, which introduces ongoing ambiguity and provides the condition for the ever-shifting nature of the case study.

In this study, the focus on possibilities for reinterpreting a case study is key; the 'slippery' quality of the genre is highlighted, as a result of the volume's vantage point with regard to the example of the history of sexuality. After Foucault, the case study genre has been identified predominantly as an anchor for new forms of disciplinary authority.[8] Scholars of homosexual and transgender history have made an invaluable contribution to revising this narrative, as part of an attempt to restore agency to those subjects who voluntarily embraced sexological discourse.[9] Yet case studies were powerfully in play beyond the milieu of specific sexual counterpublics (a term from both Michael Warner and Berlant).[10] Their wider workings in relation to a broader history of medical, legal and literary knowledge have not been analysed; neither has the agency of case writers. This volume contributes to the historiography of sexuality by contextualising the preferred case modality of historians of sexuality: the juridical case file. In her study of the 'passing' as male of Hungarian count/ess Sandor/Sarolta Vay, Dutch scholar Geertje Mak underlines the subversive nature of juridical case files, in which are gathered a range of statements that are free of editorial intervention and which do not necessarily present a clear conclusion at the end.[11] The cacophony within the historical juridical case represents a more evocative and open case modality than the typical sexological case, with the editing process seemingly reduced to a minimum, although manipulations of the reader still take place. The seemingly open nature of juridical case writing traditions also prevails in Foucault's case compilations, most famously in *Herculine Barbin: Being the Recently Discovered Memoirs of a Nineteenth-Century French Hermaphrodite*, published in French in 1978 and in English translation two years later. Here, the task of judgement is apparently left to the reader, framed only minimally by the editor-author. The case is not presented through the lens of a sexological expert seeking to present the 'true' sex of the human subject in question.

Foucault's Barbin case begins with the subject's autobiographical account, moves on to the historical dossier – including a timeline of the course of events, two accounts of sexologists and a handful of newspaper articles and surviving personal documents – and ends with 'A Scandal at the Convent', the English translation of a literary account by the German writer Oskar Panizza. Thus, Foucault moves from the intimacy of Barbin's autobiography to the depersonalisation of the medical case study, in order to ambiguously challenge his readers' propensity to find a single truth defining sexuality.[12] The apparent disjunction between autobiographical confession and the clinical language of the medical case studies disquiets the reader, who is left with the knowledge that Barbin's autobiography was literally cut short by sexologists. That Foucault himself edited the sexological case studies in order to present his publication in this way, and in doing so separated autobiography from the sexological frame narrative, is mentioned only in passing. The trajectory of Foucault's compilation clearly takes the reader from a subjective to an objective, less authentic mode, which in turn serves to exemplify Foucault's hypothesis clearly: whatever is fundamental to Barbin's sex, it is not the truth.

Foucault understood that the epistemological nature of case writings always gravitates towards a truth; his writings demonstrate his mastery of the case study genre and its predisposition towards a truth. He ingeniously creates a platform from which to launch his theories of sexuality by capitalising on the confusion that arises in the reader when faced with a range of case studies. Combined with the ongoing interest of historians of sexuality in juridical case files as a valuable resource that 'can take the researcher beyond the crime itself into the social and cultural worlds in which the act took place', Foucault's generic intervention epitomises the strengths and limits of the juridical approach.[13] He subverts the juridical case study form, retains its evocative and open aspect, and minimises its powers of judgement in order to question – with a little additional editorial effort – sexological case writings as well.

Separating the juridical case files from the narrowly defined context of the court, and opening the genre to new enquiries is a commendable and necessary task for historians of sexuality. Yet it seems ironic that during the late nineteenth century and early twentieth century, the subjects on trial, as well as the newly forming sexual public or audience for such case studies, often preferred the medical discourse to the punishment of the law. The former was less judgemental, readily accessible and even more risqué. The analysis of the human case study undertaken in this book provides the history of sexuality with a more complex account of how the sexological case was differentiated and disseminated within and across different fields of knowledge, as well as its transnational diffusion during the course of the twentieth century. Of course, the case study predates this history.

A brief history of the medical case study

Traditionally in medicine, case notes and case studies have been used to develop new categories for disease patterns. In accordance with Ludwik Fleck's notion that the fundamental problem of medical thinking lies in the need to find laws for irregular phenomena, psychiatrists such as

Krafft-Ebing sought such laws.[14] Carol Berkenkotter describes how, within psychiatry, both the move away from mainstream scientific discourse, and the central role of case histories in setting the discipline's professional discourse, produced an increasing emphasis on individual stories.[15] Ivan Crozier has noted that psychiatrists learned to interpret case studies as part of their doctoral training and that the choice to publish specific case studies represented their efforts to position themselves in a dynamic new field of knowledge.[16] By comparing similar cases, psychiatrists created concepts and categories in an attempt to classify patients and their non-normative – or non-reproductively oriented – desires and behaviours.

In these developments, the medical case study became the key form of writing, since it was singularly capable of summarising the patient statement as well as the doctor's assessment. Krafft-Ebing, for instance, arguably used the mode of the medical case study to order his thoughts on the narrative presented by a given patient, editing, omitting and evaluating what was said, while embedding this knowledge into his own theories of sexual taxonomy. The fact that the early study of sexuality was based primarily on the oral or written testimony of patients controlled their statements, but also privileged them. This underlines the possibility of patient agency, and also better explains patients' desire to participate in the Foucaultian 'perpetual spirals of power and pleasure' that defined sexological discourse.[17] In other words, the exploration of sexuality became a widely anthropological project, with a propensity to reconceptualise and rewrite patient statements.

Such a 'narrative turn' constituted a veritable shift away from the body, and presented numerous opportunities and challenges, including the potential for a new interdisciplinarity. Previously, case studies had functioned as a means of conveying and containing medical knowledge about patients' bodies (notably about their sexual anatomy). Now the focus on testimony and truth-finding forced psychiatrists like Krafft-Ebing to think more deeply about the evidentiary value of their sources. The same concern with testimony and truth-finding also made the medical case study attractive to a range of disciplines and fields of knowledge that relied on the spoken and written word, such as psychoanalysis and literature. The fact that medical interest in sexuality in the nineteenth century was 'intrinsically linked to forensic medicine' – as Harry Oosterhuis has forcefully stated – meant, furthermore, that the human case study was situated at the intersection of medical and legal discourses.[18] At the advent of sexual modernity, the accessibility of case vignettes in medical case study compilations also proved compelling for lay readers, who were more and more willing to engage with the world around them, and with literary works, through a new scientific paradigm that suited their needs with respect to identity formation.

By the 1890s the global base of psychiatry had shifted from France to the German-speaking world. This shift influenced those institutional practices that were affecting the range of emerging case modalities.

Case writings in France traditionally allowed for a greater permeability between different fields of knowledge. The legal situation in Germany and Austria, as well social and religious taboos, shaped distinctive disciplinary-based case modalities: in Germany and Austria literature had traditionally provided another way of examining 'pathological' case studies.[19] Yet in German-speaking Central Europe in the late nineteenth century, *belles-lettres* rarely explicitly portrayed sexual feelings or sexual activity, and did so mostly through suggestion. Sophisticated intellectual debates about sexuality remained sporadic, even for the most revered literary case modality, the German novella. Early psychiatrists regretted such limits in representation, and by 1900 researchers working in the life sciences controversially used the lives of certain creative writers and other 'cultural greats' to illustrate psychiatric illness to a lay audience. Due to the powerful nature of medical discourse, literature responded to this medicalisation most vehemently, by means of satire. The proponents of such mockery included: German playwright Frank Wedekind, whose polemic poem 'Perversität' ('Perversity') was originally titled 'Krafft-Ebing'; contrarian Viennese cultural critic Karl Kraus; and German entertainer Otto Reutter, whose satirical 'Hirschfeld song' (1908) made fun of the classificatory ambitions of sexologists and psychiatrists. Panizza's *Psichopatia criminalis* (1898) represents the most poignant example of such a satire, in that he ridiculed the implications of the psychiatrists' will to classify, and used the formal elements of the medical case study to subvert its meanings. Only after the First World War did writers embrace the empathetic potential of the medical case study with greater self-confidence.

The democratisation of Central Europe coincided with the peak and downfall of the case study in its medical guise after 1918. The dissemination of academic and expert knowledge to specific target audiences and, for the first time, to a mass audience returned to the genre a new sense of urgency and morality. Yet this new accessibility coincided with a wider shift in the life sciences away from the case study as an important methodological means; the result was a broad decline in the respectability of the genre. Pedagogical warnings from academic experts lost their appeal. The criminal and sexed subjects who had been the focus of the human case study for three decades now wrote and published their own cases, and found a keen readership. As elaborated in Chapter 4 of the present volume, the authors of such autobiographical texts included master thief and con man Georges Manolescu and convicted sex offenders, such as the paedophile teacher Edith Cadivec. Their autobiographical accounts could include a self-aggrandising romanticisation of sex and crime, and thus helped to foster cultural anxieties, particularly among liberal academic experts. In a politically unstable democratic milieu where the scope for effective censorship was limited, caught between profanisation and moralisation, the liberating and empowering potential of the case study became largely neglected during this period.

In the turbulent times of the inter-war years, the case modality with the most consistent methodological and academic formation remained the psychoanalytic case study – a distinct variant of the medical case study. After ambiguous beginnings, and a need to separate from psychiatric modes of reasoning, psychoanalysis came into its own as a discipline at this time. However, in the 1930s the overwhelming majority of Central European practitioners were forced into exile, from which most did not return, a pattern that continued throughout the Second World War. From 1945 onwards, the case study as a genre was conspicuously mobilised in numerous contexts, and notably in the USA, where a more open approach to sexuality helped to promote studies by Alfred Kinsey, and William Masters and Virginia Johnson.

Sexology

The rise of the human case study was shaped by two crucial and inter-related circumstances: its medical origins and its geography. The genre's prestige was underpinned by the high social status accorded to the spheres of medicine and psychiatry in Germany and Austria in the late nineteenth century. Always concerned with respectability, in their moralising discourses the middle classes focused on decency and avoided excessively detailed descriptions of sexual matters (with the exception of avant-garde theatre, which frequently pushed the limits of respectability to the brink). Erotic and pornographic writing flourished, but was published in private editions; both kinds of writing were usually censored, and on the same grounds. Within this broader discursive context, sexological case studies presented by far the most respectable framework for the depiction of sexual behaviour, even though their predominant focus on non-normative sexual conditions and identities was generally embedded in a larger forensic discourse of criminality.

Edited by medical experts, these historical case studies of sexual pathologies functioned, like medical case studies today, as an attempt to 'control the subjectivity of the observer-narrator and to stabilise and evaluate the encapsulated narrative of the patient who is its object'.[20] The closed form of the sexological case study compilation underlined the respectable nature of the undertaking. Here, case narratives – presented through the threefold structure of anamnesis, personal enquiry and diagnosis – illustrated newly emerging sexological and psychiatric theories. Since bodies did not 'speak' (at least before the onset of hormonal research), and fieldwork included sometimes insurmountable moral and practical difficulties, psychiatrists were obliged to give new levels of credibility to their patients' own statements and words. As a consequence, psychiatrists' carefully edited summaries of medical case notes were often interspersed with autobiographical material sourced directly from their patients, or from correspondents.

The formalised configuration of sexological case studies, as well as their presentation in case compilations, adhered to the structure of medical discourse and served, therefore, to rebut criticism from other medical disciplines. The quoted autobiographical materials provided rich evidence of explorations into emerging sexual subjectivities, which included some quite explicit and potentially sexually arousing passages for their readers. The subjects of these case studies sought legitimisation for their sexual preferences, life choices and identities. As Klaus Müller highlights in his account of the historical writings of male 'inverts', these individuals presented their autobiographical writings to sexologists voluntarily, and often expressed a desire to aid German science.[21] As mentioned above, Foucault has ascribed such desire to the workings of 'perpetual spirals of power and pleasure' between sexology and its informants.[22] However, sexological case studies provided for an array of emerging sexual subjectivities, subjectivities that were judged by, but also legitimised through, the respectable medical framing narrative. Hence reading offered an opportunity for recognition but also – and this was feared by sexologists and their patients – for sexual arousal. Readers' reinterpretations of particular passages written in the first person in turn influenced sexological thought, as seen with reference to Leopold von Sacher-Masoch, who was categorised as a masochist by some of his masochist readers. This readership reinterpreted Sacher-Masoch's novellas; their interpretation was then valorised through sexological discourse, and contemporaneously by cultural historians of sexuality, making the readers' views more socially acceptable at the time.

Psychoanalysis

The most powerful innovation in scientific knowledge of the human subject in the second half of the nineteenth century came from psychoanalysis. If sexology created a new platform for modern subjectivities, psychoanalysis made the relationship between analyst and patient the central scene of the (talking) cure and offered a new understanding of the reading public at large. Different from psychiatry and sexology, psychoanalysis reflected on the idealising trends of the German public in a sophisticated manner, and regularly expressed the fear that expert deliberations on genius and creativity would be interpreted as a defamation of national idols. Psychoanalyst Wilhelm Stekel sought to counter resistance to such interrogation in 1912:

> Until recently the maxim prevailed that the image of a great artist needs to be conveyed in an untainted form to posterity. Biographers saw their main task in removing dark chapters – or what they conceived to be dark chapters – from the life of their 'hero' and to convey an image of impeccable shine. We nearly retained a gallery of great human beings, a Valhalla of farouche gods, had not the accounts of one artist or the other, just like

> their works, taught us from time to time that geniuses – be they inventors, philosophers, founders of religions, poets and artists – are only human beings, with all their mistakes. What they lost in scope, they won in love and deepened insight.[23]

While analysts used the case study more self-reflexively than psychiatrists, both were vividly aware of the genre's persuasive hold as an instrument of projection and objectification. The heated nature of debates concerning artists and creativity in psychoanalytic circles owed much to the identification of psychoanalysts with creative artists. Sigmund Freud himself considered these tendencies in the German readership by developing a new case modality, the dialogic-psychoanalytic case study, which considered fragments of the life and oeuvre of creative minds. The impetus for Freud's variant of the case study was partly his wish to avoid causing offence to his middle-class readership.

Psychoanalysis was conceptualised as a life science; like literature, psychoanalysis was considered to stand astride the presumed divide between science and arts, and so it provided a bridging link between the two fields of psychiatry and literature. In the history of psychoanalysis, the years 1906–14 engendered what Frank J. Sulloway has called, by way of criticism, a literary style of reasoning.[24] While psychoanalytic case studies decisively differed from their psychiatric counterparts, the scientific self-image of psychoanalysis is undeniable. John Forrester, in his pioneering article 'Thinking in cases', best describes how psychoanalysis created 'a new way of telling a life in the twentieth century, a new form for the specific and unique facts that make that person's life their life; and at the same time, it attempts to render that way of telling a life public, of making it scientific'.[25] Received more positively than implied by Freud, psychoanalytic approaches were incorporated into other disciplinary fields, while also meeting some resistance. Overall, psychoanalysis pioneered the case study as a methodological approach and produced 'an authoritative form that is distinctly interdisciplinary, profound and enduring'.[26] In the USA, the period between 1945 and 1965 witnessed the rapid rise of psychoanalytic psychiatry. By the mid-twentieth century, psychoanalysis was becoming well accepted; increasing numbers of psychiatrists with medical backgrounds, were beginning to train in this approach.[27] Psychoanalytic writings found expression in the popular arena through films, literature and magazines, and over this period ideas from Freud's writings and his immediate circle of adherents found expression in many cultural forms.[28]

Literature

Most recently among historians of sexuality as well as literary scholars, debate about the making of sexual modernity has emphasised the interplay between the realms of science and those of literature and cultural history. While literature played an important role in the formation of sexological knowledge in England and France, the role of literature in the German lands has been understood differently.[29] French writers of the nineteenth century had already observed that the modern age urgently needed to anchor its literature in real life and to document modern maladies. The sickness of their era was hysteria, and writers such as Gustave Flaubert plumbed this topic for a voracious readership.[30] In German-speaking Central Europe the mere perusal of Krafft-Ebing's medical case study compilation *Psychopathia Sexualis* was feared to have 'psychopathic effects' on some readers. This is at least in part attributable to the belief of medical elites that masturbation had a detrimental influence on the mental health of individuals. Thus it is hardly surprising that Krafft-Ebing originally hesitated to include references to literary works in his oeuvre. Between 1886 and 1890 he discussed literary works and their authors – such as the Marquis de Sade or Jean Jacques Rousseau – only when other, mostly French sexologists had cited them beforehand.[31] Krafft-Ebing also remained within the bounds of bourgeois sexual respectability by avoiding references to the plethora of erotic fiction that could have provided a useful source for his studies. Such material – whether relatively respectable works of erotic fiction marketed to middle-class men; pulp fiction; saucy romance novels or photographs – was available to wide segments of the male population in the late nineteenth century through the black market in erotica and pornography.[32]

Initially, the moral division in the German-speaking world between erotica and *belles-lettres* prompted a turn to satire among literary writers. The most provocative example of such satire, Panizza's *Psichopatia criminalis*, represents the inversion of the case study genre. However, by the early twentieth century, bourgeois forms of cultural expression needed to adapt so as to contend with newer maladies and social ills. As the privileged cultural form of the *Bildungsbürgertum*, literature faced challenges from many quarters, challenges that an 'empirical turn' could not adequately address without a more radical reinvention of the parameters of literature itself. In the modern metropolis, the writers of *belles-lettres* found themselves confronted by the great complexity and interconnectivity of life forms, and with competing and multiplying forms of knowledge about these life forms. Any attempt to make sense of the many innovations in science and the arts felt daunting.

Indeed, especially since the rise of naturalist movements, writers of literature experienced immense pressure to move with the times. Each successive new movement or style that emerged in the first two decades of the twentieth century – expressionism, Dada, surrealism and the avant-garde – sought to address the many economic, political and social crises of the era in different ways. Expressionism, which dominated the literary scene in the years from 1910 to 1925, was advocated as a corrective to naturalism, challenging perceptions of reality far more radically than before. In the words of Marxist philosopher Ernst Bloch, the predominant way all writers adapted material from real life for literature was 'by smashing it': 'the prevailing world no longer offers them a representable illusion which may be fashioned into a story, but just emptiness and inside this some mixable rubble'.[33] Both naturalist and expressionist writers had striven to incorporate the latest findings from disciplines as disparate as medicine, psychiatry, sexology, criminology and the law. As was typical in the aftermath of the First World War, writers were unsure of the future of literary markets and of what increased competition from other media might mean for their livelihoods. In this rapidly modernising field, the case study genre arguably became for a brief time 'the answer' to 'the problem' that literature had become. Yet in the process of espousing this answer, the resultant literature became almost incomprehensible, shaped by an anxiety, if not a neurosis, about shoring up each work's epistemological foundations. Literature became a laboratory, a humanistic corollary to the laboratories of other life sciences from which it borrowed some of its inspiration. Still, in taking on the empirical world, as well as the worlds of fiction and make-believe, literature came almost entirely unstuck.

Joe Cleary has contended that the collapse of the European imperial world brought about the collapse of the Anglo-French literary world system. Until the First World War, Paris and London were the uncontested centres of world literature; bourgeois realism and the advent of the novel were considered the supreme achievements of world literature. According to this view, the 'breakup of the old London- and Paris-centred literary world-system' sparked a concomitant crisis of realism.[34] By far the greatest threat to realism, and hence to the dominant literary world system, came from the newer fashion of modernism. As Cleary points out, interestingly, the major theorists of the modern novel of the early twentieth century – as well as its main detractors – all came from the semi-periphery of the literary world system. Georg Lukács was born in the Austro-Hungarian Empire, Erich Auerbach hailed from Berlin, Mikhail Bakhtin from Oryol in Russia. Most of them cast this aesthetic crisis in catastrophic and even apocalyptic terms. Due to their personal experience of collapsing empires and regimes, these theorists and critics could not help but view the downfall of realism as the passing of a literary style. Moreover, in all but one of their accounts, modernist literature had itself become symptomatic of a more global, far-reaching trend of declining morality and value systems.[35] The antidote they envisaged was to turn the clock back to an earlier mode of representation based on realism and mimesis. For example, Auerbach praised the more moderate modernist Virginia Woolf over the more radical Irish modernist James Joyce, because of Woolf's ability to portray with 'realist depth'.[36] Lukács pitted Joyce, Döblin and Robert Musil unfavourably against Alexander Pushkin and Thomas Mann. He argued that Joyce and Döblin displayed 'a morbid preoccupation with the perversely atypical', while Mann and Pushkin confronted the spiritual problems of the German and Russian peoples.[37] Although Bakhtin's account of the rise and fall of realism differs from those offered by Auerbach and Lukács, his work, too, in the view of Cleary, is 'in the throes of the terrific European and world crisis that had erupted with devastating effect in World War I and would erupt again, even more violently, in World War II'.[38]

The return to realism that many intellectuals from Central Europe imagined as the answer to modernity's aporias involved a rethinking of the relationship between the arts and sciences. It required writers to undo the strict division of natural sciences from the arts or humanities (*Geisteswissenschaften*), which, although a hallmark of the age, cultural historians today commonly regard as obsolete. In recent years, European literary scholars such as Ottmar Ette have emphatically stressed literature's affinity with the life sciences. Ette describes literature as an 'experimental dynamic space' that is concerned with the social aspects of life, that is, our 'knowledge-of-living-together' (*ZusammenLebensWissen*).[39] Bernhard J. Dotzler argues in a similar vein. He remarks that literature itself can be an 'exploratory practice', in multiple senses of the term.[40] Latterly, rather than seeking the points of intersection between the human and the natural sciences, literary scholars have been keen to explore the particular 'poetology of knowledge' that supports literary knowledge in distinction to other forms. Before discussing ways in which the various writers and thinkers discussed in this volume grappled with these questions, it is worth recollecting that all literature simultaneously conveys knowledge and processes it.[41] As Dotzler affirms, nonetheless, not all knowledge is science.[42]

***

A History of the Case Study begins in Chapter 1 with an exploration of the influence of literature on both sexology and psychiatry in the early history of these fields during the late nineteenth century, an era in which human case studies were used to stabilise knowledge and to dismantle it. That chapter investigates the agency of the sexual public, and the indirect power wielded by these readers and patients of sexology in defending the truth of sexological case writings. Through the works and the figure of Sacher-Masoch, the chapter considers how during this period medical case studies functioned as sites of reinterpretation by doctors, and by sexological patients and other members of an emerging sexual public. Sacher-Masoch's literary case study, his novella *Venus im Pelz* (*Venus in Furs*), constitutes the first fictional account of what became known as masochism; readers' reinterpretation of the novella demonstrates how an emerging sexual public reappropriated an alleged biographical truth about the author. Ian Hacking – who has described himself as a 'philosopher of the particular case' – speaks of the 'looping effect of classifying human beings'; Hacking's phrase expresses how 'classifying changes people, but the changed people cause classifications themselves to be redrawn'.[43]

Chapter 1 describes such a looping effect and exemplifies how a newly forming sexual public, valorised through medical discourse, created an important epistemological shift in sexologists' thinking about authors.

Chapter 2 turns to another discipline that was crucial to the formation of the modern sexual subject: psychoanalysis, which was in the 1890s and into the early decades of the twentieth century a discipline 'in the making'. The chapter investigates how psychoanalysis and its proponents co-opted and adapted the medical case study as an extant and authoritative rhetorical form through which to forge a new mode of enquiry. Like sexologists, psychoanalysts were keen advocates of the case writing method, adapting techniques and writing styles from medical case histories and also from literature. Psychiatrists as well as psychoanalysts in the German-speaking world explored the discursive connection between insanity and creativity.

Additionally, Chapter 2 examines how psychoanalysts sought to incorporate and adapt sexological pathographies into psychoanalytic thought. Responses within the Vienna Psychoanalytic Society (WPV) to Isidor Sadger's psychoanalytic biographies of writers and their works fuelled a debate that directly contributed to Freud's development of psychoanalytic case writing. Much of Freud's thinking about artists and writers can be found in the works of Otto Rank. Freud advised Rank, and collaborated with him while Rank was theorising the creative personality for his book *Der Künstler* (*The Artist*), first published in 1907; the collaboration continued for many years. Freud took the debate concerning creative genius to a new methodological level. He concluded that – as intensive discussions within the WPV had shown – the life and work of artists, like the life and work of any patient, could not be encapsulated in a single case study. Rather, the psychoanalytic method could represent only a certain aspect of a patient's life. This finding freed the case study genre from its biographical focus and made it a site of explanation rather than mere illustration.[44]

Late nineteenth-century and fin-de-siècle writers first engaged with the case study genre in its psychiatric and psychoanalytic manifestations by means of satire, as recounted in Chapter 3. The chapter contrasts the interpretative powers of modern sexual publics and professional elites with the agency of the writer. It does so through enquiry into Panizza's satirical and delusional negotiation of the boundaries between the two 'cultures' of art and science (*pace* C. P. Snow). Panizza's first exposure to the case study genre was in the context of his training as a psychiatrist. More than a decade before Freud's elaborations on the psychoanalytic case, Panizza made the human case study a central form in his literary oeuvre. Panizza's case writings encompass two modalities through which literature engaged with the case study genre: he fictionalised actual patient case studies and he parodied medical case writing in his biting anti-psychiatric work *Psichopatia criminalis*. Panizza's engagement with the case study genre remains haunted by his own unruly psyche. During his psychological decline towards the end of his literary career Panizza withdrew from writing fiction. His case writings took the shape of cultural historical studies of topics related to his progressively more delusional inner world, and so they contributed to the process of Panizza's self-destruction. A short investigation into the way that psychoanalysis and psychoanalytic case studies enabled literary satire concludes the chapter.

A History of the Case Study also investigates the widely neglected field of juridical sexology, Chapter 4 showing how Wulffen's works incorporated literary knowledge into a legal and criminological framework. The chapter focuses on the pedagogical imperatives of legal reform and on Wulffen's recourse to the case study genreso that he might appeal to various coexisting professional, literary and mass audiences. His professional investment in the case study makes for a telling illustration of the rise and fall of the genre in the first decades of the twentieth century, when the increasing dissemination and accessibility of case modalities beyond the professional realms of the clinic and the court led to a change in its status. In order to popularise issues of legal reform, Wulffen exploited the accessible nature of the case study genre in an attempt to reach a wider audience, and he wrote some of the first published expert case studies that addressed both a professional and an educated public. While Wulffen's expert case studies were highly successful during the Wilhelmine era, the same approach and model for case writing met a more critical audience after 1918. Wulffen embraced the challenge of a new democratic environment by writing implicitly didactical popular crime novels. However, eventually his criminal subjects literally 'wrote back' after their sensationalised trials, using case studies in an attempt to narrate their own versions of events. The accounts of these criminals-turned-writers were often more marketable, influential and financially successful than the accounts by sexological or legal experts such as Wulffen. Thus the popularisation of sensationalist case studies written, for instance, by perpetrators of crime, was an important factor in the case study genre's loss of respectability.

After the First World War, realist literature continued to be informed by new configurations of knowledge around the criminal and pathological self. This is witnessed in Chapter 5, which concentrates on works by Döblin, a medical doctor and a main representative of the 1920s New Objectivity aesthetic movement in Germany. Other authors were preoccupied with questions of social justice, but Döblin was particularly interested in gender relations and sexually motivated violence. He represented these by drawing on contemporary psychoanalytic and sexological discourses about masochism and sadism. Many of Döblin's main characters were convicted criminals and he fashioned himself in his autobiographical writings as a literary Jack the Ripper. This coincided with the publication, for the first time, of convicted criminals' autobiographical accounts of their own lives outside the spheres of the clinic and the public of the court.

Authors with a background in the law or medicine, whose professional engagement brought them into close proximity with real criminal cases – writers such as Wulffen and Döblin – found themselves well placed to capture the imaginations of an increasingly educated and well informed reading public. The latter had developed an appetite for shocking crime stories based on empirical cases. In the lead-up to the outbreak of the First World War, writers in major cities such as Berlin, Vienna and Munich had begun to tackle several of the pressing social problems of the age, and after the war many continued to focus on war-related problems such as war trauma, shell-shock and sexually motivated violence. Readers' interest was heightened by additional anxieties of the age concerning society's decadence and the perils of accelerated modernisation and urbanisation. Somewhat to their surprise, doctors and judges also found themselves in competition with an unexpected source of knowledge about the criminal underworld. This competition was provided by the latest craze in first-person accounts penned by the con men and criminals themselves. Possibly, the writer of middlebrow to highbrow literature with insider knowledge of crime still had some advantage over criminals, but he or she needed to find fresh ways to seize the attention of an audience. If there was an unmet demand for criminal material, then Döblin, practising as a social welfare doctor in one of Germany's most seductive and dangerous metropolises, was well placed to respond.

Chapter 6 discusses the use of the psychoanalytic case study in a very different and modern form, drawing on the dramatically different historical context of post-war American politics and society, and the civil rights movement. The writing and experience of Viola Bernard, a psychoanalyst of German-Jewish background, is the subject of Chapter 6. Bernard's history allows for a close examination of the transnational and transcultural aspects of sexuality and psychoanalysis in connection with the case study genre. The chapter describes a set of circumstances in which case writing from one discipline was brought to bear directly on a landmark juridical case, and demonstrates how the wide dispersal of the rhetoric of the case study within the public domain can be placed in the service of a socio-political cause. Rather than an examination of a case modality *per se*, here the theme is a case study 'in formation'. The issue of race is brought into the expert purview of psychoanalysis, and Bernard is involved in assisting the development of a highly topical and transformative case study narrative about black subjects for and within the African-American community. Through the figure of Bernard, Chapter 6 points to the challenges involved in publicly advocating case studies that have immediate, appreciable consequences for redefining a long-institutionalised 'norm' such as racial segregation. As such, the chapter sustains the approach taken in earlier ones, referencing an individual's pioneering case writing with an attunement to its radical implications.

Laura Doan has recently argued that, for the historian of modern sexuality, the ways 'in which the normal might be seen as jostling against ... existing discourses of morality and class-inflected notions of respectability' can represent a major challenge.[45] The analysis of the case study genre presented in this volume contributes to a more multifaceted understanding of the formation of knowledge and the agency of case writers. The reinterpretation and circulation of knowledge undertaken by those foregrounded in the following chapters did not take the form of the case by chance. John Frow has argued that the work of genre 'is to mediate between a social situation and the text which realizes certain features of this situation, or which responds strategically to its demands'.[46] Case studies exemplify a norm and are measured against other norms by their readers in varying professional, cultural and historical contexts. For this reason they are bound more tightly to their interpretative framework than other genres.[47] They can often be found at the forefront of knowledge formation, since they have the ability to poignantly epitomise deviation from a presumed norm. At the same time, they rely on a framework of interpretation, however exploratory; changing frameworks and immediate historical contexts, in turn, may gravely alter or compromise the given interpretation of a case study's meaning. *A History of the Case Study* highlights this vital, generative aspect of the case study genre.

Notes

1 See Harry Oosterhuis, 'Sexual Modernity in the Works of Richard von Krafft-Ebing and Albert Moll', *Medical History*, 56 (2012), pp. 133–55; Anthony Giddens, *The Transformation of Intimacy: Sexuality, Love and Eroticism in Modern Societies* (Stanford: Stanford University Press, 1992).

2 Joy Damousi, Birgit Lang and Katie Sutton (eds), *Case Studies and the Dissemination of Knowledge* (New York: Routledge, 2015).

3 See André Jolles, *Einfache Formen. Legende, Sage, Mythe, Rätsel, Spruch, Kasus, Memorabile, Märchen, Witz* (Tübingen: Max Niemeyer, 1930), pp. 171–99.

4 On the 'abductive' nature of the case study see Charles S. Peirce, 'Lectures on Pragmatism. Lecture VI. Three Types of Reasoning', in Charles Hartshorne and Paul Weiss (eds), *Collected Papers of Charles Sanders Peirce, Vol. V* (Cambridge: Harvard University Press, 1934), pp. 151–79, p. 171.

5 Jolles, *Einfache Formen*, p. 185.

6 Umberto Eco, *The Open Work* (Cambridge: Harvard University Press, 1989), p. 7.

7 Lauren Berlant, 'On the Case', *Critical Inquiry*, 33:4 (2007), pp. 663–72, p. 664.

8 John Forrester, 'If p, Then What? Thinking in Cases', *History of the Human Sciences*, 9:3 (1996), pp. 1–25, pp. 11–12.

9 See for example Ivan Crozier, 'Pillow Talk: Credibility, Trust and the Sexological Case History', *History of Science*, 46:4 (2008), pp. 375–404; Klaus Müller, *Aber in meinem Herzen sprach eine Stimme so laut: homosexuelle Autobiographien und medizinische Pathographien im neunzehnten Jahrhundert* (Berlin: Rosa Winkel, 1991); Harry Oosterhuis, *Stepchildren of Nature: Krafft-Ebing, Psychiatry, and the Making of Sexual Identity* (Chicago: University of Chicago Press, 2000).

10 Lauren Berlant and Michael Warner, 'Sex in Public', *Critical Inquiry*, 24:2 (1998), pp. 547–66.

11 Geertje Mak, *Doubting Sex: Inscriptions, Bodies and Selves in Nineteenth-Century Hermaphrodite Case Histories* (Manchester: Manchester University Press, 2012), p. 63.

12 Michel Foucault, *Herculine Barbin: Being the Recently Discovered Memoirs of a Nineteenth-Century French Hermaphrodite* (Brighton: Harvester Press, 1980), p. xi.

13 Stephen Robertson, 'What's Law Got To Do With It? Legal Records and Sexual Histories', *Journal of the History of Sexuality*, 14:1/2 (2005), pp. 161–2.
14 Ludwik Fleck, 'Some Specific Features of the Medical Way of Thinking (1927)', in Robert S. Cohen and Thomas Schnelle (eds), *Cognition and Fact: Materials on Ludwik Fleck* (Dordrecht: Springer Netherlands, 1986), pp. 39–46, p. 39.
15 Carol Berkenkotter, *Patient Tales: Case Histories and the Uses of Narrative in Psychiatry* (Columbia: University of South Carolina Press, 2008), pp. 29, 103.
16 Crozier, 'Pillow Talk', p. 380.
17 Michel Foucault, *The History of Sexuality, vol. I: An Introduction*, trans. Robert Hurley (New York: Vintage Books, 1990), p. 45.
18 Oosterhuis, 'Sexual Modernity', p. 133.
19 See, for example, Vernon A. Rosario, *The Erotic Imagination: French Histories of Perversities* (Oxford: Oxford University Press, 1997).
20 Kathryn Montgomery Hunter, *Doctors' Stories: The Narrative Structure of Medical Knowledge* (Princeton: Princeton University Press, 1991), p. 166.
21 Müller, *Aber in meinem Herzen*, pp. 327–8.
22 Foucault, *The History of Sexuality*, p. 45.
23 The English translation of this passage is by the author of this chapter. The original German reads: 'Bis vor kurzer Zeit galt noch der Grundsatz, das Bild eines grossen Künstlers müsse der Nachwelt fleckenlos erhalten bleiben und die Biographen sahen ihre Hauptaufgabe darin, dunkle Punkte – oder was sie für dunkle Punkte hielten – aus dem Leben ihrer „Helden" zu entfernen und das Bild in tadellosem Glanze der Nachwelt zu überliefern. So hätten wir fast statt einer Galerie grosser Menschen eine Walhalla mit unnahbaren Göttern erhalten, wenn nicht Aufzeichnungen des einen oder anderen Künstlers, ebenso wie seine Werke, uns von Zeit zu Zeit belehrt hätten, dass Genies, ob sie nun Erfinder, Philosophen, Religionsstifter, Dichter oder Künstler sind, auch nur Menschen mit allen Fehlern der Menschen sind. Was sie an Distanz eingebüsst haben, haben sie an Liebe und tieferem Verständnis gewonnen'. Wilhelm Stekel, *Die Träume der Dichter. Eine vergleichende Untersuchung der unbewussten Triebkräfte bei Dichtern, Neurotikern und Verbrechern (Bausteine zur Psychologie des Künstlers und des Kunstwerks)* (Wiesbaden: Bergmann, 1912), pp. 15–16. The standard English translation of Stekel's work omits this passage. See Wilhelm Stekel, 'Poetry and Neurosis: Contributions to the Psychology of the Artist and of Artistic Creative Ability', *Psychoanalytic Review*, 10 (1923), pp. 73–96, 190–208, 316–28, and the final instalment in *Psychoanalytic Review*, 11 (1924), pp. 48–60.
24 Frank J. Sulloway, 'Reassessing Freud's Case Histories. The Social Construction of Psychoanalysis', *Isis*, 82 (1991), pp. 245–75, p. 265.
25 Forrester, 'If p, Then What? Thinking in Cases', p. 10.
26 Joy Damousi, Birgit Lang and Katie Sutton, 'Introduction: Case Studies and the Dissemination of Knowledge', in Damousi, Lang and Sutton (eds), *Case Studies and the Dissemination of Knowledge*, pp. 1–12, p. 5.
27 Nathan G. Hale, *The Rise and Crisis of Psychoanalysis in the United States: Freud and the Americans, 1917–1985* (Oxford: Oxford University Press, 1995), p. 246.
28 Hale, *The Rise and Crisis of Psychoanalysis*, pp. 276–99.
29 See Heike Bauer, *English Literary Sexology: Translations of Inversion, 1860–1930* (Basingstoke: Palgrave Macmillan, 2009); Anna Katharina Schaffner, *Modernism and Perversion: Sexual Deviance in Sexology and Literature, 1850–1930* (Basingstoke: Palgrave Macmillan, 2012).
30 See Janet Beizer, 'Emma's Daughter: Femininity, Maternity, and "Mothersickness" in *Madame Bovary*', in Suzanne Nash (ed.), *Home and Its Dislocations in Nineteenth-Century France* (Albany: New York Press, 1993), pp. 265–83, p. 266.
31 In the case of the Marquis de Sade, Krafft-Ebing seems especially dismissive. In the first edition of *Psychopathia Sexualis* he calls de Sade a monster, and refers to him merely for reasons of exhaustiveness, since de Sade is repeatedly quoted

by French writers. See Richard von Krafft-Ebing, *Psychopathia Sexualis. Eine klinisch-forensische Studie*, 1st edition (Stuttgart: Enke, 1886), p. 44. By the fourth edition of *Psychopathia Sexualis* the original seven-line reference to de Sade has grown to two short paragraphs and an extensive footnote that gives a summary of the nobleman's life. Krafft-Ebing mentions de Sade's literary works only in passing, and describes them as 'obscene novels oozing wanton and cruelty', pointing to the fact that they were later burned. See Richard von Krafft-Ebing, *Psychopathia Sexualis*, 4th edition (Stuttgart: Enke, 1889), pp. 49–50.

32 Paul Englisch, *Geschichte der erotischen Literatur* (Stuttgart: Püttmann, 1927), pp. 272–4.

33 Ernst Bloch as quoted in Georg Lukács, 'The Playful Style', in *Essays on Thomas Mann*, trans. Stanley Mitchell (New York: Howard Fertig, 1978), pp. 98–134, p. 102.

34 Joe Cleary, 'Realism after Modernism and the Literary World-System', *Modern Language Quarterly*, 73:3 (2012), pp. 255–68, p. 261.

35 Cleary, 'Realism after Modernism', p. 256.

36 Cleary, 'Realism after Modernism', p. 256.

37 Cleary, 'Realism after Modernism', p. 256.

38 Cleary, 'Realism after Modernism', p. 257.

39 Ottmar Ette, 'Vorwort', in Ottmar Ette (ed.), *Wissensformen und Wissensnormen des ZusammenLebens: Literatur – Kultur – Geschichte – Medien* (Berlin: de Gruyter, 2012), pp. i–vii, p. vi.

40 Bernhard J. Dotzler, 'Wissen in Geschichten: Zur wechselseitigen Erhellung von Literatur, Medien und Wissenschaft', *Berichte zur Wissenschaftsgeschichte*, 32:4 (2009), pp. 319–28, p. 319.

41 Dotzler, 'Wissen in Geschichten', p. 319.

42 Dotzler, 'Wissen in Geschichten', p. 319.

43 Ole Jacob Madsen, '"I am a philosopher of the particular case": An Interview with the 2009 Holberg Prizewinner Ian Hacking', *History of the Human Sciences*, 26:3 (2013), pp. 32–51, p. 39; Ian Hacking, 'Between Michel Foucault and Erving Goffman: Between Discourse in the Abstract and Face-to-Face Interaction', *Economy and Society*, 33:3 (2004), pp. 277–302, p. 279.

44 Sigmund Freud, 'Ratschläge für den Arzt bei der psychoanalytischen Behandlung (1912)', in Sigmund Freud, *Gesammelte Werke, chronologisch geordnet*, ed. Anna Freud, in collaboration with M. Bonaparte, E. Bibring, W. Hoffer, E. Kris and O. Isakower, vol. VIII (London: Imago, 1991), pp. 376–87, pp. 379–80; Sigmund Freud, 'Recommendations to Physicians Practising Psycho-Analysis', in *The Standard Edition of the Complete Psychological Works of Sigmund Freud*, ed. James Strachey, with Anna Freud, Alix Strachey and Alan Tyson, vol. XII (London: Hogarth Press and Institute for Psychoanalysis, 1964), pp. 109–20, p. 113.

45 Laura Doan, *Disturbing Practices: History, Sexuality, and Women's Experience of Modern War* (Chicago: University of Chicago Press, 2013), p. 188.

46 John Frow, *Genre* (New York: Routledge, 2006), p. 14.

47 Jolles, *Einfache Formen*, p. 179.

1

The shifting case of masochism: Leopold von Sacher-Masoch's *Venus im Pelz* (1870)

Birgit Lang

The literary, autobiographical and psychiatric case studies that accompany the making of masochism in the late nineteenth century reveal a fascinating history – that of the formation of a new language for human sexuality and love.[1] In a time of epistemological uncertainty, the case study genre became the central narrative form in a debate about the nature of masochism that included authors and their biographers, sexologists and their patients. The case remained a site of dialogue and reinterpretation for nearly thirty years, far exceeding the naming of masochism after Austrian writer Leopold von Sacher-Masoch (1836–95) by sexologist and psychiatrist Richard von Krafft-Ebing (1840–1902). The narrative of Sacher-Masoch as a masochist emerged only with the establishment of psychiatry and only after the transition within medical thought from the anatomical world of sex to that of sexual identity.[2] Generic similarities between Sacher-Masoch's novellas and the medical case study eased this transposition of ideas from the literary to the sexological realm for Krafft-Ebing's patients – and for a newly emerging sexual public that reinterpreted the original meaning of Sacher-Masoch's *Venus im Pelz* (*Venus in Furs*).

In current scholarship, the naming of masochism after Sacher-Masoch denotes the clash between the clinic and the literary world in an iconic manner. The contentious naming has a history considered at once simplistic and presumptuous; it is commonly represented as an oversimplification of the intricate relationship between Sacher-Masoch the author and his writing, and – by extension – between authors and their works in general.[3] This critique of the subjugation of literary discourse to the act of sexological classification seems particularly warranted in light of the immense academic and public success of the category of masochism – a category which, by the early twentieth century, had proven crucial to the understanding of the principles of sexual formation and human behaviour. Even the canonisation of *Venus im Pelz* as a classic text of erotic literature can be understood as a direct result of the medicalisation of Sacher-Masoch's literature.

To analyse the 'caseness' of masochism reveals a more complex picture.[4] The outcome of the struggle for new ways to debate love and sex was a distinctive discourse of sexuality that became a central feature of individual identity, as Michel Foucault first observed.[5] By the turn of the nineteenth century, masochism had evolved into an established field of truth and falsehood.[6] Patients needed to recognise themselves in such a field, while the endeavour of sexologists was to recognise the truth and falsity of their patients' statements.[7] Meanwhile, literary and medical case studies contributed to the growing understanding of a new language of love and sex.

As first observed by Harry Oosterhuis in his biography of Krafft-Ebing, during the late nineteenth century, while sexology was in its foundational phase, patients actively contributed to the construction of sexological terminology.[8] Their life experience, including their interpretation of literary works, resonates clearly in these early medical works, and its impact on sexological methodology was greater than has hitherto been acknowledged. Specifically regarding masochism, literary knowledge preceded scientific knowledge and was reinterpreted by Krafft-Ebing's patients, who functioned as the translators between the world of sex and that of sexuality. A proliferation of cases accompanies the making of masochism. And henceforth the case study became a vehicle for the transformation of literary into scientific knowledge, and vice versa.

First published in 1870, Sacher-Masoch's Darwinian novella *Venus im Pelz* represents an innovative mode of genre writing, and was part of a larger exploration of nature that allowed the author to represent the crisis of love at the dawn of the scientific age. Sacher-Masoch was the first German writer to contend with Darwinian thought, and he had a unique stance on questions concerning love. His approach contrasted with that of the generation of Darwinian writers who succeeded him from the 1890s onwards; these authors highlighted the unity of man and nature. Sacher-Masoch's Darwinian novellas presented a new literary-scientific voice, and allowed him to open the pervasive genre of the novella – the most common contemporary form for the literary case study – to highly topical matters of intimacy and sexuality. His interest was not unlike that of Krafft-Ebing, who set out to investigate sexual perversions and pathologies: Sacher-Masoch problematised the role of love and sexuality in the human world and explored its 'dark sides'.[9]

As the above terminology suggests, Sacher-Masoch's novellas refer to a Darwinian rather than a sexological discourse. That is, the literary freedom he exercised to explore the subjectivity of 'supersensualism', a formation of identity related to that of masochism, was not embedded in a sexological framework of meaning. Sacher-Masoch's literary-scientific investigation explored ways in which humankind was able to resolve the tension between natural instincts and an ethical life. In this context,

Venus im Pelz functioned as a counter-example, while his novella *Marzella* (1870) contained the idealised solution to this dilemma. Changing attitudes towards *Venus im Pelz* in subsequent decades culminated in the identification of the author with his antihero Severin von Kusiemski, and paradigmatically represent the shift from an anatomical to a psychiatric style of reasoning.

A close reading of the cases and their shifting frameworks surrounding the reception of *Venus im Pelz* sheds light on the circulation of the case study as a discursive form and on the gradual acceptance of masochism as a highly specific category for sexual proclivity. Much of this encounter was shaped by the interdependence between psychiatry and literature at the very moment when German psychiatry was founded. This is not to say that the debate about *Venus im Pelz* was confined to the realm of the clinic. Just as psychiatry relied on patient confessions and cultural histories to construct knowledge, the multitude of (auto)biographical and literary cases in public discourse were at least partly modelled on medical case studies. After Sacher-Masoch's 'outing' by his biographer, and his subsequent pathologisation in the psychiatric realm, the debate surrounding Sacher-Masoch shifted from his work to his perceived sexual identity. This was followed by autobiographical and biographical case studies that referenced medical discourse.

To analyse Sacher-Masoch's work through the lens of the case study genre is to investigate the intricate question of the development of a language of sexuality. It shows that masochist identity formation was based at least partly on the reinterpretation of a literary case, and reveals important insights concerning the construction and currency of this new language of sexuality.

The sexological case: Krafft-Ebing and the merits of literature

In his seminal work *Psychopathia Sexualis* (1886), Krafft-Ebing coined the key sexual pathologies of modernity: the homosexual, the fetishist, the sadist and the masochist. The concept of masochism became so popular that Sigmund Freud, in his 1924 study 'Das ökonomische Problem des Masochismus' ('The Economic Problem of Masochism'), declared 'it is unnecessary to quote cases to illustrate this; for the material is very uniform and is accessible to any observer, even to non-analysts'.[10] The naming of a sexual perversion after a well known author left a sour taste early on. Russian imperial prosecutor Dimitry Stefanowski, a competitor in the race to develop a sexual taxonomy, argued that Krafft-Ebing had 'covered the name of the novelist with ignominy'.[11] In his academic works, Stefanowski insisted on Sacher-Masoch's sexual normalcy, yet misinterpreted the intention of the original name-giving, which in fact paid tribute to Sacher-Masoch as an expert in the understanding of masochism. In these early years, Krafft-Ebing at no point implicated the writer but justified the naming through the fact that 'the well-known novelist Sacher-Masoch has made this sexual perversion the favourite subject of many of his novels, especially in the famous *Venus im Pelz*'.[12] As revealed by the fluctuating archive represented by successive editions of *Psychopathia Sexualis*, Krafft-Ebing's tribute to Sacher-Masoch's writing marked a methodological shift in his treatment of literature – an acceptance of literary texts as medical evidence. Krafft-Ebing owed this acceptance largely to his patients, since they referred to *Venus im Pelz* as the most accurate portrayal of their own desires. The sexologist's appreciation of Sacher-Masoch waned only after 1901, when he first identified the author as a masochist and thus subjugated him to medical norms.[13]

Case studies form the backbone of *Psychopathia Sexualis*, which was first published in 1886 and quickly revised and enlarged. The importance of the case study genre for Krafft-Ebing can be explained by his professional context. During his lifetime the renowned sexologist published eleven editions; by 1924 the seventeenth edition had been released. Krafft-Ebing's cases typically commence with a short physical description of the patient, and summarise the psychiatric family history. Reminiscent of the anatomo-clinical gaze dominant before the rise of sexology, the physical description could include genital anomalies.[14] The core of the case study consisted of the description of sexual behaviours – reported to Krafft-Ebing by the patient and rephrased by the sexologist. Over time, he relied on an increasing variety of testimonies. The first edition of *Psychopathia Sexualis* mainly comprises the collection of cases already published in the field, showing Krafft-Ebing to have been widely read in various languages.[15] In the 1890s, Krafft-Ebing sometimes privileged cases of individuals who had entered into correspondence with him, suffering from what they themselves perceived as deviant conditions and seeking an exchange with a medical expert in order to come to terms with their own feelings about their desires. Krafft-Ebing assumed that his correspondents agreed to the publication of their anonymised cases.[16] As with the collection on homosexuality, the number of masochist cases published increased considerably over the years.[17] His case correspondences concerning the more general field of neuropathology included letters from sufferers and their carers, case notes from colleagues, or other sources such as newspaper articles.[18] Comparable evidence from his masochist patients did not exist or has not survived. With his reputation on the rise, Krafft-Ebing's access to clinical and judicial cases increased, and these form the almost exclusive source of new cases in the editions of *Psychopathia Sexualis* from the late 1890s onwards.

The sexological turn from patient bodies to patient narratives constituted a paradigm shift, and attracted medical critics. In the eyes of some members of the medical profession, the entanglement of patient narratives with doctor narratives in attempts to coin new sexual taxonomies threatened to subvert professional standards, through the creation and dissemination of speculative knowledge. Moreover, it potentially undermined the steep imbalance of power between patients and the medical profession.[19] Such critique was heard from the wider medical profession, as exemplified in a comment printed in the *British Medical Journal* of 1902: 'Professor von Krafft-Ebing's book *Psychopathia Sexualis* is the largest, the most widely circulated, and we may as well at once say the most repulsive of a group of books of which it is the type'.[20] Since *Psychopathia Sexualis* proved extremely popular for an academic publication, others feared the detrimental effects upon lay readers. The American journal *Alienist and Neurologist* stated in a review of the work: 'a book to be read only by the sexually mature and psychically balanced. In its psychopathic effects it might prove dangerous in its influence over the neuropathically unstable. To the prurient curiosity of that morbid sexual element, which too extensively abounds in modern social life, its examples and personal histories would prove psychopathic poison.'[21] Krafft-Ebing's methodology was also scrutinised by his direct competitors in the field. Stefanowski's critique of the naming of masochism has already been mentioned, while in the context of homosexuality Krafft-Ebing was accused of trusting his patients too much – patients who, critics argued, were prone to lying because of the discrimination they faced and the double lives they were forced to lead.[22]

Krafft-Ebing's response to such criticism was differentiated, adhering to standards of academic credibility and bourgeois respectability; the latter had become entrenched by the beginning of the nineteenth century.[23] From the mid-1890s onwards, he used Latin for overtly explicit passages of *Psychopathia Sexualis*, in an attempt to rein in those critics who feared for the 'sanity' of his readership. This certainly made his work less accessible to the lower classes, and to women, who learned modern rather than classical languages at school. As the example of Stefanowski shows, Krafft-Ebing rebuffed academic debates within his professional publications, with direct ripostes often printed in the latest edition of *Psychopathia Sexualis*. When it came to the relationship with his patients, however, Krafft-Ebing would not open himself to scrutiny. Biographer Harry Oosterhuis has indicated that Krafft-Ebing was held in high regard by many of his patients and that his concern for patients often went beyond mere professional commitment.[24] Exactly how these relationships were structured and how Krafft-Ebing transposed his knowledge of patient 'confessions' into case studies remains difficult to reconstruct. Yet from his case vignettes it becomes clear that patients served as his 'informants'. Krafft-Ebing recognised their identificatory reading of *Venus im Pelz* – even if he did not necessarily agree with their interpretation.

Yet, and dissimilarly to comparable studies in England and France, fiction played only a minor role in the first four editions of *Psychopathia Sexualis*.[25] Krafft-Ebing considered literary works that might have met the criteria of respectability naive in the area of psychiatry. While attesting that literary writers possessed a deep understanding of the human psyche, he viewed their works as overtly idealising – a comment on the strong strand of post-Darwinian pantheism in German literature that celebrated the unity of nature and man.[26] Introducing the first edition of *Psychopathia Sexualis* he argued:

> For now poets are the better psychologists, rather than experts in psychology and philosophy. But they are emotionalists rather than rationalists and definitely biased in the depiction of their topic. This is because they only see the sunny and cozy side of the subject matter, and not its deep shadows.... To deal with the psychopathology of sexuality in an academic treatise means to be confronted with the dark side of human life and misery, in whose shadows the shining idol of the poet turns into a hideous grimace, and morality and aesthetics become insane in the face of the 'image of God'.[27]

Only four years later, Krafft-Ebing's approach to literature took a definite turn. In 1890 he published his *Neuere Forschungen auf dem Gebiet der Psychopathia Sexualis* (*Newer Research into Psychopathia Sexualis*). This can be described as a spin-off from *Psychopathia Sexualis* which presented cutting-edge research – and integrated literature methodologically into the chain of evidence. It was in this work that Krafft-Ebing first named masochism in obeisance to Sacher-Masoch, since so many of his patients referred to *Venus im Pelz* as fundamental for the understanding their own condition. The case study at the heart of *Neuere Forschungen* is that of Mr X from Berlin, a 'highly cultured man', according to Krafft-Ebing, and 'the stimulus for this study'.[28] Of good social standing, Mr X showed profound insight into his own condition and provided his autobiography voluntarily. His eloquence implied that he had overcome the shame associated with his condition, at least to the extent of being able to write about it. Having attracted the attention of a medical specialist, he entrusted Krafft-Ebing with his autobiographical account. To have been quoted in the *Neuere Forschungen* must have given Mr X some satisfaction, since he is noted as having been keen to 'serve science'.[29]

Krafft-Ebing's fascination with his Berlin correspondent is written all over the *Neuere Forschungen* volume. He does not claim Mr X as the author of the term 'masochism', as Oosterhuis has suggested.[30] Nevertheless, Krafft-Ebing's new notion of literature is intimately linked to the case of Mr X. Directly before presenting Mr X's autobiographical account, Krafft-Ebing outlines his new taxonomy of textual evidence, one that differentiates between patient statements, autobiographical accounts and literary works. Patient statements rank highest, since these have been established in a medical context and can be verified by medical authority. Autobiographies such as *Les Confessions* (1782) by Jean Jacques Rousseau rate second – even as this text is pronounced a 'superb example of good self-observation'.[31] Works of fiction are positioned last. They merit inclusion if they depict the shadowy aspects of love, exploring taboo subjects otherwise inaccessible to the medical practitioner, such as female sadism, of which Krafft-Ebing writes: 'it is of great interest if such occurrences appear in literary works. Even though they cannot be of the same value as case histories [Krafft-Ebing's term for medical case studies], they are of psychological interest since the author must have drawn from his own experience or at least must have felt in such a way'.[32]

Krafft-Ebing then introduces the case study of Mr X and describes his patient's appreciation of autobiographical and literary texts. Mr X reveals

> I was looking for connections with my preferred fantasies in all kinds of literature. Rousseau's *Confessions*, which fell to me, were a great revelation. I found experiences portrayed which at crucial points were similar to my own. I felt even more surprised when I realised how my ideas agreed with the literary works of Sacher-Masoch. I devoured them all with desire, despite the fact that many of the bloodthirsty scenes far exceeded my own fantasies.[33]

Mr X's account also offers insight into a masochist subculture in which Sacher-Masoch's text plays an important role.

> In Vienna a man of exceptional standing has undertaken trips to the Prater, dressed as a servant, on the coach box of his mistress. This was probably a deliberate imitation of *Venus im Pelz*. In general it seems to me that the works of Sacher-Masoch have contributed much to the development of this perversion in people disposed to it.[34]

The same notion is emphasised by the subject of Case 10, who 'believes he could only be attracted to women who resembled the heroines in Sacher-Masoch's novels'.[35] Consequently, in the second edition of *Neuere Forschungen* Krafft-Ebing concludes: 'as becomes clear from the above observations, many individuals afflicted with this perversion explicitly refer to Sacher-Masoch's works as typical representations of their own psychological condition'.[36]

The concept of masochism underwent marked conceptual and editorial shifts in the 1890s; as early as the second edition of the *Neuere Forschungen*, the case of Mr X begins to recede into the background.[37] Krafft-Ebing shortens the autobiographical account, removing passages that point towards a more general nervous disorder, and editing the case to fit more obviously into his suggested disease pattern.[38] Any reference to original correspondence with Mr X is omitted, and Krafft-Ebing quotes as his own the cultural history of masochism previously provided by his informant.[39] While it stands to reason that Mr X felt some disappointment at this loss of importance, such modifications were common in the practices of sexological and medical writing, and were not considered unethical in these professional contexts. Krafft-Ebing's revised concept of the role of authors, however, would remain unaltered for the remainder of his career, with literary works continuing to function as a useful means of gaining insight into taboo subjects. He explored in passing the pathologies of writers like de Sade and Rousseau, and even the canonical German writer

Heinrich von Kleist.[40] While Krafft-Ebing clearly stated that certain authors were afflicted with sexual pathologies – as Anna Katharina Schaffner has pointed out – in his view, to have convincingly portrayed certain psychological conditions in literary works did not necessarily make an author a 'psychopath'.[41]

In the case of Sacher-Masoch, Krafft-Ebing never made any explicit reference to the author's pathology. To base a key sexological category on a writer who had not made his desires public in a confessional, auto-biographical text would have been counterproductive to the success of Krafft-Ebing's project, undermining his professional credibility and possibly resulting in a defamation court case. Krafft-Ebing was nonetheless persuaded to name masochism after 'the first portrayer of masochism', because his patients were able to recognise themselves in Sacher-Masoch's literary cases. Therefore the act of naming expressed appreciation for the creator of a literary work who encouraged Krafft-Ebing's patients to reflect on their own condition. Should Krafft-Ebing have entertained any methodological doubts about the influence of literary cases on his patients, these were dispelled by the number of individuals referring to *Venus im Pelz*. Krafft-Ebing had identified an irregular phenomenon and was aiming to define its laws.

A case of 'self-intensification': early masochists

Reading Krafft-Ebing's masochist case studies, it becomes obvious that writing about sex was no easy matter. The ways in which the sexologist presents his patients, their statements and his consideration of their predicament is defined by two central elements: the interpretation of *Venus im Pelz* as an erotic text, and the moment of recognition masochist readers experienced during their perusal of Sacher-Masoch's work. Arousal and acknowledgement were likewise central to Krafft-Ebing's understanding of pathology. The former represented the symptom; the latter was the prerequisite for the treatment that some of Krafft-Ebing's patients so earnestly sought.[42] It is impossible to say what other issues his patients might have raised in their conversations with him, but clearly their knowledge of arousal and acknowledgement had been shaped by the literary text that many of them referred to as the foremost representation of their unruly desires. *Venus im Pelz* tells the story of the antihero Severin, who does not manage to establish an emancipated relationship with his partner. The confession of his submissive desires to his lover Wanda von Dunajew, and several explicit and brutal scenes that depict Severin's emotional and physical humiliation, are features of the novella. Although critical in many respects, Sacher-Masoch's relatively sympathetic and intimate portrayal of Severin, as well as the story's confessional tone, encouraged Krafft-Ebing's masochist patients to interpret *Venus im Pelz* as an expression of their own sexual identity.

Krafft-Ebing's patients undoubtedly read Sacher-Masoch's infamous novella as an erotic text. In the second edition of *Neuere Forschungen* (1891), Case 4 reports that, on reading *Venus im Pelz*, his 'semen just comes out'.[43] The subject of Case 4 was the only patient to admit so explicitly to physical arousal through his reading experience; by far the most common interpretation mentioned in the case studies was that of promoting self-awareness. Acknowledgement rather than arousal dominates descriptions of the effects of reading, a fact that might well have been imposed by Krafft-Ebing's careful editing. Hence Case 3 states:

> A most remarkable, even amazing fact is that there is an author who exposes such passions to the public at large, namely in the forms of novellas and novels, rather than others, who keep their passions to themselves in their innermost soul. In *Venus im Pelz* we find the same familiar feelings expressed, word for word, line for line, feelings which until now we believed were our own most unique experiences.[44]

In absence of other forms of acknowledgement, this first recognition of desire in a twenty-year-old literary text must have been powerful. In her long essay on the uses of literature, Rita Felski points to the power of texts through 'self-intensification': 'recognising aspects of ourselves in the description of others, seeing our perceptions and behaviours echoed in a work of fiction, we become aware of our accumulated experiences as distinctive yet far from unique'.[45] Such close identification, often sidelined in literary criticism, is not necessarily overpowering, nor must it produce an utterly uncritical reader.[46] Indeed, several of Krafft-Ebing's case narratives show subjects distancing themselves from what they perceived as the overtly pronounced, even shocking depiction of brutality in *Venus im Pelz*, a depiction which certainly surpassed their own desires. This was seen above in the response of Mr X, and is again evident in Case 3, where the patient remarks on the consequences of the unexpected transposition of fantasies from the private to the public sphere.

> Hence, maybe exactly because such secrets are dragged into the limelight, reading this book has repulsive, and hence sobering and healing effects also upon masochists. It is something different to imagine things with closed eyes in solitude and to read those same things printed in a novel. The reader can never completely suppress the critic, and hence it must seem outrageous to present such nonsense to an audience of which only a minimal part consists of masochists. It is sufficient to point to the fact that all characters involved continuously wear fur while in hot Florence, even when they are inside.[47]

For Krafft-Ebing such a critical stance towards Sacher-Masoch's text might have intimated a new consciousness on the part of the patient, a potential distancing that could lead to recovery, since the patient's acknowledgement of his own condition was central to the exchange between doctor and patient.[48] For many of Krafft-Ebing's masochist patients, it can be said that *Venus im Pelz* served, rather, as a 'coming out' novel, powerfully portraying a new sort of sexual sensibility, or one previously unmapped in medical terms. All evidence indicates that this was not the author's main intention. Within the cycle of novellas of which it was part, *Venus im Pelz* was supposed to be the author's key representation of the struggling dilettante of love who subjects himself to the forceful powers of nature – personified by his sexually domineering female lover. Sacher-Masoch envisaged the portrayal of an emerging modern subjectivity, a symptom of the crisis of modernity: a sensitive man gifted with the capacity for aesthetic pleasure, but lacking the powers to constructively convert his gifts into living an ethical and productive life.

Venus im Pelz was not the first literary text to embrace the sexual preference or the sensibility of masochists. Earlier erotic novels had likewise engaged with the sexual practices represented by Sacher-Masoch. Rousseau's *Confessions* had painstakingly and painfully described the burden of the author's sexual preferences in his own life, while Ivan Turgenev, in *Dnevnik Lishnego Cheloveka* (*Diary of a Superfluous Man*, 1850), gave an influential description of the mindset of an outsider whose explorations in the realms of love remain stunted and unsatisfactory.

When compared with erotic texts portraying similar deeds, *Venus im Pelz* was a more respectable text, written by a prized author in a key fictional form favoured by the German middle class, the novella. Having constituted the exemplary 'case' in German literature since the late eighteenth century, novellas were a popular genre, published in most middle-class journals. Their focus on one character, and their frequently expressed aspiration of unpredictability, novelty and truth, made them the key genre for the description of peculiar and remarkable people or events.[49] Different from Rousseau's *Confessions*, or from Turgenev's hero, who dies at the end of his story, *Venus im Pelz* characterises Severin as a somewhat deluded man who, through the 'inversion' of his desires, eventually finds a more commonly accepted place in society, as a misogynist. The main difference between *Venus im Pelz* and its literary predecessors lies in the relatively positive characterisation of Severin, and in its confessional power – that is, in the detail and richness of its description, which fostered the sense of acknowledgement emphasised by Krafft-Ebing's patients.

A comparison between Turgenev's *Dnevnik Lishnego Cheloveka* and *Venus im Pelz* highlights the positive thrust of Sacher-Masoch's work, and is of particular relevance since Sacher-Masoch makes several allusions to Turgenev's novella. The latter reveals the torments of the hero Chulkaturin, a social outsider. Diagnosed with a terminal illness, Chulkaturin retells the only meaningful event of his life, that of having been rejected by his beloved Elizaveta Kirillovna.[50] The parallels between *Dnevnik Lishnego Cheloveka* and *Venus im Pelz* are notable, as is Sacher-Masoch's remarkable inversion of Turgenev's plot structure. Chulkaturin is presented as a sufferer, an outsider who is rejected by the woman he loves, who fails to make sense of his life, and who is 'incompatible with the lives being led around him'.[51] Of Chulkaturin the reader knows remarkably little; nor are his sexual preferences unveiled. Chulkaturin's diary reveals a hero who pities himself and portrays a painfully conflicted self to the reader. Turgenev's achievement lay in establishing the motif of the 'superfluous man' as a key theme of Russian literature in the nineteenth century.[52] He exposes his main character to the reader without giving the latter any interpretive point of reference outside the world of the narrative. As a consequence, Chulkaturin's confession seems incomplete and unreliable, refusing to provide the reader with an interpretive framework.

Severin's diary, on the other hand, presents the reader with a detailed biography of its antihero, including a coming-of-age scene that details physical punishment inflicted by his aunt, and conversations with Wanda, his lover, during their tête-à-têtes. Sacher-Masoch provides the reader with narrative certainty through the overarching frame of his cycle of novellas, a device that delineates *Venus im Pelz* as the 'problem' novella. The author also furnishes rich background about his main character, providing Severin with the sexual biography of a 'supersensualist'. This includes an evocation of Severin's childhood, his feelings of being an outsider form the very beginning – an odd child, rejecting the milk of his wet nurse, born with a love of fur and an innate shyness around women.[53] *Venus im Pelz* describes his first sexual encounter, including the realisation of his sexual fantasies through his aunt, Countess Sobol, who has him purposefully tied up for disrespect he has shown towards her: 'what a supersensual lunatic I was! My taste for women was awakened by the blows of a beautiful and voluptuous creature in a fur jacket who looked like an angry queen. From that day on my aunt became the most desirable woman on God's earth'.[54]

Anchored in the certainty of biography, in the midst of Severin's confession to his lover, the erotic element comes into play. The above scene echoes Rousseau's description of his sexual awakening in the first book of his *Confessions*: the author's arousal during a beating by his governess, Miss Lambercier. He describes his loss of innocence as the unplanned result of punishment at the hands of a female authority figure, and laments its impact on his adult sex life.[55] Importantly, however, *Venus im Pelz* portrays a minor's subjection to sexual violence as a conscious act of cruelty. In the novella, the retelling of this act of violence turns the story of Severin's childhood and coming of age into a tale of seduction. Like masochist readers twenty years later, Wanda returns aroused; the next night she dresses as a 'Venus in Furs' and asks Severin to her room: 'your stories have disturbed me so much that I have not been able to sleep a wink'.[56] Severin's narration has served as a form of initiation and represents the beginning of an educational process – Wanda's transformation into his cruel mistress. The escalating scenarios of humiliation and violence that follow do not, however, depict a conventional sexual encounter. Instead they convey a sense of strong suppression of the sexual, perpetuating Severin's inhibited existence. In the end, Severin returns home, cured after a beating at the hands of Wanda's new lover Alexander, and he is shown able to become a productive if peculiar member of society.

This tale provided masochist readers with moments of 'self-intensification' that satisfied the human needs for recognition and the representation of erotic desire. Its confessional style and abundant detail about the life of Severin gave the novella a strong resemblance to later psychiatric case studies. The fact that Severin recovers from his 'perverse' desires might also have held some appeal in this context. At the same time, the need for identification made Krafft-Ebing's patients overlook or sideline key aspects of the story. Most seem to have been oblivious, for example, to the critical tone of the novella, expressed through its over-arching narrative, and oblivious to the irony and ridicule at the heart of *Venus im Pelz* and the cascade of humiliation to which Severin is exposed. Rather, the subjects of Krafft-Ebing's case studies express bewilderment at the cruelty conveyed in the story – a response that encapsulates the deep ambivalence felt by many patients of sexology towards their own afflictions.

A Darwinian novella: Severin, the dilettante in love

In the late 1860s, Sacher-Masoch embarked on the largest literary project of his career, a multi-volume 'natural history of humankind' collectively titled *Das Vermächtnis Kains* (*The Legacy of Cain*). This ambitious collection – a series of six volumes of six novellas each – was to circle around the themes of love, property, the state, war, work and death. Ultimately, Sacher-Masoch would complete only the first two volumes of the projected six. Shortly before the publication of the first volume, *Die Liebe* (*Love*), in 1870, Sacher-Masoch resigned from his position as a lecturer in history at the University of Graz in order to follow his literary calling. He had already published two novels, several novellas and two well received plays before first achieving wider recognition throughout Europe with the publication of *Don Juan von Kolomea* (1868).[57] This story, together with *Venus im Pelz* and the four other novellas, formed *Die Liebe*, which was published in two parts. *Die Liebe* also proved to be a literary success – two editions were published in close succession, and a third in 1878 – and the work was considered paramount in Sacher-Masoch's literary oeuvre.

Das Vermächtnis Kains signified Sacher-Masoch's unique attempt to find a new language for discussing key areas of human life, especially the realms of love and sexuality. In this context *Venus im Pelz* constitutes the key example of love 'gone wrong'. Sacher-Masoch exemplifies in Severin the struggles of a sensitive and idle man. Rather than embracing the Darwinian struggles of modern love-life – seeking to negotiate the tension between the recreational needs of humankind and a more egalitarian relationship between the sexes – he lets himself be ruled by his submissive desires alone, and fails in his love for Wanda. The first author in German literature to engage extensively with Darwinism, Sacher-Masoch reflected on the meaning of humanity's animal origins, while developing his ideas concerning a more just society. As a mode of enquiry, literature allowed him to investigate new phenomena quickly – much more quickly than medicine; after all, Krafft-Ebing was obliged to become aware of the phenomenon of masochism, find patients and steadily write up their cases.

Sacher-Masoch trusted his intellectual insights and used cutting-edge scientific and philosophical discourses to refine his aesthetic perception. In a letter to Otto von Kapf, who later became his private secretary for a time, Sacher-Masoch explained that despite his own privileged life he was a pessimist by nature and could not close his mind to the truth: 'I am not able to paint human beings in an idealised fashion…, for the very reason that I do not go by my *subjective sentiments* [Sacher-Masoch's emphasis], but only by my knowledge [Erkenntnis]'.[58] This search for truth – nowadays perhaps best described as anthropological – was shaped by Darwinian thought, contemporary moral philosophy and key works of European literature. Sacher-Masoch's critique represents a turn against idealism (especially prevalent in German literature at this period), as well as a turn towards scientific thought, specifically Darwinian method. Both strategies permitted him to see the world differently from many of his contemporaries. This was a time when writers in Germany anticipated and strived for German unification, and were inclined to aestheticise and idealise bourgeois life.[59] Inspired by Charles Darwin and philosopher Arthur Schopenhauer, among others, Sacher-Masoch was critical of such romantic tendencies within German culture.[60] Like other German writers from the Habsburg lands, Sacher-Masoch instead situated himself within a broader European literary context; his work was strongly influenced by Russian and French literature.[61] His cosmopolitan outlook was also reflected in the reception of his work: in the preamble to *Die Liebe*, well known literary critic Ferdinand Kürnberger praised Sacher-Masoch as a German Turgenev.[62] Sacher-Masoch certainly shared Turgenev's love for Eastern Europe, but where the latter focused on Russia as the setting for his novels, Sacher-Masoch focused mainly on the far east region of the Habsburg Empire.[63]

With hindsight, Sacher-Masoch's Darwinian sympathies are not surprising, since in Austrian literature Darwinism became strongly associated with liberal attitudes.[64] Political liberalism had been thwarted in 1848, and the debate about Darwinism became an *Ersatz*, a means for members of the middle class to express their beliefs – through science rather than religion.[65] Yet Sacher-Masoch differed from more conservative social Darwinians, in that he was critical of a reductionist application of Darwinian thought to human history. This can be seen from a review of contemporary cultural histories written for *Auf der Höhe*, an internationally oriented German journal he founded and edited: 'how can we separate cultural history from the history of arts and science, without being at risk of giving an inadequate, shallow and superficial account of the historical development of humanity?'[66] The question was prompted by the contemporaneous study *Kulturgeschichte in ihrer natürlichen Entwicklung bis zur Gegenwart* (*Cultural History and Its Natural Development up to the Present*), first published in 1876, and written by Friedrich von Hellwald, an ardent social and racial Darwinian who was popular among the German bourgeoisie. Hellwald argued that the struggle for existence ruled over moral considerations in natural as well as in human history.[67] With respect to these topical discourses, Sacher-Masoch aimed to combine natural and cultural history in an exploration of relationships between nature and nurture; between the Darwinian struggle for existence – without accepting biological determinism – and a new ethics that acknowledged the biological nature of human beings.[68] Applied to the realms of love, Darwinism allowed him to see lucidly the force of humanity's reproductive drive, even as he strove to imagine a more equal and just society.

Sacher-Masoch's literary response to Darwin coalesced at a point when Darwin had published *On the Origin of Species* (1859) but not yet *The Descent of Man, And Selection in Relation to Sex* (1871).[69] As such, Sacher-Masoch enjoyed a unique freedom to pursue his own ideas and to develop the new form of the Darwinian novella. This particular literary case made use of Darwinian ideas and integrated new biological understanding of human nature with insights from cultural history and contemporary ethical thought. A year before Darwin first published *The Descent of Man*, Sacher-Masoch pre-empted the English naturalist's famous statement on the relevance of evolutionary theory for understanding the origin of man and his history.[70] Sacher-Masoch's answer to the questions raised through Darwin's works was a literary anthropology of Galicia that he envisaged would stand alongside scientific discussions.[71] For Sacher-Masoch the role of literature was to 'communicate knowledge and truths ... by coining the dead gold barrels of scientific knowledge for the masses'. When it came to the 'lives and hearts of human beings', as he stressed on several occasions, literature was quite capable of 'explor[ing] new truths itself', since 'the real poet will always particularly like to make the passions and follies of humans the concern of his literary works'.[72] For him, the obligation of literature lay in reflecting on the human condition and in making society conscious of its feelings. Like many intellectuals in the nineteenth century, he was invested in the depiction of the world surrounding him.

Sacher-Masoch's worldview is succinctly encapsulated in the fable-like story that serves as the Prologue to *Das Vermächtnis Kains*, printed as front-matter in Part One of *Die Liebe*. While hunting in the Galician woods, the narrator, Leopold, encounters an ascetic wanderer, a member of a Russian Orthodox sect – Schopenhauer's Brahmane Other personified and transposed into Sacher-Masoch's Slavophilic world. Leopold orders his gamekeeper to shoot an eagle; the wanderer then steps in and accuses Leopold of having murdered, like Cain, his (feathered) brother. In the ensuing dialogue the wanderer's pessimistic outlook becomes apparent. He argues that men neither are innately good nor possess a natural sense of morality; all longing for pleasure is in vain.[73] Programmatically, the curse of Cain is apparent in the different topics of Sacher-Masoch's projected natural history of humankind: love, property, the state, war, work and death. The Prologue's wanderer is concerned specifically with the realm of love, and he elaborates the underlying reason for the inevitable battle of the sexes, arguing that natural instincts force human beings to reproduce, this being the only motive for passion between men and women.[74] He considers society's attempt to stabilise the relationship between the sexes through marriage futile, since it contradicts human nature, a topic explored fully in Part One of *Die Liebe*.[75] The wanderer admits to having played a dominant, patriarchal role as the master of women; also to having been a slave to women – bound, through their attractiveness, to work for them and their children – only to be betrayed. All these topics are explored in Part Two of *Die Liebe*.[76] For the wanderer, work for its own sake exemplifies the Darwinian view of the 'manly and bold struggle for existence'; work constitutes the only path to happiness, to the abolition of slavery and misery, gluttony and indulgence.[77] The question pivotal to the contents of *Die Liebe* becomes manifest in the Prologue at the moment of the narrator's spiritual enlightenment, when he hears nature declare, 'I am truth and life' – a selective biblical reference to John 14:6, in which Jesus states, 'I am the way, the truth and the life'.[78] Not by chance Sacher-Masoch omits the religious notion of 'the way', since from his scientific perspective the course of human action was guided by the challenge of how to lead an ethical life.[79]

Together, the two parts of *Die Liebe* present the reader with five progressively deteriorating examples of gender relations, only to resolve the conflict between the sexes in the final novella. These six Darwinian novellas are linked by their imagery of Galicia, the landscape of Sacher-Masoch's youth, and by the first-person narrator named Leopold, also Sacher-Masoch's first name. Part One of *Die Liebe* (which consists of three novellas) introduces the readers to Galicia and problematises matrimonial gender relations. Sacher-Masoch's formal innovations, such as the telegram style and the stimulating descriptions of life in Galicia, were praised by his contemporaries.[80] *Don Juan von Kolomea* (*Don Juan of Kolomea*) discusses the detrimental impact of children on married life and the main character's womanising – a situation that results in both partners finding themselves trapped in a loveless marriage. *Der Kapitulant* (*The Capitulation*) illustrates the price paid by a woman who marries for money and social standing rather than love. The man identified as her true love surrenders to what he perceives to be the nature of women, namely to women's instinct for placing the socio-economic status of a husband above genuine love. The third story, *Mondnacht* (*Moonlit Night*), portrays female infidelity and estrangement between married estate owners. This alienation is depicted as a consequence of women's exclusion from the male sphere of work.

Part Two of *Die Liebe* concentrates on more problematic areas of gender relations, as well as the suggested solution. In a letter to his publishing house, Cotta – one of few surviving personal documents – Sacher-Masoch outlines the structure of this part: its three novellas respectively symbolise intellectual love, sensual love and the happiness of moral matrimony.[81] Accordingly, *Die Liebe des Plato* (*The Love of Plato*) narrates the views of an advocate of platonic love who falls for the 'brother' of his fiancé and finally leaves the country. This represents the first articulation of 'homosexuality' *avant la lettre* and, as argued elsewhere, reflects emerging discourses about male same-sex love and desire.[82] The penultimate novella is *Venus im Pelz*, which deals with the confusion of Severin, who explains his misogynistic behaviour in the present in terms of his past masochistic experiences. *Marzella oder Das Märchen vom Glück* (*Marzella or The Fairy Tale of Love*) is the last of the three.

Venus im Pelz and *Marzella* form opposites: as is typical for cycles of novellas, the penultimate story is the so-called 'problem' novella, while the last story presents the envisaged solution. Unlike the rest of the cycle, these two novellas are bound together by the first-person narrator and by the figure of Severin. That is, the unfortunate hero of *Venus im Pelz* is introduced as a close childhood friend of Alexander, the hero of *Marzella*. This last novella focuses on Alexander's marriage to Marzella. With their respective partners, Alexander and Severin plainly represent Sacher-Masoch's ideas on 'the good' and 'the bad' of gender relations. Alexander is sensual, while Severin is supersensual, desirous not of sexual intimacy but of punishment. A seducer of women in his pre-marital life, Alexander is now happily married to the fiery daughter of his wet nurse, whom he has educated to become a (relatively) equal partner. Alexander is down-to-earth and level-headed, possessed of the moral fibre and the wealth to resolve the gender troubles of his times in the ambit of his feudal estate. Alexander is better adapted to his immediate and local environment, and signifies the survival of the fittest. For Sacher-Masoch, a strong marriage was based on mutual sensual attraction and the same cast of mind, as well as shared work. While Alexander and Marzella run their estate together, Severin educates Wanda to become a tyrant. Even after his idle adventure with Wanda in Florence and his subsequent embrace of working life, Severin dominates his new girlfriend, having only inverted his servile desires rather than overcome them. The imaginative Severin falls prey to his own mind and, for him, 'woman, as Nature created her and as man up to now has educated her, is man's enemy; she can be his slave or his despot, but never his companion. This she can only be when she has the same rights as he and is his equal in education and work'.[83]

Sacher-Masoch's contrasting portrayal of Alexander and Severin has distinct Darwinian features, in which procreation and the human struggle for existence function as the benchmarks for success. Simultaneously, because of the human subjects at their centre, his Darwinian novellas engage with a moral, emancipatory discourse. This can be seen in *Venus im Pelz*, where the intellectual inspiration for Severin's character is found in the writing of British moral philosopher John Stuart Mill – material which is then directly referenced in *Marzella*.[84] Mill's *On Liberty* (1859) famously espoused the right of humans to pursue particular tastes and activities, even if these are deemed immoral by society.[85] In keeping with this outlook, Sacher-Masoch has the protagonist of *Marzella* marry outside his own class: Alexander educates the daughter of his wet nurse to become his wife. Alexander's approach epitomises Mill's liberty of the individual and any number of individuals 'to regulate by mutual agreement such things as regard them jointly, and regard no persons but themselves'.[86] This choice coincides with Darwinian principles of adding new blood to the aristocratic family tree. In Alexander's view, the aristocratic family line is otherwise doomed, as he points out in a discussion with his friend Leopold.[87] Conversely, Severin exemplifies the very limits of such freedom, which Mill sees represented in the voluntary enslavement of man:

> In this and most other civilised countries, for example, an engagement by which a person should sell himself, or allow himself to be sold, as a slave, would be null and void; neither enforced by law nor by opinion. The ground for thus limiting his power of voluntarily disposing his own lot in life is apparent, and is very clearly seen in this extreme case.... The principle of freedom cannot require that he should be free not to be free. It is not freedom, to be allowed to alienate freedom.[88]

The example of Severin in *Venus im Pelz* represents the fate of such a 'slave' in the realm of love, and the detrimental consequences for both partners of such an unequal relationship.

In his novellas, Sacher-Masoch combined Darwinian notions of procreation and moral philosophy to challenge notions of love and sexuality for the modern era. He considered such a literary anthropology an important contribution to wider knowledge on these matters. The impact of his work was not what he expected, yet his more open-minded and liberal approach to questions of sexual deviance irrevocably challenged literary and public discourse. Twenty years before some of his readers approached Krafft-Ebing in search of legitimisation, Sacher-Masoch drew on Darwinism to depict the nether sides of love, self-consciously linking these themes to contemporary questions concerning freedom and the social position of women. Through *Venus im Pelz*, the 'problem' novella in *Die Liebe*, he showed Severin embodying the very crisis of a responsible use of freedom. Instead of pursuing an emancipated love relationship, and lifting his partner to the ethical height of man, Severin exemplifies a man's self-abasement to the ethical and intellectual level of women in their presumed equivalence to nature.

Between sex and sexuality

From the moment the first volume was published in 1870 the German response to *Die Liebe* was conflicted. Krafft-Ebing's masochist patients proved neither the first nor the last to assume Sacher-Masoch's eccentricity in sexual matters. Indeed, the reception of *Die Liebe* illuminates changing public perceptions of sexuality, and of Sacher-Masoch. In private letters the author remarked on this phenomenon with ironic bemusement. Six years after Sacher-Masoch's death, his biographer and former private secretary, Carl Felix von Schlichtegroll, had the last word. In a biography projected also as a contribution to contemporary sexological debate, Schlichtegroll confirmed the suspicion widely held among Sacher-Masoch's readers that the author of *Venus im Pelz* was a masochist. Schlichtegroll's foray into sexological discourse from the perspective of the cultural history of cruelty would enrich the genre of biography; at the same time, it compromised the reputation and image of Sacher-Masoch, helping to obscure the significance of his oeuvre and overshadowing his development of the Darwinian novella.

Part One of *Die Liebe* had been glowingly received in 1870. Yet, to the author's intense surprise, a substantial number of German literary critics took offence when Part Two appeared in the same year, particularly to the fourth and fifth novellas, that is, to *Die Liebe des Plato* and, above all, to *Venus im Pelz*. These two novellas led critics to express outright disgust at what they perceived to be obscene content. In 1870 A. von Schweiger wrote: 'one is ashamed to meet a woman on the street and to think that Sacher-Masoch's novel is a reflection of our time!'[89] The same year, in a damning review for the respectable liberal newspaper *Neue Freie Presse*, Karl von Thaler had attested that Sacher-Masoch was not alone in his proclivities: 'the sensuality of our time is sick; it is not satisfied in a harmless way, it cannot get rid of its awareness of sin.... This disease is widespread, and the best of our contemporaries are not always free of it. However, no one has caught the disease as severely as Sacher-Masoch.'[90] Those openly appreciative of the writing likewise criticised his portrayal of the shadowy side of love as far too crass, 'even for non-prudes'.[91] For these respondents, Sacher-Masoch was exceeding bourgeois respectability and with it the very boundaries of representation. Such criticism was also voiced by Rudolf von Gottschall, a stern supporter of the author, who contended that certain problems – although worth considering from a philosophical viewpoint – do not lend themselves to literary portrayal. He warned that 'in the realms of aesthetics both the psychological and the pathological involve danger': in his view such materials were both aesthetically objectionable and altogether revolting, their depiction invoking repulsion and disgust.[92]

Twentieth-century literary scholars have tended to interpret the emotive response of these literary critics in light of modern sensibilities, reading their reaction as an aversion to masochism.[93] However, the moral outrage expressed in the various contemporary reviews masks any detailed critique of what exactly was at stake. In 1878, in a rare exchange of letters with his publishers on the occasion of the third, revised edition of *Die Liebe*, Sacher-Masoch reflected on this criticism and offered a different perspective. According to his statement, the German critics had not based their rejection of *Venus im Pelz* 'on the theme of sensual love and the affinity between cruelty and sensuality ... [and] just as little on the content of the tale and the hero's love madness that makes him the slave of the beloved woman'. In Sacher-Masoch's eyes the problem lay not in Severin's 'supersensualism' but in the fact that 'the hero literally forces the heroine to mistreat him' and educates her to be his tyrant.[94]

German readers were certainly familiar with lovesick heroes on a path to self-destruction – Johann Wolfgang von Goethe's international bestseller of 1774, *Die Leiden des jungen Werthers* (*The Sorrows of Young Werther*) is probably the most famous example of such a narrative. Sacher-Masoch's suggestion that the character of Wanda was the decisive trigger for the critics' condemnation does seem plausible, particularly considering the importance of the education of women for the self-image of the German middle class. Literature had traditionally functioned to affirm the lifestyle of middle-class readers; as Jürgen Habermas has argued, it simultaneously served as entertainment and a preparation for real life.[95] Changes to middle-class households at the beginning of the nineteenth century had produced a shift in family size and had redirected female identity towards a new concept of domesticity and the virtues of modesty. In this context, the family became a place of education, one in which women could broaden their horizons under male guidance. While women were thenceforth watching over family morals, engagement with society became a joint project for both spouses and an integral part of middle-class female identity.[96] Sacher-Masoch reflected these social developments in the novellas of *Die Liebe*. In *Marzella*, he strongly advocates the education of Alexander's spouse, Marzella, while *Venus im Pelz* functions as a cautionary tale, when Severin educates Wanda to become cruel towards him. Nonetheless, German criticism was still resolutely concerned with the world of sex rather than sexuality, to the extent that Severin's condition was interpreted as physical in nature: the underlying problem structuring *Venus im Pelz* was the antihero's incapacity to perform the sexual act. Severin's impotence was thus presumed to be the basis for his distracted state of mind, and his educational and sexual aberrations were presumed to be a substitute for his suppressed sexual longings.

Sacher-Masoch clearly understood the criticism levelled at him and reacted accordingly. His response to his critics was more differentiated than commonly assumed. Firstly, he launched a belligerent counter-attack on German literary criticism in 1873. The short book *Ueber den Werth der Kritik* (*On the Worth of Criticism*) argues that personal and financial interests define the views expressed in contemporary newspapers and journals. Confidently taking the reception of his own work as the starting point, Sacher-Masoch further decries the entrenched conservative character of the criticism of his novellas, maintaining that critics apply only established literary norms, which are inevitably inadequate to works that engage with a new aesthetic.[97] Secondly, on several occasions Sacher-Masoch ineffectively pushed his publisher, Cotta, to release separate editions of the novellas from *Die Liebe*, especially *Marzella*.[98] The relevant correspondence does not reveal the author's motivation for pursuing this separate publication, but financial need could not have been the sole reason. Ultimately, Cotta did not comply with Sacher-Masoch's wishes, and the author had 171 copies of *Marzella* printed at his own expense.[99] Thus it seems likely that he wanted to emphasise the moral direction of his work, and rebuff his critics by disseminating copies of the novella that outlined the ethical and moral commitments of his writing. Thirdly, Sacher-Masoch's exchange of letters with Cotta in connection with the third edition of *Das Vermächtnis Kains* reveals a further strategy for dealing with contemporary criticism. In 1878 Cotta approached the author regarding a somewhat delicate matter. All copies of the second edition of *Die Liebe* had been sold and the publisher wished to launch a third edition – but only on the proviso that *Venus im Pelz* be omitted, or exchanged for another novella. Cotta justified this change of heart by revealing that the original novella had not been read by their literary adviser before publication; the positive reference had been based on the other novellas in the volume.[100] Replying to Cotta, Sacher-Masoch rejected the idea of a third edition of *Die Liebe* with the omission of *Venus im Pelz*; however, he proposed to rewrite the latter work. He indicated that he had been toying with this idea for at least two years. Cotta agreed to the rewrite on the condition that the new version be subject to 'in house' approval.[101] Three months later Sacher-Masoch reported on his progress, emphasising the effort necessary to rearrange his novella: many scenes had to be cut; the character of Wanda changed to an 'innately hedonistic, despotic and cruel woman'; the whip converted from a tantalising stimulus to a mere means of corporal punishment.[102] The third edition was duly published in 1878 and Sacher-Masoch's strategy of appeasement seems to have achieved its purpose. In a review of the new edition, Rudolf von Gottschall at least argued that the once offensive scenes seemed decisively toned down.[103]

But were Sacher-Masoch's Darwinian novellas steeped in the world of sex or sexuality? And is it important to consider him a *masochist*, a man whose sexual desires were pathological from the perspective of his historical time and place? These questions need to be addressed because of persistent and ongoing interest in Sacher-Masoch's sexual life and the irrefutable impact of such interest on the reception of his work. During Sacher-Masoch's lifetime, two groups had an intrinsic investment in speculating about the author's sexual desire and proclivities. On more than one occasion, critical voices, notably from the political right, accused Sacher-Masoch of writing 'degenerate' literature and of being afflicted with a pathology.[104] Probably this assumption was also made by some of Krafft-Ebing's patients, and by Sacher-Masoch's similarly inclined followers in Germany and Austria. Sacher-Masoch had claimed in 1873 that 'every aesthetic prophet, as well as any religious one, finds odd enthusiastic followers, who in their excitement and in their ardor exaggerate and outdo the master'.[105] Such followers sought contact with the author and flocked to his home in Lindheim, as evidenced in a private letter written in 1895 by his widow and second wife, Hulda von Meister: 'over and over again new enquiries regarding [new books such as] *Venus im Pelz* arrived, as if he were a factory. All those people, however, did not get in touch after his death; none of them, rich factory owners, officers, lawyers was able to express their thanks through a gift.'[106]

After his death, Sacher-Masoch's two long-term spouses attested that he was different from masochists of his time. Hulda von Meister was insistent:

> If my husband had such a 'perverse inclination', I can only [wish] every woman to have a man of such inclinations; she has heaven on earth. If my husband was driven more and more [in this direction, it was] so firstly because of his first wife and secondly because of the audience [for *Venus im Pelz*]. How beautiful and divine was this passion in my husband, how common in others.[107]

True, Wanda von Sacher-Masoch, the author's first wife, complained in her autobiography that she had been forced to wear fur coats when writing her novels at home. However, she explicitly defended her former husband against sexologists and masochists alike, accusing the former of having created a masochist fad during Sacher-Masoch's lifetime.[108] Meanwhile, masochists only 'inflame their passions through cruel fantasies', but Sacher-Masoch had shown a physiological commitment to experience his own subjugation: 'what he longed for in torture and cruelties from women, he longed for in reality – and he endured it'.[109] For Wanda von Sacher-Masoch, masochists remained 'cowardly, insipid and mentally dull'. Her criticisms seem unsurprising considering the continuing attentions she received due to the notoriety of *Venus im Pelz*. These attentions were exemplified by the letters of a Prague masochist, which she eventually forwarded to Krafft-Ebing.[110] Both Sacher-Masoch's first wife and second wife led relatively impoverished lives, Hulda von Meister because of limited copyright laws that would otherwise have protected her income. Both women were required to make a living as single mothers, while protecting their respective reputations. Despite this motivating context for the women's defence of Sacher-Masoch, it becomes clear that the writer's place was not among those perceived or defined as masochists by his contemporaries.

Nor did Sacher-Masoch perceive his own sexual proclivities as deviant. A letter to Otto von Kapf in 1876 includes the statement: 'it has always amused me, if one has accused me of frivolity or even susceptibility [to perversion], because I portray human beings the way they really are. I lead a life to which even the most rigorous Northern German or Englishman could apply their moral standards'. He points to the happiness of his marriage, the luck of having three healthy and intelligent children, and the comfort in which he and his family live.[111] He makes no reference to a desire for cruel women or comparable topics in his autobiography, which is, rather, about his fascination with science.[112] His self-image was that of a virile man and an intellectual, and the facts that he was sexually active and fathered six children made him an unlikely candidate for the nineteenth-century category of the masochist.

The most useful key to understanding Sacher-Masoch's legacy lies in the wide scope of his literary ambitions. In Pierre Bourdieu's study of Gustave Flaubert's 1869 novel *L'Éducation sentimentale* (*Sentimental Education*), the French sociologist and philosopher suggests that Flaubert separates himself from his main character, Frédéric, in an attempt to 'perceive an enterprise of ***objectification of the self***'.[113] This is a plausible interpretation through which to reflect in sociological terms on the relationship between Sacher-Masoch's life and work. Furthermore, both the year in which Flaubert's novel was first published and Sacher-Masoch's avowed admiration for Flaubert allow speculation regarding the direct influence of *L'Éducation sentimentale* on *Venus im Pelz*. Sacher-Masoch saw in Flaubert a fellow searcher for truth.[114] According to Bourdieu, Flaubert 'objectified the structure of the relationship that tied him, as a writer, to the political field', presenting only a subjective viewpoint comparable to that of Turgenev's *Dnevnik Lishnego Cheloveka*, a perspective which refused his readers an 'absolute conviction'.[115] Yet even as he admired Flaubert, Sacher-Masoch's interests lay in a distinctly different field. If Flaubert insisted on the autonomy of art and taunted his readers, Sacher-Masoch's focus was on literature as a reasoned method for the description of human behaviour. For him, literature served a scientific purpose and his literary cases remained firmly embedded in their Darwinian framework. Sacher-Masoch thus abandoned the autonomy of art, erasing the difference between fact and fiction on the pretext of finding an objective, arguable truth. His contract with his early lover Fanny von Pistor, often quoted as a proof of his masochist predisposition, succinctly outlines the difference between Severin and Sacher-Masoch.[116] Like Severin, Sacher-Masoch asks to be enslaved by his lover, but the author explicitly stipulates a need for six hours of writing time each day.[117] Severin was unable to formulate a coherent narrative of his past adventure, but Sacher-Masoch was able to document a self-conscious experiment in his own subjection to the forces of nature.[118] This experience would then inform his vivid description of Severin, his own feelings rendered unimportant as he tackled the task of writing in the self-appointed role of the scientist. If he enjoyed instigating his own sexual subjection, he conceptualised this practice by literary means through a Darwinian worldview – not a sexological one.

After Sacher-Masoch's death in 1895, and with the increasing acceptance of sexology as a field of study and investigation, the debate surrounding the author took a decisively new turn. That is, in 1901, six years after his death, and thirty-one years after the first publication of *Venus im Pelz*, Felix von Schlichtegroll published the first biography of Sacher-Masoch, titled *Sacher-Masoch und der Masochismus* (*Sacher-Masoch and Masochism*). Schlichtegroll was Sacher-Masoch's former secretary, an author and a cultural historian of cruelty; in this biography he outed his favourite author as a masochist. Schlichtegroll revealed details of Sacher-Masoch's private life, certainly awaited with curiosity by many of the latter's readers. The biography's merits as well as its parochialism are defined by the intellectual commitments of its author: Schlichtegroll's interests were centred on sexuality. He had known the man Sacher-Masoch; Sacher-Masoch's widow had permitted him access to the writer's diaries; Schlichtegroll had also edited (possibly co-authored) Sacher-Masoch's novel *Afrikas Semiramis* (*Africa's Semiramis*) and the highly successful *Hinterlassene Novellen* (*Bequeathed Novellas*) of 1907.[119] *Sacher-Masoch und der Masochismus* became the first notable success in a career that would focus predominantly on issues of masochism and sadism. This focus is obvious in Schlichtegroll's series of novels collectively titled *Die Venuspeitsche* (*The Whip of Venus*).[120] Other works followed, among them a scathing biography of Sacher-Masoch's first wife, Wanda; a historical study titled *Die Bestie im Weibe: Beiträge zur Geschichte menschlicher Verirrung und Grausamkeit* (*The Beast in Women: Contribution to the History of Human Aberration and Cruelty*), published in 1903; and a history of flagellation (*Geschichte des Flagellantismus*, 1913).[121] Writing Sacher-Masoch's biography allowed Schlichtegroll to offer insights into the life of the admired author and helped to open the genre of biography to matters of sexuality. Schlichtegroll also put forward his own views on the cultural history of masochism, although he preferred the Greek-derived term *algolagnia*.[122] Consequently, *Sacher-Masoch und der Masochismus* encompasses biographical information, several chapters on sexological discourse concerning masochism, and a survey of the depiction of masochist themes in literature and art.

Schlichtegroll's biographical description contains several key points that, by the early twentieth century, had become standard in the sexological description of masochism. He notes that Sacher-Masoch was fascinated by bloodthirsty stories; as a youth Sacher-Masoch frequently dreamed and fantasised about being controlled by a dominant woman, often a sultana who tortured him with pleasure. Moreover, Sacher-Masoch supposedly grasped the nature of these dreams after reading Rousseau's *Confessions*.[123] Schlichtegroll also provides his reader with a coming-of-age scene: apparently the young Sacher-Masoch witnessed his paternal aunt's love affair with an admirer who kissed her ermine slippers (and more). In Schlichtegroll's telling, when Sacher-Masoch's uncle discovered this and rushed into the room, he was punched by his wife, who whipped both lover and husband out of her sight.[124] Schlichtegroll's discussion of

Sacher-Masoch's life unfolds chronologically, with reference to the writer's publications, on the basis that 'the best comment [to] be made concerning Sacher-Masoch's life is that it [his oeuvre] describes the course of his life'.[125] When Schlichtegroll unveils Sacher-Masoch's long-standing affair with Anna Kottowitz, he uses Sacher-Masoch's description of Wanda von Dunajew, that is, the character Wanda in *Venus im Pelz*. The biographer suggests that Sacher-Masoch gave Kottowitz *Manon Lescaut* to read, just as Severin gives the French novel to Wanda.[126] Schlichtegroll has Kottowitz become aroused and inspired after reading *Venus im Pelz*.[127] In other words, for his biographer, Sacher-Masoch's literary works represented romans-à-clef, and were to be taken as both factual and autobiographical.

The obvious and important difference between a biography and *Venus im Pelz* – the critical distance with which Sacher-Masoch portrays Severin, his characterisation of the male protagonist as an exemplary dilettante in matters of love, and not a sophisticated writer – remains lost in Schlichtegroll's account. To structure and narrate Sacher-Masoch's biography through his works was to overstate Sacher-Masoch's consideration of the content of *Venus im Pelz* in a severely distorting manner. Since the literary estate of Sacher-Masoch was destroyed, and the surviving fragments are not readily accessible, Schlichtegroll's text has remained the key source for Sacher-Masoch's life. It is also possible that Schlichtegroll's slippage between fact and fiction affected the alleged diary entries in *Sacher-Masoch und der Masochismus*. At the time of its publication, Wanda von Sacher-Masoch insisted that the diary entries quoted by Schlichtegroll were forged.[128] Another scenario is plausible: in his will to methodically establish Sacher-Masoch as a masochist, Schlichtegroll may have interpreted or misappropriated as diary entries Sacher-Masoch's notes for *Venus im Pelz*. In independently surviving pages of his diary, Sacher-Masoch uses the first-person perspective to present his voice, while supposed 'diary' quotations are all presented in the form of dialogues – similar to those printed in *Venus im Pelz*.[129]

Whatever the factual bases of Schlichtegroll's biography, *Sacher-Masoch und der Masochismus* prompted a number of sexologists to step forward and re-evaluate images of Sacher-Masoch, and Krafft-Ebing was chief among these. For the first time, his eleventh edition of *Psychopathia Sexualis* (1901) pointed out Sacher-Masoch's masochism in a footnote. Krafft-Ebing's comment is written in a slightly defensive tone, but he also indirectly distances himself from the 'outing':

> In the last years I have, by the way, received proof that Sacher-Masoch was not only the poet of masochism but was himself suffering from this anomaly. Although this proof was given to me without any reservations, I refrain from publishing it. I have to repudiate the rebuke I have been given by some admirers of the poet and by certain critics of my book because I combined the name of a well-respected writer with a perversion of sexual life. As a human being Sacher-Masoch will surely not be less highly regarded in the eyes of any educated person just because of the fact that

> he – not through his fault – was suffering from an anomaly in his sexual life. However, as a writer he has suffered severe damages to his creative work and its reception, because he was a very talented writer – as long and as far as he did not touch on his perversion – and he would have achieved great things, if he had been a human being who felt in a sexually normal way.[130]

Reviewing Schlichtegroll's biography in 1901, Albert Eulenburg, a key figure in sexological research, retrospectively adjusted his own interpretation of Sacher-Masoch's first novel, *Der letzte König der Magyaren* (*The Last King of the Magyars*), published in 1867: 'I did not yet guess how closely the account was connected to the personal characteristics of his writer'.[131] The same review of *Sacher-Masoch und der Masochismus* also describes *Venus im Pelz* as one of Sacher-Masoch's best and most mature novellas, while implying that this work might have profited from the closeness of the writer to his 'model', Severin.[132] A year later Eulenburg published his study *Sadismus und Masochismus* (*Sadism and Masochism*) in which a chapter is dedicated to Sacher-Masoch's person. After quoting various sources, Eulenburg describes Sacher-Masoch as a weak but lovable and charming character, whose lifestyle would eventually lead to personal downfall and result in the 'unmistakably inferior quality of his late literary works'.[133] Eulenberg did not consider at all the financial strife faced by many professional writers at the time and its impact on the quality of literary production.

Emphasising the concurrence of Sacher-Masoch's alleged sexual preferences and his central literary themes, Schlichtegroll's new interpretation helped sexology to close the uncomfortable gap between Sacher-Masoch's lived life and his work; his biography was to have a profound and lasting impact on the reception of Sacher-Masoch's writing. *Sacher-Masoch und der Masochismus* also began what can only be described as a sudden fashion for masochist cultural materials: the German public was engulfed by a plethora of books, articles and illustrations in newspapers – a fact remarked upon by Freud in his elaborations on masochism quoted above. *Venus im Pelz* became a code phrase with a currency far beyond its masochist counter-public, as modernist writers such as Robert Musil and Franz Kafka turned to masochism and channelled the concept into the realms of high culture in works such as *Die Verwirrungen des Zöglings Törleß* (*The Confusions of Young Törless*) of 1906, *Die Verwandlung* (*Metamorphosis*) of 1915 and *Der Prozess* (*The Trial*), eventually published in 1925. As discussed in Chapter 5, writer and medical doctor Alfred Döblin did likewise, in works that seamlessly integrated Darwinian and scientific thought.

***

In the years following its publication, Sacher-Masoch's daring exploration of modern subjectivity from the perspective of Darwinism had garnered a group of followers who closely identified with Severin. In turn, these followers inspired Krafft-Ebing to name masochism after the author of *Venus im Pelz*. By the first years of the twentieth century the vivid content of Sacher-Masoch's problem novella, the penultimate of the six collected in *Die Liebe*, had come to haunt the author and his reputation. In a poignant and sarcastic comment, Viennese cultural critic Karl Kraus (1874–1936) noted that Krafft-Ebing owed his world fame 'to the interest in the content of novels by overheated readers, followers of his doctrine of sexual perversions', implying that only those primarily interested in sexual perversions would read Sacher-Masoch's novels.[134] Kraus pre-empted Foucault's critique of the sexologist–patient relationship, and pointed out the underlying tautology in Krafft-Ebing's methodology. When he called masochism 'a silly novel-medical term', ridiculing the fictional basis of the medical expression, he might have summarised the situation more aptly than he wished.[135] It seems unlikely that Krafft-Ebing would have included literary works in *Psychopathia Sexualis* if not for the insistence of his patients that *Venus im Pelz* described their experience so well.

The reception of *Venus im Pelz* paradigmatically depicts the shift between the worlds of sex and sexuality. Sacher-Masoch's Darwinian novella opened a new trajectory that ultimately failed to find the audience he had hoped for. Instead, the anthropological impetus behind Sacher-Masoch's Darwinian novellas made them particularly easy to reinterpret as psychiatric case studies. After his former private secretary 'outed' him as a masochist and equated literary with biographical knowledge, sexology willingly confirmed Sacher-Masoch's belonging to the world of sexuality. Sacher-Masoch became an involuntary pioneer in this respect as well. During the decade following his outing, sexological and psychoanalytic interest in pathographies of intellectuals boomed, and writers and musicians in particular found themselves at the centre of scientific debate. In the early 1900s, alongside distinct ideas about creativity, new styles of reasoning were emerging in the fields of sexology and psychoanalysis that would significantly reshape the biographical case for the twentieth century.

Notes

1 A short remark regarding the use of the term 'masochism' in this chapter: where not otherwise indicated, 'masochism' and related terms designate a current understanding of a sexual practice widely spread throughout the history of human sexuality – the receiving of predominantly sexual pleasure from acts involving the reception of pain or humiliation. Masochism does not play a central role in twenty-first-century psychiatric debate. Nevertheless, in the World Health Organization's *International Classification of Diseases* (ICD), the related term 'sadomasochism' (F65.5) is still listed under F65, 'Disorders of sexual preference' (www.who.int/classifications/icd/en/ 13/7/2011). The *Diagnostic and Statistical Manual of Mental Disorders* (DSM) published by the American Psychiatric Association lists the term under the category paraphilia. The manual's latest edition

(DSM-IV-TR) requires that, to be diagnosed as a paraphilia, the activity must be the sole means of sexual gratification for a period of six months, and either cause 'clinically significant distress or impairment in social, occupational, or other important areas of functioning' or involve a violation of consent. See Russell B. Hilliard and Robert L. Spitzer, 'Letter to the Editor: Change in Criterion of Paraphilias in DSM-IV-TR', *American Journal of Psychiatry*, 157:7 (2002), p. 1249, http://ajp.psychiatryonline.org/article.aspx?Volume=159&page=1249&-journalID =13, accessed 31 August 2012.

2 Arnold I. Davidson, 'Sex and the Emergence of Sexuality', *Critical Inquiry*, 14:1 (1987), pp. 16–48, p. 22.

3 This formulaic accusation features in many works of secondary literature and is especially pronounced in works that aim to investigate Sacher-Masoch's work as an expression of masochism. These tend to conflate the naming of masochism after the author with the legal criminalisation of masochism from the nineteenth century onwards. Key examples include John K. Noyes, *The Mastery of Submission: Inventions of Masochism* (Ithaca: Cornell University Press, 1997); Michael Gratzke, *Liebesschmerz und Textlust. Figuren der Liebe und des Masochismus in der Literatur* (Würzburg: Könighausen & Neumann, 1997).

4 Laura Doan raises the issue of 'caseness' in her book *Disturbing Practices: History, Sexuality and Women's Experience of Modern War* (Chicago: University of Chicago Press, 2013).

5 Michel Foucault, *The History of Sexuality, vol. I: An Introduction*, trans. Robert Hurley (New York: Vintage Books, 1990).

6 Compare Ian Hacking, 'Language, Truth, and Reason', in *Historical Ontology* (Cambridge: Harvard University Press, 2002), pp. 159–77.

7 Paolo Savoia, 'Sexual Science and Self-narrative: Epistemology and Narrative Technologies of the Self between Krafft-Ebing and Freud', *History of the Human Sciences*, 23:5 (2010), pp. 17–41, p. 29.

8 Harry Oosterhuis, *Stepchildren of Nature: Krafft-Ebing, Psychiatry, and the Making of Sexual Identity* (Chicago: University of Chicago Press, 2000), p. 12.

9 Birgit Lang, 'Translation as Transposition. Leopold von Sacher-Masoch, Darwinian Thought, and the Concept of Love in German Sexual Modernity', in Heike Bauer (ed.), *Sexology and Translation: Cultural and Scientific Encounters* (Philadelphia: Temple University Press, 2015), pp. 19–35.

10 Sigmund Freud, 'The Economic Problem of Masochism', in James Strachey (ed.), with Anna Freud, Alix Strachey and Alan Tyson, *The Standard Edition of the Complete Psychological Works by Sigmund Freud*, vol. XIX (London: Hogarth Press and Institute for Psychoanalysis, 1978), pp. 157–70, p. 162.

11 Dimitry Stefanowski, 'Passivism – A Variety of Sexual Perversion', *Alienist and Neurologist: A Quarterly Journal of Scientific, Clinical and Forensic Psychiatry and Neurology*, 13 (1892), pp. 650–7, p. 655.

12 Richard von Krafft-Ebing, *Neuere Forschungen auf dem Gebiet der Psychopathia Sexualis*, 1st edition (Stuttgart: Enke, 1890), p. 2. The German original reads: 'Diese im folgenden zu besprechenden Perversionen der Vita Sexualis mögen Masochismus genannt werden, da der bekannte Romanschriftsteller Sacher Masoch in zahlreichen seiner Romane, ganz besonders in seinem bekannten "Die Venus im Pelz", diese eigene Art der sexuellen Perversion zum Lieblingsgegenstand seiner Schriften gemacht hat. Dieser Masochismus stellt das Gegenstück einer nach dem Vorgang der Franzosen 'Sadismus' genannten Form sexueller Perversion dar, deren berüchtigter Vertreter der monströse Marquis de Sade war.' If not otherwise noted, all translations are by the author of this chapter.

13 Sacher-Masoch's first biographer, Carl Felix von Schlichtegroll, also underlines the fact that Krafft-Ebing named masochism in honour of Sacher-Masoch's depiction of Severin; see Schlichtegroll, the chapter titled 'Sacher-Masoch und der Masochismus', in his *Sacher-Masoch: enthaltend Sacher-Masoch und der*

Masochismus sowie 'Wanda' ohne Maske und Pelz nebst einem Dossier, ed. Lisbeth Exner and Michael Farin (Munich: Belleville, 2003), p. 34.

14 Davidson, 'Sex and the Emergence of Sexuality', p. 22.

15 Renate Hauser, 'Einleitung', in Richard von Krafft-Ebing, *Eine Studienreise durch Südeuropa 1869/70*, ed. Renate Hauser (Graz: Leykam, 2000), pp. 10–19, p. 11.

16 This happened to the British Renaissance scholar John Addington Symonds; see Seán Brady, *John Addington Symonds (1840–1893) and Homosexuality: A Critical Edition of Sources* (New York: Palgrave Macmillan, 2012), p. 24.

17 Robert Beachy, 'The German Invention of Homosexuality', *Journal of Modern History*, 82:4 (2010), pp. 801–38, p. 816.

18 Wellcome Library, London, Richard von Krafft-Ebing Papers, Case Notes 1877–1902, MSS PP/KEB/A/4: Box 1.

19 Paul Weindling, 'Bourgeois Values, Doctors and the State', in David Blackbourn and Richard J. Evans (eds), *The German Bourgeoisie* (London: Routledge, 1991), pp. 198–223, p. 198.

20 'Sexual Psychology and Pathology. Review', *British Medical Journal*, i:2145 (1902), p. 339.

21 'Review of *Psychopathia Sexualis*, English Translation of 7th Edition', *Alienist and Neurologist: A Quarterly Journal of Scientific, Clinical and Forensic Psychiatry and Neurology*, 14 (1893), pp. 526–7.

22 Ivan Crozier, 'Pillow Talk: Credibility, Trust and the Sexological Case History', History of Science, 46:4 (2008), pp. 375–404, p. 388. Crozier refers to Charles Féré, *The Evolution and Dissolution of the Sexual Instinct* (Paris: Charles Carrington, 1904), pp. 190–1, and Marc Raffalovich, 'Uranism, Congenital Sexual Inversion: Observations and Recommendation', *Journal of Comparative Neurology*, 5 (1895), pp. 33–65, p. 38.

23 George L. Mosse, *Nationalism and Sexuality: Respectability and Abnormal Sexuality in Europe* (New York: Fertig, 1985), p. 8.

24 Oosterhuis, *Stepchildren of Nature*, p. 199.

25 In late nineteenth-century England, key theorists of the study of sex often lacked a scientific background; relevant studies reflected aesthetic sensibilities, which did not necessarily make their discourse more inclusive. See Heike Bauer, *English Literary Sexology: Translations of Inversion, 1860–1930* (Basingstoke: Palgrave Macmillan, 2009), pp. 79–80. The French erotic imagination, too, was shaped by an exchange between medical and lay cultures: based on his self-assessment, writers like Gustave Flaubert were regarded as neurotic. See Vernon A. Rosario, *The Erotic Imagination: French Histories of Perversity* (New York: Oxford University Press, 1991), p. 10, p. 82. Anna Katharina Schaffner's recent study traces the interdependence between medical and literary debates on perversion; however, for her, Krafft-Ebing's work is still based in the framework of pathology. She perceives Sacher-Masoch as having been horrified by the naming of masochism. See Schaffner, *Modernism and Perversion: Sexual Deviance in Sexology and Literature, 1850–1930* (Basingstoke: Palgrave Macmillan, 2012), p. 54.

26 Peter Sprengel, *Darwin in der Poesie. Spuren der Evolutionslehre in der deutschsprachigen Literatur des 19. und 20. Jahrhunderts* (Würzburg: Könighausen und Neumann, 1998), pp. 49–50.

27 'Vorläufig dürften die Dichter bessere Psychologen sein, als die Psychologen und Philosophen von Fach, aber sie sind Gefühls- und nicht Verstandesmenschen und mindestens einseitig in der Betrachtung ihres Gegenstands. Sehen sie doch über dem Licht der sonnigen Wärme des Stoffes, von dem sie Nahrung ziehen, nicht die tiefen Schatten. Mögen auch die Erzeugnisse der Dichtkunst aller Zeiten und Völker dem Monographen einer "Psychologie der Liebe" unerschöpflichen Stoff bieten, so kann die grosse Aufgabe doch nur gelöst werden unter Mithülfe

[*sic*] der Naturwissenschaft und speciell [*sic*] der Medicin [*sic*], welche den psychologischen Stoff an seiner anatomisch-physiologischen Quelle erforscht und ihm allseitig gerecht wird.... Wer die Psychopathologie des sexualen Lebens zum Gegenstand einer wissenschaftlichen Abhandlung macht, sieht sich einer Nachtseite menschlichen Lebens und Elends gegenübergestellt, in deren Schatten das glänzende Götterbild des Dichters zur scheusslichen [*sic*] Fratze wird und die Moral und Ästhetik an dem "Ebenbild Gottes" irre werden möchte.' Krafft-Ebing, *Psychopathia Sexualis*, 1st edition, 1886, pp. iv–v.

28 Krafft-Ebing, *Neuere Forschungen*, 1st edition, 1890, pp. 25, 13.

29 'Ich schliesse [*sic*] meine Zeilen mit dem Wunsche, dass sie der Wissenschaft dienen mögen.' Krafft-Ebing, *Neuere Forschungen*, 1st edition, 1890, p. 28.

30 Oosterhuis, *Stepchildren of Nature*, p. 174f. Oosterhuis interprets the following quote from Mr X's autobiography to ascribe the authorship of the term 'masochism' to Mr X: 'I believe to have proven that what we want to call masochism is an independent occurrence'. The German original reads, 'Ich glaube somit dargethan [*sic*] zu haben, dass das, was wir Masochismus nennen wollen, als eine selbstständige Erscheinung existirt [*sic*]'. Krafft-Ebing, *Neuere Forschungen*, 1st edition, 1890, p. 25. In this context the use of 'we', however, does not imply a *pluralis modestiae*, but rather expresses familiarity between the two correspondents.

31 Krafft-Ebing, *Neuere Forschungen*, 1st edition, 1890, p. 6. At this point Krafft-Ebing also begins to reflect on the differences between the imagined and the actual wish to be caned. He would refer to the former phenomenon as 'ideational masochism'.

32 'Von grossem [*sic*] Interesse ist es, dass derlei in dichterischen Werken vorkommt. Wenn auch solche nicht den Werth von Krankengeschichten haben können, so haben sie doch mindestens psychologisches Interesse, insofern der Autor aus seiner Erfahrung geschöpft oder wenigstens derlei empfunden haben muss.' Krafft-Ebing, *Neuere Forschungen*, 1st edition, 1890, p. 29.

33 'In allerlei Lektüren suchte ich Beziehungen zu meinen Lieblingsvorstellungen. Rousseaus confessions [*sic*], die mir damals in die Hände fielen, boten mir eine grosse [*sic*] Entdeckung. Ich fand einen Zustand geschildert, der in wesentlichen Punkten dem meinigen glich. Noch mehr erstaunte ich über die Uebereinstimmung [*sic*] mit meinen Ideen, als ich Sacher-Masoch's Schriften kennen lernte. Ich verschlang sie alle mit Begierde, obwohl die blutrünstigen Scenen [*sic*] oft weit über meine Phantasien hinausgingen.' Krafft-Ebing, *Neuere Forschungen*, 1st edition, 1890, p. 17.

34 'Ein Mann in hervorragender Stellung in Wien hat, als Bedienter gekleidet, auf dem Kutschbock des Wagens seiner Maitresse Fahrten in den Prater mitgemacht. Hier dürfte eine bewusste Nachahmung der 'Venus im Pelz' vorliegen. Überhaupt scheint mir, dass die Schriften des Sacher-Masoch viel zur Entwicklung dieser Perversion bei Disponirten [*sic*] beigetragen hat.' Krafft-Ebing, *Neuere Forschungen*, 1st edition, 1890, p. 26.

35 'Er meint, es könnte ihn nur ein Weib reizen, das den Heldinnen in den Romanen von Sacher-Masoch gleiche.' Krafft-Ebing, *Neuere Forschungen*, 1st edition, 1890, p. 23.

36 'Auf Sacher-Masoch's Schriften berufen sich viele von dieser Perversion Ergriffene, wie aus den obigen Beobachtungen ersichtlich, ausdrücklich als auf typische Darstellungen ihres eigenen psychischen Zustands.' Krafft-Ebing, *Neuere Forschungen*, 2nd edition, 1891, p. 37.

37 In the sixth edition of his *Psychopathia Sexualis*, published in 1891, Krafft-Ebing differentiates the masochistic taxonomy by distinguishing between: 'maltreatment and humiliation for the purpose of sexual satisfaction – masochism'; 'disgusting acts for the purpose of humiliation and sexual satisfaction – masked masochism'; 'feet and shoe fetishists'; and 'female masochism' (already known). This greater

differentiation between masochism and masked masochism served two purposes. Firstly, Krafft-Ebing was able to unpair masochism and flagellation. For quite some time his writings had been haunted by an awareness that some people used flagellation only for sexual stimulus, while others used it as a substitute for intercourse. As of 1891, flagellation literally belonged to another chapter of *Psychopathia Sexualis*, while masochism had found a new opposite. Secondly, Krafft-Ebing was now able to integrate fetishism into his taxonomy, mentioned until this point in the context of masochism, but not properly classified.

38 Krafft-Ebing shortens part of the history of nervous disorders within the family, the strict education through his parents, and the fact that he changed his career twice without escaping general boredom and melancholia. Krafft-Ebing, *Neuere Forschungen*, 1st edition, 1890, pp. 15, 16, 18–22; *Neuere Forschungen*, 2nd edition, 1891, pp. 2–9.

39 Krafft-Ebing, *Neuere Forschungen*, 1st edition, 1890, pp. 26–7; Krafft-Ebing, *Neuere Forschungen*, 2nd edition, 1891, pp. 33–4.

40 In the fifth edition of *Psychopathia Sexualis*, published in 1890, Kleist's *Käthchen von Heilbronn* had been presented as an example of female masochism, but only a year later Krafft-Ebing judged Kleist 'undoubtedly not mentally normal'. Krafft-Ebing, *Psychopathia Sexualis*, 6th edition, 1891, p. 75. Krafft-Ebing does not name a reason for his change of heart, and the awkward phrasing in the German original remains puzzling. Krafft-Ebing presumably bases his assumption on Kleist's suicide. The first book-length study of Kleist's pathology was undertaken by psychoanalyst Isidor Sadger in 1909, as discussed in the following chapter of the present study.

41 Schaffner, *Modernism and Perversion*, pp. 48–9.

42 Ooisterhuis, *Stepchildren of Nature*, p. 195.

43 The German original reads: 'dass der Same nur so von ihm läuft'. Krafft-Ebing, *Neuere Forschungen*, 2nd edition, 1891, p. 29.

44 'Eine höchst bemerkenswerthe [*sic*], ja sogar staunenerregende Thatsache [*sic*] ist es, dass es einen Autor gibt, der den Inhalt seiner derartigen Schwärmereien, anstatt dieselben, wie Andere, im tieferstinnersten Gemüthe zu bewahren, der Allgemeinheit preisgibt und zwar in Form von Novellen und Romane. In der *Venus im Pelz* finden wir gleichempfindend Wort für Wort, Zeile für Zeile die uns so vertrauten Vorstellungen, von denen wir freilich bisher glaubten, sie seien unsere ureigensten Erfahrungen.' Krafft-Ebing, *Neuere Forschungen*, 2nd edition, 1891, p. 18.

45 Rita Felski, *Uses of Literature* (Oxford: Blackwell, 2008), p. 39.

46 Felski, *Uses of Literature*, p. 33.

47 'Daher wirkt, vielleicht gerade wegen dieser Hervorzerrung geheim zu haltender Dinge an das Tageslicht, die Lektüre dieses Buches auch auf Masochisten abstossend [*sic*], und daher ernüchternd und heilend! Ein Anderes ist es, bei geschlossenen Augen, in der Einsamkeit sich Dinge vorzustellen, und dieselben in Romanform gedruckt zu lesen. Der Leser kann den Kritiker niemals ganz unterdrücken, und da muss es empörend erscheinen, einem Publikum, das doch nur zum verschwindend geringen Teil aus Masochisten besteht, einen derartigen Unsinn vorzusetzen. Es genüge hiefür, darauf hinzuweisen, dass die betheiligte [*sic*] Personen in dem heissen [*sic*] Florenze unausgesetzt, auch im Zimmer, Pelz zu tragen.' Krafft-Ebing, *Neuere Forschungen*, 2nd edition, 1891, p. 18.

48 However, Case 3 is the only one in which such an argument prevails.

49 Hugo Aust, *Novelle* (Stuttgart: Metzler, 1990), p. 11.

50 Ivan Sergeevich Turgenev, 'The Superfluous Man', in *The Essential Turgenev*, ed. Elizabeth Cheresh Allen (Evanston: Northwestern University Press, 1994), pp. 104–51, p. 117. The timid Chulkaturin befriends Elizaveta and her family, but she falls in love with Prince N–. To his own surprise, Chulkaturin survives and defeats his rival in a duel. Little does the odious hero realise at the time that

this triggers Elizaveta's hatred. After the prince has left her, she consequently marries Bizmenkov, a minor official from the town of O– and a former servant of her lover.

51 Steven Brett Shaklan, '"So Many Foreign and Useless Words!" Ivan Turgenev's Poetics of Negation', in Robert Reid and Joe Andrew (eds), *Turgenev: Art, Ideology and Legacy* (Amsterdam: Rodopi, 2010), pp. 41–60, p. 45.

52 For a general discussion of the theme in Russian literature, see Ellen Chances, 'The Superfluous Man in Russian Literature', in Neil Cornwell (ed.), *The Routledge Companion to Russian Literature* (New York: Routledge, 2001), pp. 111–22.

53 Leopold von Sacher-Masoch, *Venus in Furs*, in Gilles Deleuze and Leopold von Sacher-Masoch, *Masochism: Coldness and Cruelty, and Venus in Furs*, trans. Jean McNeil (New York: Zone Books, 1991), pp. 143–271, pp. 173–4.

54 Sacher-Masoch, *Venus in Furs*, p. 175.

55 'In this way, then, in spite of an ardent, lascivious, and very precocious temperament, not only did I pass beyond the age of puberty without desiring, without knowing, any sensual pleasure beyond those to which Mlle de Lambercier had quite innocently introduced me; but also, when at last the passing years had made me a man, it was again the case that what should have ruined me preserved me. The taste that I had acquired as a child, instead of disappearing, became so identified with that other pleasure that I was never able to dissociate it from the desires aroused through the senses; and this vagary, in conjunction with my natural timidity, has always inhibited me in my approaches to women, because I dare not tell them everything, but nor am I able to perform everything.' Jean-Jacques Rousseau, *Confessions*, trans. Angela Scholar (Oxford: Oxford University Press, 2000), p. 16.

56 Sacher-Masoch, *Venus in Furs*, p. 177.

57 The story's importance is confirmed by its inclusion in the twenty-four-volume collection of short stories *Deutscher Novellenschatz*, edited by Paul Heyse and Hermann Kurz; the collection was published in Munich between 1871 and 1876 by R. Oldenbourg. Heyse was an acclaimed author of novels and novellas and won the Nobel Prize for Literature in 1910. Sacher-Masoch's *Don Juan von Kolomea* was republished as part of this series in 1876 and indeed formed the series' final novella. An exchange of letters between Heyse and German poet Theodor Storm, leading up to this reprint, demonstrates the rumours surrounding Sacher-Masoch. In a letter of 23 March 1870, Storm suggests that Sacher-Masoch had participated in the 1848 Revolution – Sacher-Masoch would have been only twelve years of age at the time. In a letter of March 1875, Heyse comments on Sacher-Masoch's literary capacity, pointing out that beyond the 'revolting goulash of lewdness and thirst for blood' Sacher-Masoch was not a talented writer. See *Theodor Storm–Paul Heyse. Briefwechsel. Kritische Ausgabe. Erster Band: 1853–1875* (Berlin: Erich Schmidt, 1969), pp. 33, 89.

58 '[Ich] vermag … die Menschen nicht ideal zu schildern, weil ich mich nicht … von meinen subjektiven Empfindungen, sondern ganz nur von meiner Erkenntniß [*sic*] leiten laße [*sic*].' Wellcome Library, London, Western MS 6909, Sacher-Masoch to Otto von Kapf, 6 March 1876, folio 2 of 6.

59 Larissa Polubojarinowa, 'Österreichischer Realismus als ein Problem der Literaturgeschichte (Leopold von Sacher-Masoch, Maria von Ebner-Eschenbach)', in Werner Wiesinger (ed.), *Akten des X. Internationalen Germanistenkongresses Wien 2000. Epochenbegriffe. Grenzen und Möglichkeiten* (Bern: Lang, 2002), pp. 477–82, pp. 479–80.

60 Werner Michler, *Darwinismus in der Literatur. Naturwissenschaftliche und literarische Intelligenz in Österreich, 1859–1914* (Vienna: Böhlau, 1999), p. 130.

61 Polubojarinowa, 'Österreichischer Realismus als ein Problem der Literaturgeschichte', p. 478.

62 Ferdinand Kürnberger, 'Vorrede zum Don Juan', in Leopold von Sacher-Masoch,

Das Vermächtnis Kains. Novellen. Erster Theil. Die Liebe. Erster Band (Stuttgart: Cotta, 1870), p. 49.

63 If Turgenev belonged to those Russian writers open to Western influences, especially from Germany, Sacher-Masoch revealed Austrian Galicia to his German-speaking readership. Sacher-Masoch also shared with Turgenev a persuasion that writers needed to reproduce 'the reality of life accurately and powerfully', even if this did not correspond with the author's sympathies. See Hermann Menkes, 'Leopold von Sacher-Masoch (1890)', in Michael Farin (ed.), *Leopold von Sacher-Masoch. Materialien zu Leben und Werk* (Bonn: Bouvier, 1987), pp. 121–7, p. 127; Ivan Turgenev, 'Apropos of Fathers and Sons', in *Fathers and Sons*, trans. Michael R. Katz (New York: Norton, 1989), pp. 167–73, p. 171. It remains unclear whether Turgenev and Sacher-Masoch corresponded. However, a letter between German writer Theodor Storm and Ivan Turgenev indicates that the latter knew Sacher-Masoch's novella *Mondnacht in Galizien*: see Karl Ernst Laage, *Theodor Storm und Iwan Turgenjew* (Heide in Holstein: Westholst-Verlag, 1967), pp. 104–5. In a letter to the German painter, writer and art critic Ludwig Pietsch, Turgenev disparagingly mentions Sacher-Masoch's penchant for the depiction of aristocratic women. Ivan Turgenev, *Iwan Turgenjew: Briefe an Ludwig Pietsch* (Berlin: Aufbaum, 1968), p. 84.

64 Michler, *Darwinismus und Literatur*, p. 12.

65 Alfred Kelly, *The Descent of Darwin: The Popularization of Darwinism in Germany, 1860–1914* (Chapel Hill: University of North Carolina Press, 1981), p. 5.

66 'Wie kann man die "Culturgeschichte" von der "Geschichte der Künste und Wissenschaftentrennen", ohne sich der Gefahr auszusetzen, eine mangelhafte, flache und oberflächliche Auffassung von der historischen Entwicklung der Menschheit zu geben?' Jenny Marr, 'Darwinismus und Culturhistorik', *Auf der Höhe. Internationale Revue* (ed. Leopold von Sacher-Masoch), 2:8 (1883), pp. 462–4, p. 463. Two years later, Oswald Zimmermann and Marr, Sacher-Masoch's former lover, were instrumental in denouncing the journal as anti-German and philo-Semitic. Financial difficulties forced Sacher-Masoch to close down the journal, despite winning a libel case against Zimmermann in May 1886 – see Lisbeth Exner, *Leopold von Sacher-Masoch* (Reinbeck bei Hamburg: Rowohlt, 2003), p. 109.

67 Richard Weikart, *From Darwin to Hitler: Evolutionary Ethics, Eugenics, and Racism in Germany* (Basingstoke: Palgrave Macmillan, 2009), p. 169.

68 Michler, *Darwinismus und Literatur*, p. 22.

69 *On The Origin of Species* – and other works – were translated into German by palaeontologist H. G. Bronn soon after first being published in English. On the politics of this translation see Sander Gliboff, *H. G. Bronn, Ernst Hackel, and the Origins of German Darwinism: A Study in Translation and Transformation* (Cambridge: MIT Press, 2008).

70 Charles Darwin, *The Descent of Man, and Selection in Relation to Sex, Vol. II* (London: John Murray, 1871), p. 385.

71 In 1870, seven years before the showdown between Ernst Haeckel and his former professor Rudolf Virchow at the Fiftieth Congress of the Association German Scientists and Physicians in Munich, Sacher-Masoch aimed to popularise Darwinian ideas in an area about which Darwin had said little; *The Descent of Man* would be more forthcoming in that respect. Kelly, *The Descent of Darwin*, p. 58.

72 'Die Poesie soll eine bilderreiche "Naturgeschichte des Menschen" sein, wo sie dies nicht ist, wo sie abstrakte Phantome oder ideale Phantasiegebilde bietet, erfüllt sie ihre sittliche Aufgabe nicht.... Der echte Dichter wird immer mit Vorliebe die Leidenschaften und Thorheiten der Menschen zum Gegenstande seiner Dichtung machen.' Sacher-Masoch, *Das Vermächtnis Kains. Novellen. Erster Theil. Die Liebe. Erster Band*, p. 32.

73 Sacher-Masoch, *Das Vermächtnis Kains. Novellen. Erster Theil. Die Liebe. Erster Band*, pp. 12–13.
74 Sacher-Masoch, *Das Vermächtnis Kains. Novellen. Erster Theil. Die Liebe. Erster Band*, pp. 16–17.
75 Sacher-Masoch, *Das Vermächtnis Kains. Novellen. Erster Theil. Die Liebe. Erster Band*, pp. 16–17.
76 Sacher-Masoch *Das Vermächtnis Kains. Novellen. Erster Theil. Die Liebe. Erster Band*, p. 10.
77 Sacher-Masoch, *Das Vermächtnis Kains. Novellen. Erster Theil. Die Liebe. Erster Band*, p. 22.
78 Sacher-Masoch, *Das Vermächtnis Kains. Novellen. Erster Theil. Die Liebe. Erster Band*, p. 29.
79 In the final (unwritten) novella of the planned cycle, Jesus was to function as a symbol of overcoming egoism. Sprengel, *Darwin in der Poesie*, p. 58.
80 Fritz Lemmermeyer, 'Leopold von Sacher-Masoch', in Farin (ed.), *Leopold von Sacher-Masoch*, pp. 127–37, p. 136.
81 Deutsches Literaturarchiv, Marbach, Cotta Br. (letters to the Cotta publishing house), Sacher-Masoch to J.-G. Cottasche Buchhandlung, 7 March 1870.
82 Birgit Lang, 'Translation as Transposition', pp. 42–4. Sacher-Masoch tells the story of the first marriage of Count St–, who had served as a model for *Die Liebe des Plato*. When he first meets his wife he tells her that he 'would be quite capable of falling head over heels in love if only she were a man'. Leopold von Sacher-Masoch, *Die Messalinen Wiens. Geschichten aus der guten Gesellschaft* (Leipzig: Ernst Julius Günther, 1873), p. 139.
83 Leopold von Sacher-Masoch, *Das Vermächtnis Kains. Novellen. Erster Theil. Die Liebe. Zweiter Band* (Stuttgart: Cotta, 1870), p. 367. The translation here is by Birgit Lang. The standard English translation deviates from the original and reads 'woman, as Nature created her and as man up to now has found her attractive, is man's enemy; she can be his slave or his mistress, but never his companion. This she can only be when she has the same rights as he and is his equal in education and work'. Sacher-Masoch, *Venus in Furs*, p. 271.
84 Sacher-Masoch, *Das Vermächtnis Kains. Novellen. Erster Theil. Die Liebe. Zweiter Band*, p. 516.
85 John Stuart Mill, 'On Liberty', *Essays on Politics and Society. Collected Works of John Stuart Mill*, vol. XVIII (Toronto: University of Toronto Press, 1977), pp. 213–310, p. 261.
86 Mill, 'On Liberty', p. 299.
87 Sacher-Masoch, *Das Vermächtnis Kains. Novellen. Erster Theil. Die Liebe. Zweiter Band*, p. 511.
88 Mill, 'On Liberty', pp. 299–300.
89 'Man schämt sich auf der Gasse einem Weibe zu begegnen, denkt man, daß Sacher-Masoch seinen Roman einen Spiegel der Zeit nennt!' A. von Schweiger, 'Literarische Streifzüge. Sacher-Masoch', in Farin (ed.), *Leopold von Sacher-Masoch*, pp. 40–3, p. 43.
90 'Die Sinnlichkeit der Gegenwart ist *krank*; sie freut sich nicht harmlos, sie kann das Bewußtsein der Sünde nicht loswerden.... Die Krankheit ist allgemein, und die Besten unter unseren Zeitgenossen sind nicht immer frei davon. So arg aber wie Sacher-Masoch hat sie noch Keinen erfasst.' Karl von Thaler, 'Nihilismus in Deutschland', in Farin (ed.), *Leopold von Sacher-Masoch*, pp. 43–50, p. 44.
91 Lemmermeyer, 'Leopold von Sacher-Masoch', p. 136.
92 Rudolf von Gottschall, 'Sacher-Masoch als Novellist (1878)', in Farin (ed.), *Leopold von Sacher-Masoch*, pp. 114–21, p. 115.
93 The same can be argued for the case of the *Die Liebe des Plato* with regard to homosexuality: see Birgit Lang, 'Translation as Transposition', pp. 37–52, pp. 43–4, 48–9.

94 'Nicht an dem Thema der sinnlichen Liebe und der Verwandtschaft von Wollust und Grausamkeit hat man Anstoß genommen, ebensowenig an der Fabel, an dem Liebeswahnsinn des Helden, der ihn zum Sklaven der Geliebten macht…. Man war nur von der Entwicklung und Motivierung peinlich berührt, es widerte an, daß die Heldin von dem Helden förmlich gezwungen wurde ihn zu mißhandeln.' Deutsches Literaturarchiv, Marbach, Cotta Br., Sacher-Masoch to J.-G. Cottasche Buchhandlung, 2 July 1878.

95 Jürgen Habermas, *The Structural Transformation of the Public Sphere: An Inquiry into Category of Bourgeois Society*, trans. Thomas Burger (Cambridge: MIT Press, 1989), pp. 50–1.

96 Rebekka Habermas, *Frauen und Männer des Bürgertums. Eine Familiengeschichte (1750–1850)* (Göttingen: Vandenhoeck und Ruprecht, 2000), pp. 399–400.

97 Leopold von Sacher-Masoch, *Ueber den Werth der Kritik. Erfahrungen und Bemerkungen* (Leipzig: Ernst Julius Günther, 1873), pp. 6–7.

98 Deutsches Literaturarchiv, Marbach, Cotta Br., Sacher-Masoch to J.-G. Cottasche Buchhandlung, 12 April 1878.

99 Deutsches Literaturarchiv, Marbach, Cotta Br., Sacher-Masoch to J.-G. Cottasche Buchhandlung, 16 October 1878.

100 Deutsches Literaturarchiv, Marbach, Copierbuch IX (handwritten copies of letters from the Cotta publishing house, in chronological order), J.-G. Cottasche Buchhandlung to Sacher-Masoch, 30 March 1878.

101 Deutsches Literaturarchiv, Marbach, Copierbuch IX, J.-G. Cottasche Buchhandlung to Sacher-Masoch, 8 April 1878.

102 'von Haus aus eine genußsüchtige und despotische grausame Frau.' Deutsches Literaturarchiv, Marbach, Cotta Br., Sacher-Masoch to J.-G. Cottasche Buchhandlung, 2 July 1878.

103 Gottschall, 'Sacher-Masoch als Novellist (1878)', p. 120.

104 For example, Oswald Zimmermann, 'Ein Pamphlet. Sacher-Masoch's *Auf der Höhe*', in Farin (ed.), *Leopold von Sacher-Masoch*, pp. 342–56.

105 'Bald findet aber der ästhetische Prophet, eben so gut wie der religiöse, einzelne schwärmerische Jünger, welche in ihrer Begeisterung und ihrem Feuereifer über die Schnur hauen, den Meister überbieten, den "Tyrann übertyrannisieren" um mit Shakespeare zu sprechen….' Sacher-Masoch, *Ueber den Werth der Kritik*, p. 27.

106 'Immer wieder von neuem kamen Anfragen an ihn wegen einer Venus im Pelz als ob er eine Fabrik davon hätte, diese alle haben sich aber nicht gemeldet bei seinem Tode, diese alle, reiche Fabrikanten, Offiziere, Rechtsanwälte, können nicht ihre Dankbarkeit durch ein Geschenk beweisen.' Deutsches Literaturarchiv, Marbach, Hulda von Sacher-Masoch to Anton Lampa, 5 April 1895.

107 'Wenn mein Mann diese "perverse" Neigung gehabt hat, so ich jeder Frau einen mit diesen Neigungen behafteten Mann, sie hat dann den Himmel auf Erden: Wenn mein Mann aber immermehr hineingehetzt worden ist, so ist erstens seine erste Frau, zweitens das Publikum Schuld…. Wie schön und göttlich war diese Passion bei meinem Mann und wie gemein trat sie bei Anderen auf.' Deutsches Literaturarchiv, Marbach, Hulda von Sacher-Masoch to Anton Lampa, 5 April 1895.

108 Wanda von Sacher-Masoch, 'Masochismus und Masochisten', in *Lebensbeichte. Meine Lebensbeichte. Memoiren (1905) sowie Masochismus und Masochisten. Nachtrag zur Lebensbeichte (1908). Mit einem Dossier*, ed. Lisbeth Exner and Michael Farin (Munich: Belleville, 2003), pp. 315–47, p. 336.

109 '[W]as er sich an Qualen und Grausamkeiten vom Weib erträumte, sehnte er sich in der Wirklichkeit auch zu erdulden – und erduldete es.' Wanda von Sacher-Masoch, 'Masochismus und Masochisten', p. 336.

110 Wanda von Sacher-Masoch, 'Masochismus und Masochisten', pp. 337–43.

111 'Es ist mir stets erheiternd, wenn man mir Frivolität oder gar Anfälligkeit vorwirft, weil ich die Menschen so schildere[,] wie Sie in der That [*sic*] sind, ich

selbst habe ein Leben an das selbst der rigoroseste Norddeutsche oder Engländer seinen moralischen Maßstab legen könnte.' Wellcome Library, London, Western MS 6909, Sacher-Masoch to Otto von Kapf, 6 March 1876, folio 1 of 4.

112 Leopold von Sacher-Masoch, 'Eine Autobiographie', *Deutsche Monatsblätter. Centralorgan für das literarische Leben der Gegenwart*, 2:3 (1879), pp. 259–69.

113 Pierre Bourdieu, *The Rules of Art: Genesis and Structure of the Literary Field*, trans. Susan Emanual (Stanford: Stanford University Press, 1996), p. 25; Bourdieu's emphasis.

114 On the other hand, according to Sacher-Masoch, Émile Zola had only replaced the idealisation of beauty with that of ugliness. See Gottschall, 'Sacher-Masoch als Novellist (1878)', p. 127.

115 Pierre Bourdieu, *The Field of Cultural Production: Essays on Art and Literature*, ed. Randal Johnson (New York: Columbia University Press, 1993), p. 207, p. 210.

116 In contemporary scholarship, Albrecht Koschorke's detailed biography similarly presupposes Sacher-Masoch's masochism and consequently falls short in the assessment of Sacher-Masoch's literary works. See Albrecht Koschorke, *Leopold von Sacher-Masoch. Die Inszenierung einer Perversion* (Munich: Piper, 1988). This view is also expressed in Exner, *Leopold von Sacher-Masoch*, p. 64.

117 'Contract between Mrs Fanny von Pistor and Leopold von Sacher-Masoch', as reprinted in Deleuze and Sacher-Masoch, *Masochism*, p. 277.

118 This is further underlined by the fact that the homodiegetic narrator, Leopold, who befriends Severin, explores his successful entanglement with Venus in the introduction to the novella. Sacher-Masoch, *Venus in Furs*, p. 144.

119 Exner, *Leopold von Sacher-Masoch*, pp. 128f.

120 The series was published by the Dresden-based publishing house Dohrn between 1901 and 1906. It encompassed the following volumes: *Die Hexe von Klewan* (1901); *Satans Töchter* (1905); *Die Wölfin* (1906).

121 The most extensive bibliography of Schlichtegroll's oeuvre can be found in Schlichtegroll, *Sacher-Masoch*, pp. 409–11.

122 On the larger debate around the naming of the category masochism and contemporary alternatives, see Ivan Crozier, 'Philosophy in the English Boudoir: Havelock Ellis, Love and Pain, and Sexological Discourses on Algophilia', *Journal of the History of Sexuality*, 13:3 (2004), 275–305.

123 Schlichtegroll, 'Sacher-Masoch und die Masochisten', p. 25.

124 Schlichtegroll, 'Sacher-Masoch und die Masochisten', p. 26.

125 Schlichtegroll, 'Sacher-Masoch und die Masochisten', p. 86.

126 The short French novel by Abbé Prévost was first published in 1731. It is set in France and Louisiana, and tells the story of the Chevalier Des Grieux and his lover, Manon Lescaut. The chevalier forfeits his family wealth in order to be with his young and hedonistic lover. Her taste for extravagance bankrupts him on several occasions. The pair settle in Louisiana; however, when the Governor's nephew discovers that they are not married he woos Manon. The chevalier challenges him to a duel and flees with Manon after he believes he has killed the man. Manon dies during the flight and the chevalier returns to France to join an abbey. The novel was controversial at the time, and a toned-down version was reprinted in 1754. The text is referenced in many key works of nineteenth-century literature, for example in Stendhal's *Le Rouge et le Noir* (1830); in *La Dame aux camélias* (1848) by Alexandre Dumas and perhaps most famously in Oscar Wilde's novel *The Picture of Dorian Gray* (1890).

127 Schlichtegroll, 'Sacher-Masoch und die Masochisten', p. 100.

128 Wanda von Sacher-Masoch argued that Sacher-Masoch had written her a letter in which he threatened publish a diary that would 'destroy' her if she did not do as he pleased. Wanda von Sacher-Masoch, 'Masochismus und Masochisten', p. 321.

129 Seven pages relating to the death of Sacher-Masoch's son Alexander from 7 May to 27 December 1877 survived in London: Wellcome Library, London, Western

MS 6909, folio 75. Two further diary pages, from 1869, presented by Exner, are also written in the first person. Exner considers these proof of Sacher-Masoch's masochist predisposition – see Exner, *Leopold von Sacher-Masoch*, pp. 62–4.

130 'In den letzten Jahren wurden mir übrigens Beweise dafür beigebracht, dass S.-Masoch nicht bloss der Dichter des Masochismus gewesen, sondern auch selbst mit der in Rede stehenden Anomalie behaftet gewesen sei. Obwohl jene mir ohne Vorbehalt zukamen, nehme ich gleichwohl Abstand, sie zu veröffentlichen. Den Tadel, den einzelne Verehrer des Dichters und gewisse Kritiker meines Buches mir dafür zu Theil werden liesen [*sic*], dass ich den Namen eines geachteten Schriftstellers mit einer Perversion des Sexuallebens verquickte, muss ich zurückweisen. Als Mensch verliert S.-Masoch doch sicher nichts in den Augen jedes Gebildeten durch die Thatsache [*sic*], dass er mit einer Anomalie seines sexuellen Lebens schuldlos behaftet war. Als Autor hat er aber dadurch in seinem Wirken und Schaffen schwere Schädigung erfahren, denn er war, solange und soweit er sich nicht auf dem Boden seiner Perversion bewegte, ein sehr begabter Schriftsteller und hätte gewiss Bedeutendes geleistet, wenn er ein sexuell normal fühlender Mensch gewesen wäre.' Krafft-Ebing, *Psychopathia Sexualis*, 11th edition, 1901, pp. 95f. Mr Z, Case 78 in the 11th edition, allowed Krafft-Ebing access to his private correspondence with Sacher-Masoch, from which Krafft-Ebing quotes as part of the case notes. According to Krafft-Ebing, Sacher-Masoch argued that the 'passion to play the slave' was widespread in Germany and Russia. Sacher-Masoch had also conveyed to Mr Z the story of a Danish woman who insisted that her lovers lick her feet and her anus, and Krafft-Ebing used Latin to reproduce this passage. If the lovers did not obey, they were chained and whipped until they did so. The passage fascinated Krafft-Ebing, especially for its mention of a man in chains who was forced to watch his rival make love to the woman. Krafft-Ebing points out that if what was said was true – 'which cannot be readily assumed of the poet of masochism' – this would constitute a remarkable example of female sadism. *Psychopathia Sexualis*, 11th edition, 1901, p. 138. The 12th edition of *Psychopathia Sexualis* (1906), which was continued in Krafft-Ebing's name after his death in 1902, additionally refers to Eulenburg's study, without changing the argument; the same holds true for further editions.

131 '[I]ch ahnte noch nicht, in wie engem Zusammenhang diese Schilderung mit der persönlichen Eigenart ihres Autors standen.' Albert Eulenburg, 'Sacher-Masoch', *Die Zukunft*, 3 (1901), pp. 197–201, p. 199.

132 Eulenburg, 'Sacher-Masoch', p. 200.

133 '[D]ie unverkennbare Minderwerthigkeit [*sic*] seines späteren, literarischen Schaffens.' Albert Eulenburg, *Sadismus und Masochismus* (Wiesbaden: Bergmann, 1902), p. 50.

134 '[D]em stofflichen Interesse ... das überhitzte Romanleser seiner Lehre von den sexuellen Perversitäten abgewannen.' Karl Kraus, 'Irrenhaus Österreich', *Die Fackel*, 6:166 (1904), pp. 1–21, p. 5.

135 '[E]in alberne[s] Roman-Medizinerwort.' Karl Kraus, 'Die Büchse der Pandora', *Die Fackel*, 7:182 (1905), pp. 1–18, p. 6.

2

Fin-de-siècle investigations of the 'creative genius' in psychiatry and psychoanalysis

Birgit Lang

In Victorian society, admiration for the 'creative genius' abounded. It was based on stereotypical notions of the Romantic artist, who, 'by the neat and necessarily contradictory logic of aesthetic elevation and social exclusion, [was] both a great genius and greatly misunderstood'.[1] In Germany the propensity to idealise the artist as a creative genius was further propelled by intellectuals' and writers' contribution to imagining the German nation throughout the nineteenth century, and by the tendency of literary works to aestheticise and idealise bourgeois life.

By the late nineteenth century, this Romantic image of genius began to transform, despite much resistance from parts of the German public. For over two decades from the late 1890s onwards – roughly until the First World War – psychiatrists, psychoanalysts and the reading public were particularly captivated by the mental health and sex life of German creative writers, artists and intellectuals. For the sake of simplicity, all such individuals are throughout this chapter collectively referred to as creative artists. Both psychiatric discourse and the more conservative strand of psychoanalytic discourse provided a powerful new lens through which to interpret biographies of exceptional human beings. Artist pathographies, or psychiatric case studies of creative artists, expanded the case study genre towards biography and presented readers with new insights into the private lives of particular creative artists.

Sigmund Freud and his pupil Otto Rank brought contrasting approaches to enquiring into aspects of artistic personality, creativity and oeuvre, partly in an attempt to curb the idealising tendencies of the German reading public. The differing biographical and artistic studies reproduce what Christian von Zimmermann has identified as the two main biographical narratives characteristic of modernity, namely anthropologisation and idealisation, that is, either an attempt to underline similarities between exceptional and average human beings, or an admiring elevation of biographical subjects that emphasises their status as exceptional individuals.[2] As discussed in Chapter 1, in the instance of the reinterpretation of Leopold von Sacher-Masoch's life and oeuvre, in the late nineteenth century anthropologisation arose from specific needs related to readers' sexual identities and contributed to the making of sexual modernity. Underlying this new, highly specific, sexualised account of Sacher-Masoch's life was a need among his readers to humanise their own subject position, a need that was powerfully projected onto Sacher-Masoch as a creative writer. To psychiatrists and psychoanalysts of the fin de siècle, interrogation of the lives and works of creative artists contributed significantly to the appreciation of certain medical, psychiatric and psychological phenomena. Such an undertaking was supported by readers who were variously invested in medical discourse – perhaps as patients of sexologists, or as cultural critics, such as Max Nordau, who popularised and generalised degeneration theory to serve his own pessimistic views of contemporary society.

At the same time, the idealising majority of Germany's educated middle class perceived the psychiatrists' deliberations on genius and creativity as defamation of national idols. This led Freud in particular to consider new ways of writing about artists, which took into consideration such idealising tendencies. The response to anthropologisation extended from repudiation to hesitation, and is epitomised in the pages of *Geschlecht and Gesellschaft* (*Sex and Society*), a popular middle-class journal concerned with sexual reform that clearly targeted the progressive educated middle class. Before the First World War, literary works provided the journal with a window onto the past and an opportunity to argue against contemporary restrictive mores, in an attempt to develop a new sexual ethics.[3] Refusing to discuss pathographies of eminent writers and artists, the journal preferred to hold such figures in continued high esteem. The medicalisation of talented individuals and their works was repudiated, and psychoanalytic insights were given very limited room in the journal's pages.

For the purposes of analysing the case study genre, in nineteenth-century German biographical writing the greatest difference between strategies of anthropologisation and idealisation lay in a penchant for generalisation versus particularisation. Psychiatrists and psychoanalysts were predisposed towards generalisation, in that they considered their studies of creative artists as illustrations of their own theories. This holds true for researchers identified with the fields of psychiatry, sexology and psychoanalysis alike, although the methodological finesse of their approaches varied markedly, as did their understanding of the tastes of their respective readerships. Yet Paul Julius Möbius, Isidor Sadger, Rank and Freud all shared a complex and ambivalent relationship to creative artists. The psychiatrist Möbius attempted to map signs of degeneration onto the oeuvre, bodies and genes of selected creative artists in his pathographies. Sadger, an early pupil of Freud, presented a mixture of arguments centred on degeneration and psychoanalysis which aimed to form a bridge between psychiatric and psychoanalytic discourse. Freud – founder of psychoanalysis – and his close collaborator Rank understood the creative process as an insightful but limited method for revealing the workings of the human psyche that, unlike psychoanalysis, was not scientific in nature. Conversely, the idealising tendencies of German intellectuals and readers advanced a notion of creative artists as extraordinary human beings, and insisted on their exceptionalism. These narratives of exceptionalism were intimately connected to middle-class lifestyle, works of art and literature, engendering a sense of belonging in their publics.[4]

The bulk of all these deliberations took the shape of case studies. Scholars of nineteenth-century Europe have identified the new case modality of pathography with the development of notions of normality and abnormality, as well as the appropriation of literary modes of interpretation by the medical disciplines. Meanwhile, psychoanalysis is usually credited with a more playful and less normative approach to the analysis of literature and the creative arts.[5] Detailed study of the generic influence of the case study reveals a new, more diverse and complex picture. By mapping the divergence of case study modalities, this chapter shows that methodological rather than disciplinary differences fashioned both psychiatric and psychoanalytic approaches to case writing on creative genius. The crucial methodological difference was that of rhetorical form, specifically whether the form was 'closed' or 'open'. The closed form considered the life narrative of creative artists as an illustration of a psychiatric, sexological or psychoanalytic theory, never considering the creative contributions that made their objects of study exceptional in the first place. This caused insult to middle-class sensibilities, as exemplified by the case studies written by Möbius and Sadger around the turn of the century.

By contrast, Möbius's early pathographies and Freud's later dialogic-psychoanalytic case studies considered artists' biographies *and* their oeuvres. In psychoanalysis, the rift between supporters of closed and open case studies added to the competitive streak characteristic of early psychoanalysts. Their discussions provided a forum in which a scientific model for explaining creativity could first emerge. In this context, Freud can be credited for anticipating the workings of the unconscious in his readers, and for developing the most nuanced strategies through which to convince his readers. As a consequence, Freud's case studies have continued to retain much higher currency in the humanities and among the reading public more generally. Such techniques of manipulation – towards a higher scientific aim – make Freud's case studies extremely evocative, contributing to their ongoing appeal to psychoanalysts, as well as readers in the humanities more generally.

The art of pathography: from open beginnings

The importance of the pathography as a new case modality in the late nineteenth and early twentieth centuries cannot be overestimated. In the field of psychiatric discourse, pathographies legitimated exhaustive studies of members of the intellectual elite. In biographical writing – so long predominated by idealising norms of respectability – pathographies made admissible matters of mental health and sexuality.

At the same time, these new case writings opened the door for overgeneralisation and even stigmatisation of their objects of study. In the twentieth century, this propensity of pathography has been analysed by Foucaultian scholars, and identified with the politics of biopower that aim to control individual subjects via normalising discourses and techniques.[6] As argued in Chapter 4, such forceful discourses directly impacted upon society's understanding of criminality and mental health. Jutta Person has paradigmatically identified pathography with the overcoming of literature's interpretative power through scientific and medical discourse, and a renewal of the early modern mapping of physical features to character traits.[7] Such normalising discourses were also effective in relation to creative artists. Nonetheless, pathographies of artists were not written with the explicit intent of belittling their objects of study; rather, the authors of such studies often show a keen interest both in literary and psychological phenomena. Pathographies with a focus on prominent individuals represented a diversion from the sinister world of psychiatric illness, and allowed for a compassionate stance, while their main function was to communicate scientific insights to a wider audience. These were surely conflicted accounts, driven by academic self-interest and institutional traditions, but to identify pathography solely as a product of biopower is to produce a distorted image of such writing.

A different view of pathography has emerged in the history of popular medicine. In her innovative study *Reconstructing Illness*, Anne Hunsaker Hawkins has discovered a new facet of the generic effects of pathography.[8] Through analysis of autobiographies and biographies, she outlines the assumptions, myths and attitudes that individuals brought to the medical encounter in the USA during the late twentieth century. The publication of patient narratives beyond the confines of clinical casuistry was made possible, however, only by the increased dissemination of such writing at certain points in history: in this instance, after the 'scientific turn' in medicine in the 1960s, which brought discredit to the case study as an academic genre.[9] Weimar Germany represents another historical precedent: as outlined in Chapter 4, during the Weimar Republic, intensified general interest in the case study led to a popularity that furthered the eventual decline of its academic merit.

Fin-de-siècle case studies of creative artists were still powerfully embedded in psychiatric discourse. They aimed to illustrate the effects of degeneration on society's elite, even though this case variant shifted in its consideration of the artistic oeuvre. Early pathography was intended to disseminate medical knowledge to educated burghers, often by analysing works of art. Modern pathography concentrated on a more specialised psychiatric discourse and benefited from considerable advances at the beginning of the twentieth century, notably in the area of differential diagnosis of psychopathic personality traits. Those who took this psychiatric approach became increasingly concerned with ways in which diagnostic criteria could be mapped onto patient bodies. For reasons of popularity, modern pathography retained its focus on creative artists, but the pathographical interest in the artworks expressed earlier vanished. In the German-speaking world, pathography as a case modality and distinctive kind of biography originated with Möbius.

The shift from early to modern pathography is very pronounced in Möbius's writings, and his works serve as the main representatives of early and modern pathography in this chapter. Having begun his academic career with a doctorate of philosophy (1873), Möbius graduated as a medical doctor in 1877. His studies of creative artists fall into a period during which he had returned to private practice, renouncing his affiliation with Leipzig University, despite groundbreaking work in neurology.[10] As for Freud several decades later, the move away from the university system produced a focus on patients outside psychiatric institutions who were able to function in everyday life, and furthered his interest in the indeterminate area between normality and insanity.

Yet unlike Freud, Möbius throughout his career insisted on a solely biological explanatory framework for insanity. This view was strongly shaped by Munich-based reformer and professor of psychiatry Emil Kraepelin (1856–1926), who was also Möbius's lifelong friend.[11] The publication in 1899 of the sixth edition of Kraepelin's *Psychiatrie: ein Lehrbuch für Studirende und Aerzte* (*Clinical Psychiatry. A Textbook for Students and Physicians*) would prove profoundly important for Möbius's pathographies. Kraepelin differentiated between four types of psychopathic personalities: born criminals, pathological liars, querulous persons and compulsive personalities. His re-categorisation of psychopathology brought about a pronounced shift in pathographical writing and contributed significantly to the development of modern pathography as well as a modern psychiatric diagnostics.[12] Early on, his ideas encountered much resistance in psychiatric circles within Europe, and Möbius's shift in pathographic writing can be seen as an important and previously unrecognised means of advocating Kraepelin's position to an educated readership.[13]

The shift between early and modern pathography is best demonstrated in Möbius's studies of Johann Wolfgang von Goethe. Germany's national poet was a subject well chosen to give currency to Möbius's own psychiatric interests, not least because Goethe himself was innately interested in the representation of psychologically testing situations: the psychological motivations of his characters allowed Goethe to represent and explain human behaviour in general.[14] Möbius's 1898 study *Über das Pathologische bei Goethe* (*On Pathology in Goethe*), the first pathographical study of Goethe, was his key contribution to early pathography.[15] In this study, he explicitly seeks to popularise psychiatric knowledge by arguing that the majority of human beings are degenerate to a degree.[16] The book discusses Goethe's approach to mental illness and the representation of mental illness in a selection of Goethe's works; it also narrates a biography of Goethe and his family, structured by the same theme of degeneration. Presenting the reader with a medically informed cultural and personal history, *Über das Pathologische bei Goethe* constitutes an attempt to delineate the vast area of uncertainty between 'debility and normal behaviour'.[17] The longest section of this study focuses on the depiction of insanity in a representative selection of Goethe's writings, from the Sturm und Drang *Die Leiden des jungen Werther* (*The Sorrows of Young Werther*), first published in 1774, to Goethe's autobiographical *Aus meinem Leben: Dichtung und Wahrheit* (*From My Life: Poetry and Truth*), written and published 1811–33.

Möbius could use his own retelling of Goethe's life to destigmatise mental health problems. He claimed that the mental suffering of the celebrated 'prince of poets' in his youth could be situated in the grey area between insanity and normality – a normality that the Möbius of early pathography conceded as 'boring', due to the 'complete balance' of such a personality.[18] About Goethe himself Möbius cautiously stated that while pathology was minimal in Goethe's mature years, his spontaneous and intense periods of writing coincided with phases of general agitation that were followed by long phases of clarity and stillness. Hence the neurologist suggested a first, tentative connection between creativity and degeneration, a connection he would explore in his second pathography of Goethe, published five years later.[19]

This second study of Goethe made Möbius the first proponent of modern pathography, which took hold from the turn of the century onwards. Published in Leipzig in 1903, *Goethe* centred on the physical person, without consideration of artistic creation, and thus announced a pronounced shift in pathographic methodology. The conceptual vocabulary developed in *Goethe* was new and allowed Möbius to combine biological detail with biographical information. The three-part study begins with an opening portrait outlining 'the form and movement' of Goethe the person: his anatomical features, the movement of his body and face, as well as his linguistic utterings and actions. The second part provides evidence for this portrayal, mainly through letters and descriptions of Goethe by the poet's contemporaries. The third part investigates the relationship between Goethe and neuroanatomist and craniologist Franz Joseph Gall (1758–1828). Gall pioneered the study of the localisation of mental functions in the human brain; a contemporary of Goethe, he crafted one of his famous life-masks – today lost – from Goethe's face. Gall plays an important role in Möbius's interpretation, since he provided the pathographer with a system of classification through which to map biological detail onto biographical information. In *Goethe*, Möbius expands and adapts Gall's mapping system to include a series of motivators, and simplifies some of Gall's categories.[20] The new system, in turn, provides

Möbius with the headings that structure his contemplation of Goethe's mental powers and includes a long list of criteria: from 'life instinct' to 'sex drive' and from personal character traits such as bravery and vanity to various aspects of intellectual giftedness.[21]

In other words, Möbius's discussion changes direction to survey Goethe's body, personality and intellect rather than his oeuvre. Similar studies followed on Friedrich Nietzsche (1902), the composer Robert Schumann (1906) and poet and novelist Joseph Victor von Scheffel (1907). Except for the works on Goethe and Schopenhauer, Möbius's aim in these volumes was to portray a specific disorder through the relevant biography. These and other pathographies self-evidently adhered to the new methodology. Available biographical information was sifted through and a posthumous diagnosis given, which pinpointed a range of psychiatric and other medical conditions pertinent to the subject's life history; the oeuvre of the creative artists in question was not considered. This method also applied to the studies discussed in the foregoing chapter, in which Richard von Krafft-Ebing and Albert Eulenburg redefined their view of Sacher-Masoch from expert writer to masochist.

In consonance with such psychiatric reinterpretation, Möbius now began to explore in a more abstract manner the subject of creative artists, and embraced a cultural history based on this new psychiatric footing. As part of a response to Charles Darwin's theories of degeneration, Möbius viewed the cultural elite as a threatened group. In the aftermath of Darwinian thought, social Darwinism, as a public rhetoric, considered that cultural sophistication had come at the price of degeneration. Kraepelin's system of differential diagnostics allowed Möbius to present underlying pathologies, and to present behavioural advice intended to counteract individual predispositions. In this context Möbius underlined that unwise choices, for example in marriage, meant that degenerative processes would be furthered. For instance, in his contentious essay of 1900, *Über den physiologischen Schwachsinn des Weibes* (*Concerning the Physiological Feebleness of the Female*), he emphasised that 'intellectuals' should marry women who were physically and mentally robust rather than educated – 'healthy women, not brainy ladies' – in order to maintain sufficient numbers of healthy offspring.[22] Accordingly, Möbius's view of Christiane Vulpius, Goethe's mistress and later his wife, was comparatively favourable, since she was not a *Gehirndame*. In 1901 Möbius published a generalising treatise titled *Über Kunst und Künstler* (*On Art and Artists*), in which he portrayed creative artists as individuals with high aspirations, who belonged to 'a sensual and carnally excitable race [while being] highly anomalous in their lifestyle'.[23] In *Über Kunst und Künstler* Möbius sought to prove that genius is a singularly biological trait – and, except for the writing of poetry, a trait inherited in a patrilinear fashion.

On publication, these popular pamphlets elicited a range of reactions. *Über den physiologischen Schwachsinn des Weibes* situates the maturity of women between that of children and men, and outlines ways in which the emancipation of women represents a sociological threat. The outcry it prompted came from representatives of the women's movement and from the educated middle class.[24] The former felt attacked; the latter 'had heard it all before', and in a more progressive fashion. As discussed in Chapter 1, thirty years before, a presumed link between women and degeneration of the social fabric had guided Sacher-Masoch's protagonist Alexander in his choice of Marzella as his bride. In the same novella, the narrator, Leopold, expressed ambiguity concerning the suitability of such explanations for Germany. Here, Venus lectures the narrator of *Venus im Pelz* on the nature of love in the European North by stating 'To you Nature is an enemy'.[25] Yet, in medicine the discussion surrounding intellectual elites occurred thirty years later, and from a perspective of social Darwinism.[26] Again, readers from the educated middle class were critical of such a stance.

Regardless of this critique, Möbius's studies of such celebrated German individuals as Goethe and Nietzsche provided a model for a number of similar volumes, successfully forging the modern pathography as a new approach to biography, and a new case modality in which consideration of a creative artist's oeuvre became fundamentally irrelevant. For instance, pathographies dominated the biographical studies in the important series of monographs titled 'Grenzfragen des Nerven- und Seelenlebens. Einzeldarstellungen für Gebildete aller Stände' ('Intersecting Issues of Nervous and Inner Life. Monographs for the Educated of all Classes'). Munich-based sexual pathologist Leopold Löwenfeld and psychiatrist Hans Kurella had founded this enterprise in 1902. Under Löwenfeld's editorship, 130 volumes were published over three decades. The series tackled a wide array of topics, from somnambulism to discussion of abnormal characteristics and the occurrence of delusional ideas in different nation states. The first volume to embrace the topic of creative artists was the above-mentioned study of Nietzsche by Möbius, published in 1902; thenceforth, a range of authors undertook studies of prominent writers, such as Conrad Ferdinand Meyer, Heinrich von Kleist and Guy de Maupassant.[27]

A related project with a more literary focus was Sigismund Rahmer's shorter-lived series titled 'Grenzfragen der Literatur und Medizin' ('Intersecting Issues of Literature and Medicine'), published between 1906 and 1908, with volumes on the pessimistic dramatist Christian Grabbe; Swedish playwright, novelist and poet August Strindberg; and American Romantic writer Edgar Allan Poe.[28] In these modern pathographies, the biographies of artists serve to illustrate medical phenomena and classifications, again with very little or no consideration of the creative oeuvre. Thus the attempt to educate readers through depicting and humanising psychiatric illness came at great cost to the esteem in which the artists and their works were generally held.

Isidor Sadger's psychoanalytic pathographies

Modern pathographies stressed the biological foundations of pathology and genius, and sidelined the oeuvre of the creative artist. Among the critics of Möbius's pathographies were disgruntled literary historians and members of the educated middle class; other critics included medical colleagues who condemned as unscientific his foray into literature. The most immediate challenge arose from medical colleagues who were competitors in the field of pathography and who aimed to carve a niche in a similar academic market. Sadger, who was an early psychoanalyst and physician in his own right, developed Möbius's work methodologically. He maintained the focus on the biographies of creative artists, but also scrutinised the solely biological explanatory framework given by Möbius, and attempted to combine psychiatric and psychoanalytic approaches. Sadger felt keenly that the disagreement among medical experts concerning Kraepelin's 'hair-splitting psychiatric differential diagnostics' was detrimental to pathography as a project. He contended that modern pathography led to a general confusion among lay readers, since diagnostic categories were subject to rapid change – and he promoted his own psychoanalytic pathographies as studies in which this problem was resolved.[29]

By the 1920s, Sadger considered himself to be the oldest of Freud's practising students.[30] Already a medical doctor with established interests in pathography, and in the emerging field of hydrotherapy for the treatment of psychiatric patients, Sadger listened to Freud's lectures on neurosis (in the winter semester of 1895–96) and on hysteria (in 1896 and again in 1898). Soon afterwards he began to use psychoanalytic methods in his own practice, yet Sadger remains one of the lesser-known early analysts.[31] Ulrike May was the first to examine Sadger's personality and his work, and has characterised the relationship between Sadger and Freud as one of ambivalence.[32] Despite Sadger's enthusiastic response to Freud's theories, for example, the latter was slow to invite Sadger to join the Wiener Psychoanalytische Vereinigung (the WPV, or Vienna Psychoanalytic Society, discussed below), and did so only in 1906, four years after its inauguration. Sadger soon became a controversial figure within this group, partly due to his rejection of the more symbolic manifestations of sex that were so central to Freud's theories in this period.[33] Freud was well aware of Sadger's theoretical limitations; however, he also appreciated Sadger's work with openly homosexual patients at a time when no other analyst acknowledged the needs of such individuals in their practice.[34] Moreover, Freud valued Sadger's role in the early dissemination of psychoanalytic knowledge.

The importance of understanding Sadger's early explorations into the realm of literature cannot be overstated, since these forays explain much about his later standpoint in the debates about authorship within the WPV during the early 1900s. Secondary literature perceives Sadger predominantly as a conservative force within these debates, as the contrarian pathographer either unable or unwilling to understand Freud's perspective – and who, according to Alan Elms, was even bullied by Freud.[35] These perceptions are commonly grounded in the frank style of discussion that took place in the WPV, as portrayed in the Society's minutes. There, Sadger's penchant for impassioned dialogue becomes clear, and his rhetoric is brusque at times. Where Freud promoted a differentiated style of argumentation, and much of his persuasiveness stems from ambiguity and understatement, Sadger tended to present his theories in black and white, to reinforce his line of reasoning. He was certainly a pathographer first among this group, since his investigations into the realm of literature began a decade earlier than those in psychoanalysis, but his approach was not quite as dull as suspected by twenty-first-century criticism.[36]

Much of Sadger's early work on creative genius was devoted to the representation of degeneration in modernist literature. In an article from 1896, he criticised Norwegian playwright Henrik Ibsen, the founder of modernism in theatre, for depicting heredity in a purely negative manner as degeneration, and for giving no value to the role of education in the play *Nora*. Furthermore, Sadger declares the life-threatening sickness of Nora's husband and the eye condition of the character Hedwig in *The Wild Duck* 'figments of poetic phantasy', and he judged the narrated progression of both diseases to be unconvincing from a medical perspective. Instead of conceding the naturalist author's poetic licence, Sadger deemed Ibsen a failure in diagnostic skills.[37] From the perspective of the medical practitioner, such a contention seems fitting, in particular since Ibsen had studied medicine before taking up his career as a writer. Sadger's article was published in the liberal daily *Neue Freie Presse*, with a purpose to inform; after all, Ibsen worked within a realistic paradigm capable of misleading the wider theatre audience about matters of disease.

In a later article titled 'Kranke Dichter und Krankendichtung' ('Sick Poets and Literature on Illness', 1897) Sadger underlines a similar point by arguing that there was no necessary connection between the actual degeneration of authors and their choice to depict degeneration. Here he points to the role of literature in the dissemination of Darwinist ideas, and insists that Ibsen's drama *Ghosts* popularised notions of heredity more than 'all books and treatises of Darwinism'.[38] Sadger contends that, paradoxically, many poets who garnered fame before 1870 were 'degenerate', although their work failed to acknowledge or discuss matters of degeneration, while the modernist writers were predominantly healthy but posed as sick, and thus misled their audiences.[39] According to Sadger, the 'nervousness' supposedly characteristic of poets was a result of modernist literature's love affair with mental illness, and became a key factor in writers' strategies for self-representation in the literary field.[40] This flavouring of sickness, he argues, was only furthered by Cesare Lombroso's attempts to declare illustrious writers such as Émile Zola to be degenerate – and by the writings of Nordau on degeneration.[41] Regardless of such speculations, very few biographical studies of modernist writers had been undertaken, Sadger elaborates, and a dearth of facts made it difficult to develop scientific theories about contemporary writers and artists. Like Möbius in his first study of Goethe, Sadger maintained that, during an author's lifetime, only limited archival sources could be unearthed if the writer had not published a reflective autobiography such as Jean-Jacques Rousseau's *Les Confessions* (*The Confessions*, 1782), or August Strindberg's *Le Plaidoyer d'un fou* (*The Confession of a Fool*, 1895).[42] To Sadger, the reading public's obsession with nervousness, like literary writers' obsession with degeneration, had no ground in medical reality. He did not believe that these phenomena were on the rise, but rather that the zeitgeist of modernity fed public discourse about both trends.[43]

As would seem timely, Sadger embraced the pathographical model to consider the life stories of authors. In brief, his purpose was to shed new light on 'real' degeneration, and to illustrate this for a lay audience through the study of a highly select group of 'afflicted' poets. Sadger's tactic is documented in the phrase 'pathographical-psychological study' – the subtitle of his 1909 study of Kleist, which was published in Löwenfeld's aforementioned influential series. Sadger's new approach shared with psychiatric pathographies a chief interest in tracing degeneration through the arc of a writer's life story, in an attempt to popularise new medical concepts for a lay readership.

The main intellectual aim Sadger strove to fulfil was the destigmatisation of creative artists as a group; he saw that their reputation suffered from the negative connotations associated with the term *Entartung* (degeneration). Sadger retranslated the term anew from the original French into German – with reference to French psychiatrist Jacques Joseph Valentin Magnan (1835–1916) – into *dégénéré supérieur* and *dégénéré inférieur*. The latter he translated into the German *Belastung* ('burden'), which impacts upon genius, and the former he translated as *Schwachsinn* ('imbecility'), with reference to 'real' degeneration, as prevalent in criminals.[44] The key symptoms of *Belastung* Sadger saw as recurrent major depressive episodes, combined with the inability of afflicted subjects to connect to 'their ego' (Sadger's phrase). This implies that afflicted individuals are keen to make changes in their lives as soon as a certain degree of familiarity has been established. According to Sadger, this familiarity can include their immediate surroundings, living quarters, cities, but also professions and circle of friends.[45] Other symptoms of *Belastung* include self-indulgence, 'abnormal cerebral reactions', or a high degree of emotivity, especially a violent temper, and an abnormal sexual constitution.[46]

Sadger's renovated terminology smoothly resolved a key conceptual problem inherent to debate about degeneration: quite elegantly he rejected Lombroso's clumsy model in which genius is drawn into a parallel connection with criminality – and which explains any negative character traits in genius as an atavistic phenomenon. In effect, Sadger was writing against Lombroso and Nordau, and the great popularity of their culturally pessimistic theories in the German-speaking world.[47] To Sadger no genius existed without *Belastung*, but he expressed the hope that this new term would destigmatise creative artists by removing the taint of the term 'degeneration'.

Sadger's reference to degeneration represented only one part of the equation. Where Möbius relied exclusively on biology as an aetiological explanation for the phenomenon of degeneration, Sadger considered psychoanalytic explanations more important, but he did not grant them an exclusive status. In other words, rather than sidelining a preceding explanatory model, Sadger sought to combine the old and the new. The five parts of Sadger's psychoanalytic pathography of Kleist, for instance, concern the latter's hereditary *Belastung*, especially his depressive mood, his inability to form long-term relationships, and a geographical restlessness that Sadger had previously identified as typical of this condition. The added psychoanalytic framework allowed Sadger to consider the role of repressed homosexuality in the poet's life, including a complex that Sadger terms Kleist's underlying 'erotic fixation on the mother', a view shared by several present-day Kleist biographers.[48] In order to explain Kleist's fixation, Sadger references his contemporaneous work on homosexuality, in which he argued that homosexual men desired the qualities and characteristics of their own mother in their male partner.[49] In the third and fourth part of his study Sadger outlines Kleist's relationship to his fiancée and the importance of male friendship in his life. The final chapter offers a psychoanalytic interpretation of the specific requirements for Kleist's double suicide with Henriette Vogel. Sadger argues that Henriette's roles as wife and mother, and her willingness to die with Kleist, fulfilled the poet's inverted longing for unification with his mother.

Sadger's attempt to destigmatise the figure of the creative genius entailed a move away from Möbius's biological framework. Yet there emerges a remarkable contradiction at the heart of Sadger's assumption: he introduces the term *Belastung* to dissociate creativity from the negative connotations surrounding the term 'degeneration' but, in comparison with Möbius, Sadger seems wholly concerned with negative character traits. Where Möbius underlines positive character traits in genius, such as bravery, wit, acquisitiveness and love of children, Sadger sees no need to categorise the positive traits of genius; they are never discussed in his many psychoanalytic pathographies.[50] Nor did Sadger ever posit any possible links between creativity and resilience.

Methodological similarities between psychiatric and psychoanalytic pathographies therefore consisted in their biographical focus, in their neglect of the subject's creative oeuvre and achievements, and in interpreting certain character traits as an expression of an underlying medical symptomatology. Sadger remained true to Möbius's closed case study format, in that he used creative artists solely as a means to illustrate his theories. Psychoanalysis allowed him to hypothesise about the early lives of creative artists, and about their psychological conflicts, more convincingly and in more detail than Möbius. However, he retained the same blind spot, namely the inability to see and affirm the artists' gift for creation – the reason why artists became illustrative cases in the first place.

Creative artists and the Vienna Psychoanalytic Society

The most vehement critique of pathography originated from inside Freud's immediate circle of psychoanalysts in Vienna. To the members of the WPV Sadger became the contested representative of pathography, despite his avowed intermediary position between psychiatric and psychoanalytic reasoning.[51] As a proxy for psychiatric pathographies, his contributions stood at the heart of the question that, beginning in 1906, engulfed the Vienna group for almost a decade: the question of whether the open or the closed case modality was best suited to the task of analysing creative artists. Open dialogic-psychoanalytic case studies considered both the life and the oeuvre of such individuals and granted some agency to the creative artist, while closed case studies were illustrations of pathography.

The ripostes in these debates proved complex and long-winded, and have since been attributed with far-ranging implications. Freudian and literary scholar Peter Rudnytsky has argued that they contributed to the growing maturity of the psychoanalytic movement.[52] Historian of psychoanalysis Louis Rose contends that they laid the groundwork for Freud's cultural theoretical writings of the inter-war period, while to American psychologist and Freud critic Frank Sulloway the literary style of reasoning developed in this period came at the cost of objectivity and scientificity.[53]

In a manner of speaking, all these commentators were right, at least partly. The heated debates inside the WPV concerning the use of psychoanalytic pathographies as mere illustrations of psychological phenomena in general, and the relative merits of dialogic-psychoanalytic case studies for representing creative artists, became a means of articulating views on creative agency; issues surrounding methodology; claims to scientificity. More specifically, these discussions provided a forum in which a scientific model for explaining creativity could first emerge. In this ultimately stunted attempt, the case study genre played a pivotal role, since Freud's preferred method for investigating creative art and artists was through writing dialogic-psychoanalytic case studies. These allowed for controlled play between specific details and general observations, and were aimed at overcoming resistance in his readers. Nonetheless, in the introduction to his 1919 treatise on the evolution of the *Volksepik*, or 'folk epic', Otto Rank conceded:

> Coming from pathology, psychoanalysis has shed piercing light on the little-understood part of the unconscious formation of fantasy, yet was

> only able to provide isolated insights into the complex process of creative production; up until now these have not blossomed into a concluding delineation.[54]

In his thoroughgoing study of the WPV, Rose portrays the organisation as a 'new center of cultural activity'.[55] It might be more accurate to say that in 1906 Freud instigated in psychoanalysis a turn towards analysis of creative artists; he wished to outline the relationship between psychoanalysis, psychiatry and creativity, and saw his chance to use such case studies to promote the cause of psychoanalysis as a discipline. Not by chance were the early popularisers of psychoanalysis, Sadger and Rank, the key figures in this debate about genius and creativity.[56]

During the summer of 1906 Freud read *Gradiva* by German novelist Wilhelm Jensen (1837–1911) and his literary case study about the novella was published the following year.[57] In 1906 he also met the young Rank, who, upon being introduced to Freud, had three manuscripts ready to show: eventually published in 1907, Rank's two-chapter theoretical-psychoanalytic case study *Der Künstler* had been inspired by Freud's 1905 *Drei Abhandlungen zur Sexualtheorie* (*Three Essays on the Theory of Sexuality*). Also honed by 1906 was Rank's first draft of his study on the incest motif (published in 1912), as well as an unpublished manuscript on the motif of homosexuality in literature. Rank's biographer E. James Lieberman explains how the young Rank had gained considerable insight into his own psyche through engagement with literary and philosophical works before he became a devout disciple of Freud.[58] Rank's drafts on the topic made such a favourable impression upon Freud that he appointed Rank as the paid secretary of the WPV and the editor of its minutes. Also in 1906 Freud invited Sadger, Sadger's nephew Fritz Wittels and bookseller Hugo Heller to join the society. Wilhelm Stekel, a gifted analyst of symbols, and professor of musicology Max Graf – the father of 'Little Hans' – had already been part of Freud's circle since its inception in 1902.[59] With Graf and lawyer Hanns Sachs, Rank was part of a younger generation of psychoanalysts who were not physicians and who were interested to open psychoanalysis to the consideration of culture and society.

In other words, although the members of the WPV belonged to a range of professions, the 1906 expansion and subsequent consolidation of the group brought in several avid culture enthusiasts and experts. Lectures about creative artists and aspects of their oeuvre became commonplace during the weekly meetings of the WPV. The content of these lectures established a precedent, such that a range of newcomers to the WPV presented on topics related to the sphere of cultural and artistic activity.[60] For example, Rank's three inaugural lectures to the society in October 1906 discussed the representation of incest in selected works of German and world literature, while one month later Sadger gave his initial lecture, speaking on the relationship between Austrian poet

Nikolaus Lenau (1802–50) and his passion for Sophie von Löwenthal, the wife of a friend. These lectures and the ensuing discussions had the great advantage of facilitating dialogue between old and new members of the WPV; as learned members of the middle class, all were easily familiar with the subject matter to hand. There was no need to present lengthy case histories; speakers were free to concentrate on the details important for their particular reflections.

The new psychoanalytic investigations of artists and their oeuvre filled the members of the WPV with a joyful inquisitiveness. Freud described the 'connection between the impressions of the artist's childhood and his life-history on the one hand and his works, as reactions to those impressions, on the other' as 'one of the most attractive subjects of analytic examination'.[61] These debates also attracted animated attention further afield, particularly from Swiss circles interested in psychoanalysis. Carl Gustav Jung wrote to Freud in 1907, wishing him to know that

> the history of Jensen's childhood is now clear to me. A very beautiful solution is to be found in the stories 'The Red Umbrella' and 'In the Gothic House'. Both, particularly the first, are wonderful parallels of 'Gradiva', sometimes down to the finest details. The problem is one of brother–sister love. Has Jensen a sister? I refrain from expatiating on the details, it would only spoil the charm of discovery.[62]

Yet the deliberations of members of the WPV were also defined by much ambivalence. Many members of the circle had dabbled in writing literature during puberty (as was common for middle-class male youth at the time) and contributors to the WPV meetings regularly made comments about their emotional rapport with writers and their works. Still, it is safe to assume that many would have explained the overcoming of their artistic inclinations in psychoanalytic terms, as personal psychological progress. The passion that the psychoanalysts brought to debates concerning genius and creativity was fuelled by a complex subcurrent of competitiveness with writers of literature and poetry in particular, and creative artists in general.

Perhaps the best example of this atmosphere of competitiveness can be found in the debate that followed a presentation to the WPV on 12 January 1910 by Wittels, concerning Austrian writer and journalist Karl Kraus. Wittels, a former friend of Kraus, had shared with him a love for underage actress Irma Karczewska, a fact known to the members of the WPV. In his talk Wittels gave a relatively insightful and reflective psychoanalytic account of Kraus's character and career. The response in the ranks of the WPV was divided, but positive overall. However, Freud pointed out the need for tolerance in such an analysis, since otherwise it would rightfully incur the charge of inhumanity – and, one could add, border on character assassination. Reform pedagogue Karl Furtmüller agreed vehemently with Freud; he found Wittels's talk overly dogmatic, and insufficient in explaining why Kraus did not fit the journalistic mould epitomised by the middle-class Viennese daily *Neue Freie Presse*. Wittels inferred that, to Kraus, the newspaper symbolised his father. Freud also gently warned Wittels to avoid publicising his analysis outside the scientific realms of the WPV.[63] Freud's hunch about Wittels's need for a wider audience, and by implication, for a narcissistic triumph over his former friend, turned out to be correct. In the year of his talk Wittels published a satirical roman-à-clef titled *Ezechiel. Der Zugereiste* (*Ezechiel. The Newcomer*) which depicts Kraus in a highly ironic light. As a result, Wittels was evicted from the ranks of the WPV and joined forces with Freud again only in 1925. Unsurprisingly the novel heightened Kraus's outspoken criticism of psychoanalysis.[64]

As already flagged, the matter of creativity and genius formed an important theme of the weekly gatherings of the WPV from the time when Rank began minuting the meetings in 1906. At its centre remained the question of whether creativity could be understood as an inherited trait or as a function of the psyche. Sadger introduced the term *Belastung* on the occasion of his first lecture at the WPV (on Lenau), and from the beginning Freud objected to the genetic implications created by such a focus. In Freud's view it deflected attention from the formation of symptoms. Sadger, Freud suggested, had not considered the fact that Lenau was an onanist throughout his life.[65] As Katja Guenther has succinctly argued, Freud's contribution to neurology consists of the discovery that lived experience can contribute to symptom formation, which is not necessarily caused by physical lesions (as previously assumed).[66] Nonetheless, Sadger insisted that some proclivities cannot be explained by psychosexual causes.[67]

During the two and a half years between Sadger's talks on Lenau and Kleist, his presentations on poets to the same 'inner circle' of psychoanalysts became increasingly contested, mainly because others in the group, including Freud, had developed an interest in artists that was distinctly different from Sadger's. Among his colleagues in the WPV, a shift from pathography to exploration of the creative process as the main goal of psychoanalytic thinking took place in exactly this timeframe.[68] The ambitious and productive methodological debates that ensued occurred against the backdrop of Freud's as well as Rank's research and publications on the topic. While sometimes discussed critically in secondary literature, these debates are usually outlined from a Freudian perspective.[69]

Three aspects of Sadger's works sparked repeated criticism: his aim, his methodology and the impact of his studies on the lay reader. Sadger intended to use a select group of poets to illustrate his contribution to the theory of degeneration; although his self-attested aim was to humanise the poets, this project met with increasing resistance inside the WPV. Deliberations concerning the case modality most apposite for writing about creative artists became emotional on more than one occasion. Early on, fellow physician Max Steiner supported Sadger's pathographical approach to Swiss writer Conrad Ferdinand Meyer.[70] Wittels also considered Sadger's position sympathetically; he spoke against the emotive character of the discussions and supported a biographical approach, fearing that the new suggested methodology was too subjectively focused on analysis of an artist's oeuvre, and allowed projection of subconscious interpretations onto literary works.[71] Yet, after the Kleist paper in 1909, even the gentle Rank declared – with some exasperation – his 'in principle', personal dislike of pathography.[72] In response to Sadger's 1907 lecture on Meyer, Freud had explicitly stated that he saw no need to write pathographies at all: 'theories can only suffer, and subject matter does not gain anything by it'.[73] Rudolf Reitler, Stekel, Freud, Graf, Hugo Schwerdtner, Rank and Ernst Federn all spoke out against pathography (some more than once) and Sadger's reliance on it as a form of enquiry.[74]

Graf commented thoughtfully on the debate. He confirmed pathology to be pertinent to biographical studies of authors, but affirmed the average artist to be 'healthy'. Graf also provided a reason for this argument, namely that the creative process enables artists to overcome their psychological impediments and resolve their inner conflicts, as both Freud and Rank had already stated. Graf further maintained that 'the purely medical analysis, the pathography, does not contribute to the understanding of the creative process, because it only deals with such inhibitions, and not with the positive creative forces'.[75] In 1909 Freud commented in a similar vein when he poignantly declared that 'poets are too precious to us to simply [serve to] illustrate that every human being has such typical fundamental impulses'.[76] His statement hones in on the significant difference between the two case modalities that were contested in the WPV: at stake was the overgeneralisation about the nature of creative artists versus investigation of the creative process – mastery of which provides artists with the agency to help themselves and their audience in psychological terms.

On a methodological level, two criticisms were levelled at Sadger's approach. Firstly, Graf contended that Sadger's understanding of autobiographical sources was naive. Like Möbius, Sadger had argued that autobiographical texts made available a form of evidence more reliable than literary representation: in a work of fiction, he claimed, it remains impossible to identify an authentic truth about the author, as distinct from a figment of his or her imagination.[77] Similarly to Krafft-Ebing, Sadger argued in his lecture on Meyer that the literary oeuvre does not reveal with any certainty 'what the poet really experienced, since nothing differentiates the real from illusion'. Consequently, to Sadger it seemed impossible to decide 'where truth ends and poetry begins'.[78] Graf objected by arguing that the reliability of autobiographical sources is also compromised, as artists already think about posterity while writing, and subsequently gloss over issues, especially when they claim to speak the truth.[79]

The members of the WPV raised a second, related objection in the context of Sadger's biographical treatment of Kleist, in which he daringly explored Kleist's family constellations and homosexual leanings. Sadger drew his conclusions indirectly, which earned him much criticism for a lack of biographical evidence that might verify his hypothesis. Eduard Hitschmann stated that biographical materials were unavailable for the first twenty years of Kleist's life and, as such, an attempt at a pathography was nonsense. It followed, argued Federn, that Kleist's subconscious homosexuality and his overly close bond to his mother represented figments of Sadger's imagination. Freud's exasperation focused on the missing evidence and the wrong interpretations.[80]

The problem of limited sources has remained a long-standing issue for biographers of Kleist, as demonstrated by the wave of biographies occasioned by the two-hundredth anniversary of Kleist's death in 2011. In the book version of Sadger's study of Kleist (his lecture can be accessed only indirectly, through the WPV minutes) Sadger did reference relatively recently discovered materials in his elaborations, including Kleist's emotive letter to his admired friend Ernst Heinrich Adolf von Pfuel. Kleist biographer Sigismund Rahmer had unearthed this document only in 1902, in the Pfuel family archive. Rahmer had a great interest in pathographical studies – he edited the aforementioned series 'Grenzfragen der Literatur und Medizin', and published two pathographies, on Strindberg and Lenau.[81] Yet when it came to Kleist, Rahmer refused such an approach – at one with Sadger's opponents in the WPV – due to the dearth of sources, and because of his declared esteem of the poet. By contrast, Sadger saw Rahmer's refusal as a chance missed.

From a twenty-first-century perspective, Sadger's study of Kleist has at least in part stood the test of time, prompting the question of what else Sadger's fellow WPV members found challenging about his ideas and expression. Why did psychoanalysts fail to appreciate the potential of psychoanalytic pathographies to further their cause through the dissemination of psychoanalytic vocabulary and concepts? The criticism most consistently voiced was the perceived unpopularity of pathography, both within the WPV and among the imagined readers of Sadger's work. At the same time, this deep resentment that pathography triggered in the WPV seems astounding, considering that Sadger's interest in poets presumably played a crucial role in his admission to the circle. Yet it is most enlightening in this context that Federn remarked that Stekel had expressed a fear that Sadger's publications would shed a negative light on the discipline of psychoanalysis as a whole.[82] This alarm was not entirely unfounded within the reasoning of the group: Sadger published his studies in the Löwenfeld series, which had already been instrumental in the dissemination of Freud's ideas to scientific readers, as Freud stated in a letter to Jung on 1 January 1907.[83] If Freud's turn towards investigating creative artists and their works was an attempt to popularise psychoanalysis beyond his immediate circle of followers, then within the WPV the heavy-handed reaction to Sadger's attempts to write pathography were also related to a fear that Sadger's works might successfully monopolise the topic, both to the outside world and within psychoanalytic circles.

Regrettably, there is little indication as to how Sadger's pathographies, and indeed pathographies in general, were received in the years between 1907 and 1912. While his works on Meyer and Kleist were published in Löwenfeld's renowned series, none of Sadger's volumes was reprinted after the first edition. If we see Sadger's work in a localised psychoanalytic context, however, it has to be pointed out that the heavy-handed Viennese viewpoint was not matched by others. The available reviews of Sadger's Meyer study, written by Jung, and by theologian and future lay psychoanalyst Oscar Pfister, were overwhelmingly positive. Jung was Freud's disciple at the time when he wrote his review; his essay underlines the special place this psychoanalytic study held within the genre of pathography, and emphasises Sadger's striving to 'encompass the development of the whole personality psychologically, to truly understand it'. As a psychiatrist he judged Sadger's efforts accurately. Four years later Pfister called the same study 'a valuable, tactful and scientific monograph'.[84]

Negative emotion and attempts to defend Freud's position seem to have coalesced in resistance to Sadger's pathographic writing, even though many of the alternatives presented by other members of the WPV likewise failed to follow Freud's model of an open case study. Actually, those writings by Stekel, Rank and Freud that did not encompass contemplation of the author's oeuvre garnered little attention. Meanwhile, at least in print, Sadger modified his position only in 1912, in an essay for the first volume of *Imago* titled 'Von der Pathographie zur Psychographie' ('From Pathography to Psychography'), when he finally integrated analysis of a poet's work with a biographical account. This essay also represents Sadger's last endeavour on the topic of creative genius.

The dialogic-psychoanalytic case study

Anticipating the workings of the unconscious in his readers, it was Freud who developed the most nuanced strategies for engaging with the creative arts. Freud was also the main proponent of the dialogic-psychoanalytic case study. Besides 'Der Wahn und die Träume in W. Jensens "Gradiva"' ('Delusions and Dreams in Jensen's "Gradiva"'), the key texts of this case modality are Freud's analysis of a childhood memory written down by Leonardo da Vinci (1910), 'Eine Kindheitserinnerung des Leonardo da Vinci'; the discussion of William Shakespeare's theme of the three caskets (1913); and his analysis of Michelangelo Buonarroti's marble statue of Moses (1914). The last was published anonymously, in the psychoanalytic periodical *Imago*.[85] The method behind Freud's analyses of creative artists and their oeuvres differed from that of psychiatric and psychoanalytic pathographies. Rather than illustrating psychiatric or psychoanalytic theories, the dialogic-psychoanalytic case study correlated a facet of an artist's biography with a particular aspect of the oeuvre, or with one of the artist's works in particular.

Freud's investigation of the relationship of creative artists to the subconscious began with an informal talk of 1907 titled 'Der Dichter und das Phantasieren' ('Creative Writers and Day-Dreaming', published in 1908), which portrays the artist as an intermediary between the neurotic and the dreamer. In his study of Freud's readings of literature and art, Michael Rohrwasser submits that Freud viewed the artist as his 'unsanctified opponent'.[86] If Freud's position appears positively mellow in the context of the WPV, nevertheless such underlying competitiveness was present, and productively so. It allowed Freud new methodological insights into the workings of the case study genre, and instigated an adaptation of the closed case study modalities of psychiatry and psychoanalysis.

May 1907 saw publication of Freud's first major analysis of a work of literary fiction, the essay 'Der Wahn und die Träume in W. Jensens "Gradiva"', centred on Wilhelm Jensen's story *Gradiva*. Here Freud outlines his understanding of the relationship between psychiatry, art and psychoanalysis, and showcases a new case modality, termed throughout the present volume the dialogic-psychoanalytic case study. This form of case study includes analysis of a specific part of a creative artist's oeuvre, and considers it either with reference to an aspect of the artist's life history, or with reference to the workings of art – as occurs in the *Gradiva* case study. Freud's development of this new case modality was motivated by the desire to tempt his readers away from their resistance to the closed case modalities that were characteristic of psychiatry and psychoanalysis. His dialogic-psychoanalytic case study of *Gradiva* functions like other pathographical studies to the extent that it serves to illustrate a generalised rule; more precisely, it demonstrates the essential result of his earlier book *Die Traumdeutung* (*The Interpretation of Dreams*) – that dreams represent wish fulfilment. At the same time, Freud's account of *Gradiva* adapted the case study genre in a self-conscious attempt to maintain middle-class readers' interest in his insights into the workings of art.

As becomes apparent in 'Der Dichter und das Phantasieren', Freud was fascinated by the ways in which poets '[manage] to make such an impression on us with [their works] and to arouse in us emotions of which, perhaps, we had not even thought ourselves capable'.[87] He outlines two crucial strategies in this regard: the softening of the writer's egotistic day-dreams through alterations and disguise, and the enticement of the reader through the reward of aesthetic pleasure, which in turn allows the reader the release of greater pleasure from deeper sources.[88] Arguably Freud also wished to reduce the distance he felt between his own writerly nature 'and that of the common run of humanity' (his readers), as part of an attempt to popularise psychoanalytic theories.[89] His rhetorical strategies curbed the attack on creative artists that readers had come to expect. He persuasively sought to overcome readers' resistance by providing aesthetic reading pleasure, by using a rhetoric of humility, and, most importantly, by introducing a controlled dissonance between the particulars of the case study and the surrounding theory based on his understanding of the workings of the unconscious.

Freud's *Gradiva* case study exemplifies his sophisticated insights and his manipulations of readers, revealing his motivation for such a writing project. Early on in this study Freud hypothesises that, within the discipline of psychiatry, Norbert Hanold, the protagonist of Jensen's story, would be classified as degenerate. Freud notes that the diagnosis of degeneration – 'whether it is right or wrong' – distances the reader from the main character, because to classify somebody as 'degenerate' seems removed from the reader, who sees him- or herself as 'an average human being and as the norm'.[90] In the discussions of the WPV this argument was generally accepted. Freud, Rank and Stekel repeated this assessment early on; Stekel reaffirmed his view on the occasion of Sadger giving his Kleist paper, in 1909.[91] On the same occasion, Freud outspokenly essayed why listeners felt like resisting Sadger, even when Sadger presented correct statements: in Freud's opinion, academic discussion of creative artists without consideration of their oeuvres alienated the audience.

Seeking the opposite of alienation with his audience, in his pioneering analysis of Jensen's *Gradiva* Freud mitigates the generalisations developed in *Die Traumdeutung* in three substantial ways. Firstly, like creative artists, he cultivates aesthetic pleasure. Freud's biographer Ernest Jones observed that Freud's da Vinci dialogic-psychoanalytic case study was 'written with such delicacy and beauty of language as to rank high and to compel admiration for its literary qualities alone. In fact some reviewers, such as Moritz Necker in the Munich *Allgemeine Zeitung*, praised above all [Freud's] masterly prose, "which many professional writers must envy"'.[92]

A second quality of the *Gradiva* study is Freud's stance of humble self-reflexivity that similarly undermines the distance between psychoanalyst and reader. This self-reflexivity is at play, for instance, where Freud promotes sympathy for Hanold's experience of temporary delusion. The protagonist of Jensen's story is fascinated by a female figure in an antique bas-relief whom he names Gradiva. Zoe Bertgang is Hanold's childhood friend who wishes to marry him, and when she appears as Gradiva, Hanold believes the encounter to be real. Freud likens this incident to that of a physician who experienced a similar phenomenon when visited by the sister of a diseased patient. Freud then admits to being this physician.[93] Moreover, to refer to readers Freud uses the first-person plural pronoun 'we', thereby including himself in this broad category.

Almost inevitably, such a personal disclosure and intimate address has a levelling effect on the relationship between psychoanalytic specialist and reader. Freud's admission in the *Gradiva* essay went hand in hand with an outspoken appreciation of creative artists and expression of tolerance towards their failures. In various comments to Sadger, Wittels and Stekel after their respective lectures in the WPV, Freud stressed the importance of tolerance in understanding artists. His attempts to curb the competitive, projective streak in these analyses was based on a fundamental appreciation of the uniqueness of creative artists – and by extension of human beings in general. Freud underlines this position again in 1929 when elaborating on Goethe and da Vinci: 'but human images can never be repeated, and profound differences between the two great men are not lacking'.[94] In 'Der Wahn und die Träume in W. Jensens "Gradiva"', he goes so far as to describe Jensen's story, or novella, as a 'perfectly correct psychiatric study'.[95] In a similarly receptive vein he addresses 'our readers' and anticipates his audience to be capable of formulating certain questions, and of critiquing his position. Hence he takes the opinions of his readers very seriously.

The third, and greatest, incentive for Freud's readers to warm to his case studies of creative artists lay in the methodological realm. Scholars of rhetoric Gert Üding and Bernd Steinbrink have argued that the close alignment of framework and illustrative example defines the rhetorical power of case studies in argumentative discourse, and that in the literary realm the oscillation between framework and example creates the fictitious tone needed to entice readers and create ambiguity.[96] By setting in play a controlled dissonance between the matter of the case study and his framing theory, Freud was able to balance the generalisations of the closed case study with particularisation. The meandering quality of Freud's dialogic-psychoanalytic case studies reflects Freud's understanding of cognitive processes, and derives from the texts' intermediary position between argumentative and poetic discourses.

Freud developed two techniques in this context. Like Möbius in his early pathographies, he explored both biography and artistic works, yet instead of concentrating on the complete biography and oeuvre of a given creative artist, he focused on snippets of both that he contrasted with one another. This represented a further particularisation in light of the generalising nature of his theories. His readers could explore his insights further given their own broader background knowledge and understanding of the subject matter. In this way he allowed his readers to generate new insights along psychoanalytic principles. Where Möbius's early case studies, for example, worked on the basis of comprehensiveness, the fact that Freud's theories were generally applicable and accessible played in his favour. This meant that, ideally, readers who were familiar with the subject matter or his theories could further explore their understanding of both.

Freud also sidestepped the logic of the medical case study in another way, namely by inverting the importance of framing theory and example. This method resembles therapeutic techniques used to alleviate – in psychoanalytic terms – the resistances of the superego. Freud applies his insights into the workings of unconscious displacement (substitution of originally dangerous and unacceptable thoughts) through a new aim or a new object, by working with the logic of the unconscious, and by inverting the role of framing theory and example. The framing theory in his dialogic-psychoanalytic case studies is rhetorically weak, but captures the reader's attention with a question or proposition. Meanwhile, the reader is absorbed by an interesting and often roundabout example that does not quite fit the theory outlined. This gives Freud's case writings an evocative character and well explains readers' ongoing fascination with his writing.

In the *Gradiva* study, for instance, Freud's framework for the case seems straightforward enough – he seeks to illustrate a paradigm developed in *Die Traumdeutung* (his most famous work at the time), namely that dreams represent fulfilled wishes rather than commonly believed future prognostications.[97] The explanation of this paradigm he provides succinctly in the final paragraph, almost as an addendum, while the main focus of the case study is on the analysis of the short novel and his associative explorations of the relationship between psychoanalysis and the arts. The body of his discursive case study, then, provides the reader with an understanding of the terminology involved, and with new reflections, while not allowing the reader to oppose either the creative writer or the psychoanalyst in question. Thus the case study tricks the unconscious of its readers in order to enable them to enjoy and understand the workings of associative thought consciously as well as unconsciously.

To invoke Freud's own words in relation to genius, a mere generalisation creates a distance which underlines the human fallibility of the creative artists in question and, by extension, the fallibility of the reader who identifies with the artist. It thus insults the reader's superego, creating resistance. This effect is all the more powerful since Freud also concedes that ambivalence towards the genius is already a given among admirers of creative artists. Hence readers can project their innate ambivalence towards the father and other figures of authority such as the creative artist onto the closed-form pathographies of psychiatry and psychoanalysis.[98] From this perspective, middle-class readers' tendency towards idealisation revealed a decidedly immature streak.

By creating a case study modality that permitted readers to contain their ambivalence, rather than project it onto creative artists or expert writers of pathography, Freud sought to do justice to creative artists. By outlining not their abnormality but their capacity for insight, he drew his reader into a more complex narrative that marked the differences between the scientific endeavour of psychoanalysis and the humanist potential of literary writing.[99] Rather than being mere illustrations of a psychoanalytic theory, Freud's case studies seemingly 'run away with him': his meandering associations are perceptive and insightful, yet they do not always obviously connect to the question he set out to answer. Through reference to Jensen's story and an explanation of the workings of art, Freud provided middle-class readers with the intellectual and emotional rewards that were needed for their embrace of his theories.

If, for Freud, art led to 'a region in which, as it were, primitive man's strivings for omnipotence are still in full force', the question arises of how his insights from case studies of creative artists influenced his case writings in general.[100] Indeed, Freud conceded what psychiatry could ot: that creative artists are distinguished from psychoanalysts by their methodology, but share a similar understanding of the workings of the human mind:

> The author no doubt proceeds differently. He directs his attention to the unconscious in his own mind, he listens to its possible developments and lends them artistic expression instead of suppressing them by conscious criticism. Thus he experiences from himself what we learn from others – the laws which the activities of this unconscious must obey. But he need not state these laws, nor even be clearly aware of them; as a result of the tolerance of his intelligence, they are incorporated within his creations. We discover these laws by analysing his writings just as we find them from cases of real illness; but the conclusion seems inescapable, that either both of us, the writer and the doctor, have misunderstood the unconscious in the same way, or we have both understood it correctly.[101]

The foregoing discussion has placed Freud's writing into a much wider context of case writing, and has underlined how specific discourses as well as the attempt to communicate psychoanalytic results to a wider audience shaped his dialogic-psychoanalytic cases. Much has been said about the methodological contradictions between Freud's published case histories and his therapeutic practice. Sulloway even contends that the reasoning of the former remains pseudo-scientific camouflage.[102] In this context it is important to acknowledge that Freud's preferred method of investigating creative art and artists was not confined to the dialogic-psychoanalytic case study. As sketched in his 1907 study of *Gradiva*, methodologically Freud envisaged two ways of pursuing analysis of literature. These differed from methods championed by psychiatrists and fellow psychoanalysts:

> One [way] would be to enter deeply into a particular case, into the dream-creations of one author in one of his works. The other would be to bring together and contrast all the examples that could be found of the use of dreams in the works of different authors. The second method would seem to be far the more effective and perhaps the only justifiable one, for it frees us at once from the difficulties involved in adopting the artificial concept of 'writers' as a class. On investigation this class falls apart into individual writers of the most various worth – among them some whom we are accustomed to honour as the deepest observers of the human mind. In spite of this, however, these pages will be devoted to an enquiry of the first sort.[103]

In line with the psychoanalyst's focus on a single patient, Freud viewed psychoanalytic studies of creative genius as intensive analysis of a particular case, and as a broader, thematic and more generalising psychoanalytic literary history. On publication of the *Gradiva* case study Freud already knew that such works existed, written by his devout pupil and protégé

Rank. By 1906, Freud was familiar with Rank's three manuscripts mentioned earlier: the first draft of *Der Künstler*, and two preliminary versions of thematic analyses, one concerned with the literary motif of incest and the second focused on the motif of the homosexual.[104]

Das Inzest-Motiv in Dichtung und Sage (*The Incest Theme in Literature and Legend*, 1912) has been called the 'most important single work of psychoanalytic criticism' in relation to literature.[105] Already in his 1914 essay on the history of psychoanalysis, Freud acknowledged the importance of Rank's 'exhaustive work on the theme of incest', which he saw 'easily tak[ing] the first place' in psychoanalytic studies focused on literature, trumping his own works.[106] Over 700 pages, with an encyclopaedic scope consisting of two parts and twenty-four chapters, Rank sets forth an overview of the literary depiction of subconscious incest phantasies between parents and children, and between siblings. His literary examples belong to the classical and Western canon, but also include observations concerning myth, legends and fables, and on the role of incest throughout history. Unlike Freud's dialogic-psychoanalytic case studies, this work analyses the life histories and oeuvres of writers only occasionally. As Rank outlines in his introductory chapter, more thorough, more specific investigations needed to be postponed until after his study, which, he argues, explores the general and major findings. Indeed, some of Rank's later works, particularly his evocative study of the doppelgänger motif – written in 1914 and published in 1925 – might be understood as instances of the 'more thorough investigations' he had envisioned.[107] The sheer breadth of *Das Inzest-Motiv in Dichtung und Sage*, and its generalising impetus, pushed the case study genre to its limits. Driven by Rank's need to arrive at an exhaustive explanation of the phenomenon in question and as a case compilation of sorts, it did not allow readers an easy identification through autobiographical case vignettes. Such commitment to generalisability had been manifest years earlier, in his comprehensive attempt to explain the nature of creative sublimation in *Der Künstler*.

Almost nothing is known about the contemporary reception of *Das Inzest-Motiv in Dichtung und Sage*. Freud predicted that the study's 'subject [was] bound to arouse the greatest unpopularity'.[108] If Freud was correct, his assessment might explain why Rank decided against publishing his follow-up volume on homosexuality. It was with limited success, then, that Rank – with Freud's support – tried to lead the psychoanalytic case study genre beyond Freud's dialogic-psychoanalytic case study into new territory of the thematic case compilation, and it remains intriguing to ponder why Freud left it to Rank to develop the open-form case study to a more comprehensive level. Rank's more schematic attempts to explore the nature of genius met a fate similar to psychiatric and psychoanalytic pathographies: these more generalising studies failed to attract the attention of either the psychoanalytic movement or the educated reading public.

***

This chapter has examined the styles of reasoning adopted in biographical case studies of creative artists in the early twentieth century. In psychiatric pathographic writing, the shift from the open- to the closed-form case study developed chronologically, whereas in psychoanalytic writing the same shift occurred simultaneously. This caused friction in Freud's inner circle of fellow psychoanalysts and a fragmentation of psychoanalytic knowledge about creative artists and their work that continues to haunt the psychoanalytic investigation of literature and artworks.

Writers of the closed-form case studies utilised only the life histories of prominent cultural figures in an attempt to explain certain theories and to normalise specific behaviours. These case writings include the modern psychiatric pathographies of the early twentieth century; the majority of Sadger's psychoanalytic pathographies (before his late turn to psychography in 1912); and the typologies of artists written by Stekel, Rank and Freud. In very different ways, these closed case studies written by psychiatrists and psychoanalysts provided readers with generalisations concerning literary authors and other artists that did not include consideration of their creative oeuvres. This generated resistance among educated middle-class readers, who, after all, admired 'cultural greats' first and foremost for their works, and who had come to admire, idealise and even fetishise their personae through engagement with the results of their creative efforts.

On the other hand, the open-form case studies integrated information about creative artists with consideration of their oeuvre. These examples were thus characterised by a dialogic structure and an appreciation that – as articulated by Möbius for the very first pathography – literary and artistic works belong to a wider educated public, not only to medicine.[109] To Freud, Möbius was the forefather of psychotherapy. He was a neurologist and his early pathographies constituted a new kind of medical-biographical expert case study, outlining ways in which hereditary influences shaped the life of a genius as much as the average burgher.[110] Due to their open form, and their acknowledgement of the literary or artistic oeuvre, his pathographies encountered much less resistance among the intellectual elite and middle-class readers. Discussion of the oeuvre gave Möbius the opportunity to integrate new insights about his subject, and so afforded a more balanced picture of the gifted individual, one that did not rely on generalising statements alone. A comparable specificity and dialogic structure are inherent in Freud's famous studies of literary or artistic works and in Rank's literary historical investigations.

Perhaps the greatest difference between these contributions to debate about creative artists within psychiatry and psychoanalysis lay in the interest shown by Rank and Freud in the mystery of the creative process. In many ways this enabled Freud to carve out what he perceived as a scientific middle ground between psychiatry and literature, which entailed a dissociation from both fields of knowledge. The discursive parameters of psychiatry did not favour interest in the workings of the psyche in general, nor in the workings of creative minds in particular; literature and the other arts, according to Freud, produced these insights intuitively rather than scientifically. To psychiatrists and psychoanalysts of the fin de siècle, interrogation of the lives and works of creative artists contributed significantly to the humanisation of certain medical, psychiatric and psychological phenomena. By way of significant contrast, Chapter 3 explores the satirical means through which the creative writer Oskar Panizza resisted psychiatric narratives of genius and madness, and also how these narratives intimately fashioned concepts of the writerly self.

Notes

1 Rob Pope, *Creativity. Theory, History, Practice* (New York: Routledge, 2005), p. 236.
2 Christian von Zimmermann, *Biographische Anthropologie. Menschenbilder in lebensgeschichtlicher Darstellung (1830–1940)* (Berlin: de Gruyter, 2006), p. 8.
3 See Birgit Lang and Katie Sutton, 'The Aesthetics of Sexual Ethics: *Geschlecht und Gesellschaft* and Middle-Class Sexual Modernity in Fin-de-Siècle Germany', *Oxford German Studies*, 44:2 (2015), pp. 177–98.
4 Jürgen Habermas, *The Structural Transformation of the Public Sphere: An Inquiry into Category of Bourgeois Society*, trans. Thomas Burger (Cambridge: MIT Press, 1989), pp. 50f.
5 Important titles of a general nature are Marilyn Charles, *Psychoanalysis and Literature: The Stories We Live* (Lanham: Rowman & Littlefield, 2015); Shoshana Felman, *Literature and Psychoanalysis: The Question of Reading, Otherwise* (Baltimore: Johns Hopkins University Press, 1982); Lilian R. Furst, *Just Talk: Narratives of Psychoanalysis* (Lexington: University Press of Kentucky, 1999); Jean-Michel Rabaté, *The Cambridge Introduction to Literature and Psychoanalysis* (New York: Cambridge University Press, 2014); Shlomith Rimmon-Kennan, *Discourse in Psychoanalysis and Literature* (Routledge Revivals) (Hoboken: Taylor & Francis, 2014); Steve Vine, *Literature in Psychoanalysis: A Reader* (New York: Palgrave Macmillan, 2005); Linda Ruth Williams, *Critical Desire: Psychoanalysis and the Literary Subject* (London: Edward Arnold, 1995); Paul Williams and Glen O. Gabbard, *Key Papers in Literature and Psychoanalysis* (London: Karnac, 2007).
6 Michel Foucault, *The History of Sexuality, vol. I: An Introduction*, trans. Robert Hurley (New York: Vintage Books, 1990), p. 140; Susanne Hilken, Matthias Bormuth and Michael Schmidt-Degenhard, 'Psychiatrische Anfänge der Pathographie', in Matthias Bormuth, Klaus Podoll and Carsten Spitzer (eds), *Kunst und Krankheit. Studien zur Pathographie* (Göttingen: Wallstein, 2007), pp. 11–26; Jutta Person, *Der pathographische Blick. Physiognomik, Atavismustheorien und Kulturkritik* (Würzburg: Königshausen & Neumann, 2005), p. 11. In the context of criminality, a Foucaultian approach was influentially first promoted in Peter Becker, *Verderbnis und Entartung. Eine Geschichte der Kriminologie des 19. Jahrhunderts als Diskurs und Praxis* (Göttingen: Vandenhoeck & Ruprecht, 2002).
7 Person, *Der pathographische Blick*, pp. 11–12.
8 See Anne Hunsaker Hawkins, *Reconstructing Illness: Studies in Pathography*, 2nd edition (West Lafayette: Purdue University Press, 1999).

9 Burkhard Madea, 'Case Histories in Forensic Medicine', *Forensic Science International*, 165 (2007), pp. 111–14, p. 111.

10 On the complex history of Möbius's departure from his university employer see Holger Steinberg, *'Als ob ich zu einer steinernen Wand spräche'. Der Nervenarzt Paul Julius Möbius. Eine Werkbiografie* (Bern: Huber, 2005), pp. 58–112.

11 Holger Steinberg, *Kraepelin in Leipzig. Eine Begegnung von Psychiatrie und Psychologie* (Bonn: Narrenschiff, 2001).

12 Emil Kraepelin, *Psychiatrie: ein Lehrbuch für Studirende und Aerzte*, 6th edition (Leipzig: Barth, 1899). Möbius discusses Kraepelin's new categories in Paul Julius Möbius, "Über Entartung", in Leopold Löwenfeld and Hans Kurella (eds), *Grenzfragen des Nerven- und Seelenlebens* (Wiesbaden: Bergmann, 1900), pp. 95–123, p. 102.

13 Ulrich Palm and Hans-Jürgen Möller, 'Reception of Kraepelin's Ideas 1900–1960. Review Article', *Psychiatry and Clinical Neurosciences*, 65 (2011), pp. 318–25, p. 318. On Kraepelin's status in the history of psychiatry see Paul Hoff, *Emil Kraepelin und die Psychiatrie als klinische Wissenschaft* (Berlin: Springer, 1994); Richard Noll, *American Madness: The Rise and Fall of Dementia Praecox* (Cambridge: Harvard University Press, 2011), pp. 66–73.

14 Paul Julius Möbius, *Über das Pathologische bei Goethe* (Leipzig: Barth, 1898), p. 16.

15 Möbius's special interest in creative artists of outstanding cultural importance began with a study of Jean-Jacques Rousseau in 1889. In the opening pages of this study, he refers to the merit of Rousseau's works, which, he points out, belong to the educated public, not only to medicine. Möbius justifies his project by noting that the biographical literature available in French and German clearly lacks an understanding of Rousseau's medical history. If anything, Möbius acknowledges concerns about the propriety of bringing medical knowledge to a wider public. Paul Julius Möbius, *J.-J. Rousseau's Krankheitsgeschichte* (Leipzig: Vogel, 1889), p. v. His monograph on philosopher Arthur Schopenhauer, first published in 1899, represents another example of an early pathography. Paul Julius Möbius, *Über Schopenhauer* (Leipzig: Barth, 1903).

16 Paul Julius Möbius, *Über das Pathologische bei Goethe* (Leipzig: Barth, 1898), p. 6.

17 Paul Julius Möbius, *Über den physiologischen Schwachsinn des Weibes*, 5th edition (Halle a.S.: Marhold, 1903), p. 43.

18 Möbius, *Über das Pathologische bei Goethe*, p. 15.

19 Paul Julius Möbius, *Goethe* (Leipzig: Barth, 1903), pp. 37–66.

20 Gall's categories are simplified to the following: 'life instinct, drive to eat, group sense and sense of order'. Möbius, *Goethe*, p. 39.

21 The complete list encompasses life instinct, drive to eat, sex drive, love of children, friendship and attachment, group sense, bravery, activity (in the sense of both thirst for action and vehemency of character), cunningness, acquisitiveness, vanity, thoughtfulness, religion, wit, power of judgement, sense of order, sense for mimicry, poetry, philology, philosophy, visual arts, architecture, music and mathematics.

22 '[G]esunde Weiber und nicht Gehirndamen.' Möbius, *Über den physiologischen Schwachsinn des Weibes*, p. 43; Steinberg, *'Als ob ich zu einer steinernen Wand spräche'*, pp. 225–6; Heinz-Jürgen Voß, *Making Sex Revisited. Dekonstruktion des Geschlechts aus biologisch-medizinischer Perspektive* (Bielefeld: Transcript, 2010), pp. 178–80.

23 'Die Dichter und Künstler sind im Allgemeinen Leute von hohem Streben, indessen sind sie eine sinnlich, geschlechtlich reizbare Rasse und höchst unregelmässig in ihrer Lebensweise.' Paul Julius Möbius, *Über Kunst und Künstler* (Leipzig: Barth, 1901), p. 79.

24 The expressions of outrage included but were in no way limited to works of German suffragettes such Hewig Dohm's *Die Antifeministen* (1902), Oda Olberg's

Der Weib und der Intellectualismus (1902) and Johanna Elberskirchen's treatise *Feminismus und Wissenschaft* (1903). Steinberg discusses Möbius's understanding of gender and its reception through second-wave feminism in '*Als ob ich zu einer steinernen Wand spräche*', pp. 225–6.

25 Leopold von Sacher-Masoch, Prologue to *Venus in Furs*, in Gilles Deleuze and Leopold von Sacher-Masoch, *Masochism: Coldness and Cruelty, and Venus in Furs*, trans. Jean McNeil (New York: Zone Books, 1991), pp. 143–271, p. 145.

26 See in particular Richard J. Evans, 'In Search of German Social Darwinism. The History and Historiography of a Concept', in Manfred Berg and Geoffrey Cocks (eds), *Medicine and Modernity: Public Health and Medical Care in Nineteenth- and Twentieth-Century Germany* (Cambridge: Cambridge University Press, 1997), pp. 55–80; also Alfred Kelly, *The Descent of Darwin: The Popularization of Darwinism in Germany, 1860–1914* (Chapel Hill: University of North Carolina Press, 1981). In Germany, Max Nordau directed his critique against selected modernist artists in his controversial *Entartung* (1892); much of this thought was inspired by Cesare Lombroso's attempts to conceptualise the effects of degeneration in men of genius.

27 In chronological order, the relevant titles are: Paul Julius Möbius, *Über das Pathologische bei Nietzsche* (Wiesbaden: Bergmann, 1900); Albert Eulenburg, *Sadismus und Masochismus* (Wiesbaden: Bergmann, 1902); Ferdinand Probst, *Der Fall Otto Weininger* (Wiesbaden: Bergmann, 1904); Isidor Sadger, *Konrad Ferdinand Meyer. Eine pathologisch-psychologische Studie* (Wiesbaden: Bergmann, 1908); Gaston Vorberg, *Guy de Maupassants Krankheit* (Wiesbaden: Bergmann, 1908); Isidor Sadger, *Heinrich von Kleist. Eine pathographisch-psychologische Studie* (Wiesbaden: Bergmann, 1909); Oswald Feis, *Hector Berlioz. Eine pathographische Studie* (Wiesbaden: Bergmann, 1909); Alfred Storch, *August Strindberg im Lichte seiner Selbstbiographie* (Munich: Bergmann, 1921); Adolf Heidenhain, *J. J. Rousseau* (Munich: Bergmann, 1924); Walther Riese, *Vincent van Gogh in der Krankheit* (Munich: Bergmann, 1926). Other titles that relate more generally to the arts: Leopold Löwenfeld, *Über die geniale Geistesthätigkeit mit besonderer Berücksichtigung des Genies für bildende Kunst* (Wiesbaden: Bergmann, 1903); Ernst Anton Jentsch, *Musik und Nerven*, 2 vols (Wiesbaden: Bergmann, 1904 and 1911); Leopold Löwenfeld, *Hypnose und Kunst* (Wiesbaden: Bergmann, 1904); Leopold Löwenfeld, *Über die geistige Arbeitskraft und Hygiene* (Wiesbaden: Bergmann, 1905); Otto Hinrichsen, *Zur Psychologie und Psychopathologie des Dichters* (Wiesbaden: Bergmann, 1911); Otto Hinrichsen, *Sexualität und Dichtung. Ein weiterer Beitrag zur Psychologie des Dichters* (Wiesbaden: Bergmann, 1912).

28 The published titles were: Erich Ebstein, *Chr. D. Crabbos Krankheit* (Munich: Reinhardt, 1906); Ferdinand Probst, *Edgar Allan Poe* (Munich: Reinhardt, 1906); Sigismund Rahmer, *August Strindberg. Eine pathologische Studie* (Munich: Reinhardt, 1907); Alfred Lichtenstein, *Der Kriminalroman. Eine literarische und forensisch-medizinische Studie mit Anhang: Sherlock Holmes zum Fall Hau* (Munich: Reinhardt, 1908).

29 '[S]pitzfindige psychiatrische Differentialdiagnostik.' Isidor Sadger, 'Von der Pathographie zur Psychographie', in Jens Malte Fischer (ed.), *Psychoanalytische Literaturinterpretationen* (Tübingen: Niemeyer, 1980), pp. 64–85, p. 65.

30 Alan Dundes, 'Introduction', in Isidor Sadger, *Recollecting Freud*, ed. Alan Dundes (Madison: University of Wisconsin Press, 2005), p. 8. Sadger had arrived in the Austrian capital from Galicia aged sixteen to study at the prestigious medical faculty of the University of Vienna, from which he graduated eight years later, in 1891.

31 Ulrike May, 'Ein Traum (1897) und ein Brief (1902): Zur frühen Beziehung zwischen Freud und Isidor Sadger', *Luzifer-Amor. Zeitschrift zur Geschichte der Psychoanalyse*, 12:24 (1999), pp. 25–48, p. 27.

32 See Ulrike May-Tolzmann, 'Zu den Anfängen des Narzißmus: Ellis-Näcke-

Sadger-Freud', *Luzifer-Amor. Zeitschrift zur Geschichte der Psychoanalyse*, 4:8 (1991), pp. 50–88; May, 'Ein Traum (1897) und ein Brief (1902)'.

33 May-Tolzmann, 'Zu den Anfängen des Narzißmus', pp. 67–8.

34 Birgit Lang and Katie Sutton, 'The Queer Cases of Psychoanalysis: Rethinking the Scientific Study of Homosexuality, 1890s–1920s', *German History*, 34:3 (2016), pp. 419–44, p. 431.

35 Alan C. Elms, 'Sigmund Freud, Psychohistorian', *Annual of Psychoanalysis*, 31 (2003), pp. 65–78, pp. 68–71; Charles B. Strozier and Daniel Offer, 'Freud and His Followers', in Charles B. Strozier and Oliger Abdyli (eds), *The Leader: Psychological Essays* (New York: Springer, 2011), pp. 13–30, pp. 14–15; Edward Timms, *Karl Kraus, Apocalyptic Satirist. Culture and Catastrophe in Habsburg Vienna* (New Haven: Yale University Press, 1986), p. 104.

36 Davis Whitney, for example, has argued that 'Sadger essentially offered documentation and reportage, not analysis and interpretation. It was Freud who took this rich and often remarkably contemporary raw material and reshaped it to reflect his own philosophy'. Davis Whitney, *Queer Beauty: Sexuality and Aesthetics from Winckelmann to Freud and Beyond* (New York: Columbia University Press, 2010), p. 210.

37 Isidor Sadger, 'Henrik Ibsen. Eine pathologische Studie', *Neue Freie Presse* (4 February 1896), pp. 1–2.

38 Isidor Sadger, 'Kranke Dichter und Krankendichtung', *Deutsche Revue*, 22:4 (1897), pp. 36–44, p. 38.

39 Sadger, 'Kranke Dichter', p. 39.

40 Sadger, 'Kranke Dichter', p. 40.

41 Sadger, 'Kranke Dichter', pp. 41–2.

42 Sadger, 'Kranke Dichter', p. 43.

43 Sadger, 'Kranke Dichter', p. 44.

44 Isidor Sadger, *Belastung und Entartung. Ein Beitrag zur Lehre vom kranken Genie* (Leipzig: Demme, 1910), p. 73. Möbius translated many of Magnan's works into German, but used the term 'Entartungsirresein' for the French 'dégénéré supérieur'. For the translation of these terms see 'Psychopathie – psychopathische Persönlichkeiten', in Christian Müller (ed.), *Lexikon der Psychiatrie: Gesammelte Abhandlungen der gebräuchlichsten psychopathologischen Begriffe* (Berlin: Springer, 2013), pp. 402–6, p. 402.

45 Sadger, *Belastung und Entartung*, p. 15.

46 Sadger, *Belastung und Entartung*, pp. 10–65.

47 'Schließlich kann man "belastet" sein, d. h. ein Päckchen ins Leben mitbringen, und doch von außerordentlicher Begabung, sowie in den Augen vieler Menschen "nervös" zu sein fast gleichbedeutend ist mit dem Anerkennungsdiplom für höhere Intelligenz.' Sadger, *Belastung und Entartung*, p. 73.

48 Sadger, *Heinrich von Kleist*, p. 12. Sigismund Rahmer was well aware of the appeal that Kleist's biography held for the emerging homosexual public of the fin de siècle, as shown by his publication of a letter by an openly homosexual literary critic in his second Kleist volume. Even so, Rahmer deemed Sadger's elaborations too speculative. Sadger found it possible to legitimate his interpretation through his particular theory of degeneration, which took account of both hereditary and environmental arguments (the latter founded in psychoanalytic theory) and his own groundbreaking psychoanalytic work with openly homosexual patients. Rahmer's first Kleist volume was *Das Kleist-Problem auf Grund neuer Forschungen zur Charakteristik und Biographie Heinrich von Kleists* (Berlin: Reimer, 1903); the second, *Heinrich von Kleist als Mensch und Dichter. Nach neuen Quellenforschungen* (Berlin: Reimer, 1909) (letter appears pp. 348–9).

49 Sadger, *Heinrich von Kleist*, p. 28.

50 Sadger, *Belastung und Entartung*, p. 71. Paradoxically, Sadger's opposition to the more populist notions of degeneration overemphasised negative traits, sacrificed

the positive aura attributed to genius and highlighted that which the genius shared with more ordinary members of the human race. Earlier in his work Sadger outlines how the subjects of his research relate to the norms that they deviate from. Unlike Möbius, he chooses quite crass examples of *Belastung*, and concludes that his choice of severe cases is justified, since he found in 'lesser' cases a less pronounced symptomatology. To him, these negative qualities in the genius represent the commonality between genius and imbecility; that is, they represent the character traits common to *dégénéré supérieur* and *dégénéré inférieur*. Sadger, *Belastung und Entartung*, p. 9.

51 Zimmermann, *Biographische Anthropologie*, p. 240; Steinberg, '*Als ob ich zu einer steinernen Wand spräche*', pp. 257–63.

52 Peter Rudnytsky, *Reading Psychoanalysis: Freud, Rank, Ferenczi, Groddeck* (Ithaca: Cornell University Press, 2002), p. 59.

53 Louis Rose, *The Freudian Calling: Early Viennese Psychoanalysis and the Pursuit of Cultural Science* (Detroit: Wayne State University Press, 1998), p. 14; Frank J. Sulloway, 'Reassessing Freud's Case Histories. The Social Construction of Psychoanalysis', *Isis*, 82 (1991), pp. 245–75, p. 265.

54 'Die Psychoanalyse hat zwar, von der Pathologie her, den wenig durchschauten Anteil der unbewußten Phantasiebildung grell beleuchtet, vermochte es jedoch in dem an mancherlei Unfaßbarkeiten grenzenden Bereich der Kunst zu vereinzelten Einsichten in den komplizierten Vorgang der dichterischen Produktion zu bringen, die noch zu keiner abschließenden Darstellung gediehen sind.' Otto Rank, 'Das Volksepos. Psychologische Beiträge zu einer Entstehungsgeschichte. II. Die dichterische Phantasiebildung', *Imago*, 5 (1919), pp. 372–93, p. 372.

55 Rose, *The Freudian Calling*, p. 52.

56 Sadger was the first to promote psychoanalysis to a wider medical audience in the prestigious *Centralblatt fuer Nervenheilkunde und Psychiatrie* (*Central Journal for Neurology and Psychiatry*) and his writing of popular scientific articles may well have helped to attract Freud's invitation to join the WPV. See Isidor Sadger, 'Die Bedeutung der psychoanalytischen Methode nach Freud', *Centralblatt für Nervenheilkunde und Psychiatrie*, 30 (1907), pp. 41–52. In the same volume, Sadger also favourably reviewed Rank's *Der Künstler*, published the same year, calling the study 'the shortest, most compendious yet best summary of Freud's teachings'.

57 Ernest Jones claims the book was suggested to Freud by C. G. Jung; Peter Rudnytsky argues that Wilhelm Stekel recommended the novella to Freud. See Ernest Jones, *Sigmund Freud Life and Work, vol. 2: Years of Maturity 1901–1919* (London: Hogarth Press, 1955), p. 382; Rudnytsky, *Reading Psychoanalysis*, p. 2.

58 E. James Lieberman, *Acts of Will: The Life and Work of Otto Rank* (New York: Free Press, 1985), p. 26.

59 Like Freud, Stekel and Sadger had graduated from the renowned Medical Faculty at the University of Vienna (Sadger ten years after Freud, in 1891, Stekel in 1897).

60 Other examples are: Hanns Sachs's talk on 15 February 1911 on the applicability of psychoanalysis to literary works, and Bernhard Dattner on 8 March 1911 on the psychoanalytic problems of Raskolnikov, the main character in Fjodor Dostoevsky's *Crime and Punishment* (1866).

61 'Zusammenhang zwischen den Kindheitseindrücken und Lebensschicksalen des Künstlers und seinen Werken als Reaktionen auf diese Anregungen gehört zu den anziehendsten Objekten der analytischen Betrachtung.' Sigmund Freud, 'Das Interesse der Psychoanalyse für die nicht psychologischen Wissenschaften (1913)', in Sigmund Freud, *Gesammelte Werke, chronologisch geordnet*, ed. Anna Freud, in collaboration with M. Bonaparte, E. Bibring, W. Hoffer, E. Kris and O. Isakower, vol. VIII (London: Imago, 1957), pp. 403–20, p. 416; Sigmund Freud, 'The Claims of Psycho-analysis to Scientific Interest', in *The Standard Edition*

of the Complete Psychological Works of Sigmund Freud, ed. James Strachey, with Anna Freud, Alix Strachey and Alan Tyson, vol. XIII (London: Hogarth Press and Institute for Psychoanalysis, 1955), pp. 163–90, p. 186.

62 C. G. Jung, 'Letter from C. G. Jung to Sigmund Freud, November 2, 1907', in William McGuire (ed), *The Freud/Jung Letters: The Correspondence Between Sigmund Freud and C. G. Jung* (Princeton: Princeton University Press, 1974), pp. 95–6. The stories mentioned comprise Jensen's volume *Übermächte* (1892). Rank later confirmed the importance of sibling relationships in his study of the incest theme in literature and legend. See Otto Rank, *Das Inzest-Motiv in Dichtung und Sage: Grundzüge einer Psychologie des dichterischen Schaffens* (Leipzig: Deuticke, 1912) and, in English, Otto Rank and Gregory C. Richter, *The Incest Theme in Literature and Legend: Fundamentals of a Psychology of Literary Creation* (Baltimore: Johns Hopkins University Press, 1992).

63 Hermann Nunberg and Ernst Federn (eds), *Protokolle der Wiener Psychoanalytischen Vereinigung*, vol. II (Gießen: Psychosozial-Verlag, 2008), pp. 354–6.

64 Fritz Wittels's novel about Kraus was titled *Ezechiel, der Zugereiste* (Berlin: Fleischel, 1910). For details on the Kraus affair see (in alphabetical order): Leo Lensing, '"Freud and the Child Woman" or "The Kraus Affair"? A Textual "Reconstruction" of Fritz Wittels's Psychoanalytic Autobiography', *German Quarterly*, 69 (1996), pp. 322–32; Margarete Mitscherlich-Nielsen, 'Sittlichkeit und Kriminalität. Psychoanalytische Bemerkungen zu Karl Kraus', *Psyche*, 29:2 (1975), pp. 131–53; Lutz D. H. Sauerteig, 'Loss of Innocence: Albert Moll, Sigmund Freud and the Invention of Childhood Sexuality Around 1900', *Medical History*, 56:2 (2012), pp. 156–83; Edward Timms (ed.), *Freud and the Child Woman: The Memoirs of Fritz Wittels* (New Haven: Yale University Press, 1995); Edward Timms, 'The "Child–Woman": Kraus, Freud, Wittels, and Irma Karczewska in Fin-de-Siécle Vienna', in Edward Timms and Ritchie Robertson (eds), *Vienna 1900: From Altenberg to Wittgenstein* (Edinburgh: Edinburgh University Press, 1990), pp. 87–107; Harry Zohn, *Karl Kraus and the Critics* (Columbia: Camden House, 1997).

65 Nunberg and Federn (eds), *Protokolle*, vol. I, p. 62.

66 Katja Guenther, *Localization and Its Discontents: A Genealogy of Psychoanalysis and the Neuro Disciplines* (Chicago: University of Chicago Press, 2015), pp. 84–5.

67 Nunberg and Federn (eds), *Protokolle*, vol. I, p. 65.

68 Nunberg and Federn (eds), *Protokolle*, vol. II, p. 203.

69 See, for example, Michael Rohrwasser, *Freuds Lektüren. Von Arthur Conan Doyle bis zu Arthur Schnitzler* (Gießen: Psychosozial-Verlag, 2005).

70 Nunberg and Federn (eds), *Protokolle*, vol. I, p. 249.

71 Nunberg and Federn (eds), *Protokolle*, vol. I, p. 249; vol. II, p. 252.

72 Nunberg and Federn (eds), *Protokolle*, vol. II, p. 201. In 1907 Wilhelm Stekel and Ernst Federn had reacted aggressively enough to Sadger's elaborations on Conrad Ferdinand Meyer that Fritz Wittels felt the need to distance himself from their emotional reaction. Nunberg and Federn (eds), *Protokolle*, vol. I, p. 249.

73 'Die Theorien können nur Schaden leiden, und für den Gegenstand schaut dabei nichts heraus.' Nunberg and Federn (eds), *Protokolle*, vol. I, p. 250.

74 Nunberg and Federn (eds), *Protokolle*, vol. I, pp. 172–8, 240–4, 249–53; vol. II, pp. 198–204.

75 'Die rein medizinische Analyse, die Pathographie, trägt zur Erkenntnis des dichterischen Prozesses deshalb wenig bei, weil sie sich nur mit jenen Hemmungen beschäftigt, nicht mit den positive dichterischen Kräften.' Nunberg and Federn (eds), *Protokolle*, vol. I, p. 249.

76 The German original reads: 'Um nachzuweisen, dass jeder Mensch diese typischen Fundamentalregungen habe, sind uns die Dichter zu gut.' Nunberg and Federn (eds), *Protokolle*, vol. II, p. 202.

77 For example Nunberg and Federn (eds), *Protokolle*, vol. I, p. 243.

78 'Aus den Werken lasse sich nichts mit Sicherheit konstatieren, was der Dichter Reales erlebte, weil nichts das Reale vom Illusionierten unterscheide; man wisse nicht, wo die Wahrheit aufhöre und die Dichtung beginne. Der Weg aus den Werken sei also sehr unverläßlich.' Nunberg and Federn (eds), *Protokolle*, vol. I, p. 243.

79 Nunberg and Federn (eds), *Protokolle*, vol. I, pp. 246–7.

80 Nunberg and Federn (eds), *Protokolle*, vol. II, pp. 200–2. Rudolf Reitler had already raised the issue of evidence in the context of Sadger's Meyer pathography. See Nunberg and Federn (eds), *Protokolle*, vol. I, p. 174.

81 Rahmer, *August Strindberg*; Sigismund Rahmer, *Nikolaus Lenau als Mensch und Dichter. Ein Beitrag zur Sexualpathologie* (Berlin: Curtius, 1911).

82 Nunberg and Federn (eds), *Protokolle*, vol. I, p. 240.

83 McGuire, *The Freud/Jung Letters*, pp. 17–19. As McGuire also states, Löwenfeld published Freud's monograph *Über den Traum* in 1901 in the series 'Grenzfragen des Nerven- und Seelenlebens', and included contributions by Freud in two other books: 'Freud's Psycho-analytic Procedure' in *Die psychischen Zwangserscheinungen* (1904); and 'My Views on the Part Played by Sexuality in the Aetiology of the Neuroses' in the fourth edition of *Sexualleben und Nervenleiden* (1906).

84 C. G. Jung, 'Besprechung von Sadger *Konrad Ferdinand Meyer. Eine pathographisch-psychologische Studie.* Das symbolische Leben. Verschiedene Schriften', in C. G. Jung, *Gesammelte Werke*, vol. XVIII (Stuttgart: Patmos, 2011), pp. 795–6, p. 795. The text was originally published in 1909, and reads: 'Sadger bestrebt sich vielmehr, die Entwicklung der ganzen Persönlichkeit psychologisch zu erfassen, das heißt wirklich innerlich zu verstehen'. Oskar Pfister, *The Psychoanalytic Method*, trans. Charles Rockwell Payne (Milton Park: Routledge, 1999 [German original 1913]), p. 117.

85 Sigmund Freud, 'Eine Kindheitserinnerung des Leonardo da Vinci', in *Gesammelte Werke*, vol. VIII, pp. 128–211; Sigmund Freud, 'Leonardo Da Vinci and a Memory of His Childhood', in *The Standard Edition of the Complete Psychological Works of Sigmund Freud*, vol. XI, pp. 57–138; Sigmund Freud, 'Das Motiv der Kästchenwahl', in *Gesammelte Werke*, vol. X, pp. 24–37; Sigmund Freud, 'The Theme of the Three Caskets', in *The Standard Edition of the Complete Psychological Works of Sigmund Freud*, vol. XII, pp. 289–302; Sigmund Freud, 'Der Moses des Michelangelo', in *Gesammelte Werke*, vol. X, pp. 172–201; Sigmund Freud, 'The Moses of Michelangelo', in *The Standard Edition of the Complete Psychological Works of Sigmund Freud*, vol. XIII, pp. 209–38.

86 Rohrwasser, *Freuds Lektüren*, pp. 225–7.

87 '[U]ns mit [ihren Werken] so zu ergreifen, Erregungen in uns hervorzurufen, deren wir uns vielleicht nicht einmal für fähig gehalten hätten.' Sigmund Freud, 'Der Dichter und das Phantasieren', in *Gesammelte Werke*, vol. VII, pp. 213–23, p. 223; Sigmund Freud, 'Creative Writers and Day-Dreaming', in *The Standard Edition of the Complete Psychological Works of Sigmund Freud*, vol. IX, pp. 141–54, p. 153.

88 Freud, 'Der Dichter und das Phantasieren', p. 223; Freud, 'Creative Writers and Day-Dreaming', p. 153.

89 Freud, 'Der Dichter und das Phantasieren', p. 213, translated here by Birgit Lang. Strachey's translation reads 'their kind and the common run of humanity'. Freud, 'Creative Writers and Day-Dreaming', p. 141.

90 '[E]in Normalmensch und das Maß der Menschheit.' Sigmund Freud, 'Der Wahn und die Träume in W. Jensens "Gradiva"', in *Gesammelte Werke*, vol. VII, pp. 31–122, p. 72. The English translation given here is by Birgit Lang, since Strachey translates too decisively 'for we readers are the normal people and the standard of humanity'. Sigmund Freud, 'Delusions and Dreams in Jensen's "Gradiva"', *The Standard Edition of the Complete Psychological Works of Sigmund Freud*, vol. IX, pp. 1–96, p. 44.

91 Nunberg and Federn (eds), *Protokolle*, vol. I, p. 249; vol. II, p. 176.

92 Jones, *Sigmund Freud, vol. II: Years of Maturity*, p. 381.

93 Freud, 'Der Wahn und die Träume', p. 73; Freud, 'Delusions and Dreams in Jensen's "Gradiva"', p. 46.

94 'Aber Menschenbilder können sich nicht wiederholen, es fehlt auch nicht an tiefgehenden Unterschieden zwischen den beiden Großen.' Sigmund Freud, 'Brief an Dr. Alfons Paquet', in *Gesammelte Werke*, vol. XIV, pp. 545–50, p. 547; Sigmund Freud, 'The Goethe Prize', in *The Standard Edition of the Complete Psychological Works of Sigmund Freud*, vol. XXI, pp. 205–14, p. 208.

95 Freud, 'Der Wahn und die Träume', p. 69; Freud, 'Delusions and Dreams in Jensen's "Gradiva"', p. 42.

96 Gert Üding and Bernd Steinbrink, *Grundriss der Rhetorik. Geschichte – Technik – Methode* (Stuttgart: Metzler, 2011), pp. 268–9.

97 Another example is Freud's essay 'Der Dichter und das Phantasieren', where he closes with an apology for not having resolved the original question.

98 Freud, 'Brief an Dr. Alfons Paquet', p. 550; Freud, 'The Goethe Prize', p. 211.

99 Nunberg and Federn (eds), *Protokolle*, vol. II, p. 201.

100 '[E]in Gebiet, auf dem die Allmachtbestrebungen der primitiven Menschheit gleichsam in Kraft verblieben sind.' Freud, 'Das Interesse der Psychoanalyse für die nicht psychologischen Wissenschaften', p. 417; Freud, 'The Claims of Psycho-analysis to Scientific Interest', p. 187.

101 'Wir schöpfen wahrscheinlich aus der gleichen Quelle, bearbeiten das nämliche Objekt, ein jeder von uns mit einer anderen Methode, und die Übereinstimmung im Ergebnis scheint dafür zu bürgen, daß beide richtig gearbeitet haben. Unser Verfahren besteht in der bewußten Beobachtung der abnormen seelischen Vorgänge bei anderen, um deren Gesetze erraten und aussprechen zu können. Der Dichter geht wohl anders vor; er richtet seine Aufmerksamkeit auf das Unbewußte in seiner eigenen Seele, lauscht den Entwicklungsmöglichkeiten desselben und gestattet ihnen den künstlerischen Ausdruck, anstatt sie mit bewußter Kritik zu unterdrücken. So erfährt er aus sich, was wir bei anderen erlernen, welchen Gesetzen die Betätigung dieses Unbewußten folgen muß, aber er braucht diese Gesetze nicht auszusprechen, nicht einmal sie klar zu erkennen, sie sind infolge der Duldung seiner Intelligenz in seinen Schöpfungen verkörpert enthalten. Wir entwickeln diese Gesetze durch Analyse aus seinen Dichtungen, wie wir sie aus den Fällen realer Erkrankung herausfinden, aber der Schluß scheint unabweisbar, entweder haben beide, der Dichter wie der Arzt, das Unbewußte in gleicher Weise mißverstanden, oder wir haben es beide richtig verstanden.' Freud, 'Der Wahn und die Träume', pp. 120–1; Freud, 'Delusions and Dreams in Jensen's "Gradiva"', p. 91.

102 Sulloway, 'Reassessing Freud's Case Histories', pp. 265–6; Marina Leitner, *Ein gut gehütetes Geheimnis. Die Geschichte der psychoanalytischen Behandlungs-Technik von den Anfängen in Wien bis zur Gründung der Berliner Poliklinik im Jahr 1920* (Gießen: Psychosozial-Verlag, 2001), p. 13–19; David J. Lynn and George E. Vaillant, 'Anonymity, Neutrality, and Confidentiality in the Actual Methods of Sigmund Freud: A Review of 43 Cases, 1907–1939', *American Journal of Psychiatry*, 155:2 (1998), pp. 163–71, pp. 169–70; Anne Sealey, 'The Strange Case of the Freudian Case History. The Role of Long Case Histories in the Development of Psychoanalysis', *History of the Human Sciences*, 24:1 (2011), pp. 36–50, p. 37.

103 Freud, 'Delusions and Dreams in Jensen's "Gradiva"', p. 32.

104 The Otto Rank Papers held in the Rare Book & Manuscript Library at Columbia University in New York City date the fragments of the relevant manuscripts to 1906. Judging from a footnote in the 1912 study, Rank still planned to publish this work. Rank, *Das Inzest-Motiv*, p. 31.

105 James M. Ford, *Patriarchy and Incest from Shakespeare to Joyce* (Gainesville: University Press of Florida, 1998), p. 2; see also Rudnytsky, *Reading Psychoanalysis*, pp. 58–85.

106 Sigmund Freud, 'On the History of the Psycho-Analytic Movement', *The Standard*

Edition of the Complete Psychological Works of Sigmund Freud, vol. XIV, pp. 1–66, p. 36. These remarks are also proof of the close collaboration between Freud and Rank at this point, also reflected in the fact that *The Interpretation of Dreams* contained, from its fourth to its seventh editions (1914–22), two essays by Rank: 'Dreams and Creative Writing' and 'Dreams and Myths'. These were printed at the end of Chapter 6, but were subsequently omitted. See also the relevant remark by James Strachey in Sigmund Freud, 'The Interpretation of Dreams', *The Standard Edition of the Complete Psychological Works of Sigmund Freud*, vol. IV, pp. ix–627, p. xii. On the relationship between Freud and Rank see Marina Leitner, *Freud, Rank und die Folgen. Ein Schlüsselbegriff für die Psychoanalyse* (Vienna: Turia & Kant, 1998); Lieberman, *Acts of Will*; E. James Lieberman and Robert Kramer (eds), *The Letters of Sigmund Freud and Otto Rank. Inside Psychoanalysis* (Baltimore: Johns Hopkins University Press, 2011); Esther Menaker, *Otto Rank: A Rediscovered Legacy* (New York: Columbia University Press, 1982); Peter Rudnytsky, *The Psychoanalytic Vocation: The Legacy of Otto Rank and Donald Winnicott* (New Haven: Yale University Press, 1991); Rudnytsky, *Reading Psychoanalysis*, pp. 58–85; Jessie Taft, *Otto Rank* (New York: Julian, 1958); Anton Zottl, *Otto Rank: Das Lebenswerk eines Dissidenten der Psychoanalyse* (Munich: Kindler, 1982).

107 Rank, *Das Inzest-Motiv in Dichtung und Sage*, p. 3.

108 'Inhalt [ist] der größten Unliebsamkeit sicher.' Sigmund Freud, 'Zur Geschichte der psycho-analytischen Bewegung', in *Gesammelte Werke*, vol. X, pp. 44–113, p. 77; Freud, 'On the History of the Psycho-Analytic Movement', p. 36.

109 Möbius, *J.-J. Rousseau's Krankheitsgeschichte*, p. v.

110 Pathography in this context does not mean a description of a personal experience of illness – as Anne Hunsaker Hawkins defines the genre – but a specific medical and psychiatric expert case study that mapped signs of degeneration to the artistic mind. See Hawkins, *Reconstructing Illness*, p. 1.

3

'Writing back': literary satire and Oskar Panizza's *Psichopatia criminalis* (1898)

Birgit Lang

Oskar Panizza's *Psichopatia criminalis* (1898) constitutes the most biting parody of the psychiatric case study genre in German literature, and has been praised as a subversive work in the broader context of the anti-psychiatry movement of the 1960s and 1970s.[1] As a former psychiatrist who had been designated for priesthood and later prosecuted in court for blasphemy, Panizza (1853–1921) had intimate knowledge of 'the three great professions of the Western tradition – law, medicine, and theology – [that] developed practices centred on cases'.[2] *Psichopatia criminalis* for the first time and in literary form problematised the overlapping of legal and medical discourse, as well as the interdisciplinary nature of forensics. A short work, *Psichopatia criminalis* echoes the deterministic reasoning that characterised the psychiatric discourse about creative artists explored in Chapter 2. Panizza's text is of satirical and even dystopian character. A site of casuistric mastery, it is also the site of the first appearance of Panizza's doppelgänger, the German Emperor, who became the central figure in the author's increasingly delusional system of thought. The intrinsic element of judgement that is inherit to the case study genre suited both of these 'objectives' well.

For a range of reasons *Psichopatia criminalis* has remained deeply uncomfortable for readers from the very beginning. As this chapter explores, the text has found varying and disparate reading publics. German playwright Heiner Müller (1929–95) affirmatively claimed Panizza as a textual terrorist, and over time various audiences have felt drawn to the theme of political repression in *Psichopatia criminalis*, without necessarily being able to reflect on the link between their attraction and Panizza's perceived victimisation. For other readers, Panizza's late literary oeuvre in particular seems tainted by the fact that the eccentric writer was committed to a mental asylum, never to leave the confines of the asylum again. These readers remain haunted by Panizza's psychotic illness, which seems to call into question his literary abilities. Literary scholar Michael

Bauer remarks that *Psichopatia criminalis* does not always succeed in 'remain[ing] within the boundaries of satire, and sometimes descends to a direct polemic against the politics of its addresses'.[3]

The following analysis agrees with Bauer's assertion that *Psichopatia criminalis* pushes the workings of satire to its dystopian limits and questions the comprehensibility of intent in *Psichopatia criminalis* from the reader's point of view. It considers whether Panizza's *Psichopatia criminalis* was indeed conceptualised as a satire and, as such, whether the work helped its author and readers to release aggression against authorities – or whether the work reinforced Panizza's system of delusion and contributed to his demise. Again, if Panizza's text was also an expression of a self-destructive will, readers are left to question their attraction to Panizza's writings in the first place, and to ask how their acts of reading and interpretation deflect and become complicit in Panizza's enterprise. The present chapter aims to unravel these complex issues of authorial and readerly intent; of agency and ethics; of the role of the case study genre in this context, with its generic tendency to point towards one truth and to contain an intrinsic element of judgement.

Psichopatia criminalis

Throughout the twentieth century, *Psichopatia criminalis* received continuous attention from German intellectuals. To date, however, literary and historical scholars have devoted only a few fleeting remarks to Panizza's forty-eight-page work.[4] This satire of the German state sees Panizza purportedly diagnosing a new psychiatric disorder, the eponymous 'psichopatia criminalis'. He proceeds to suggest that the authorities should commit all sufferers (by which he means all dissidents) to a mental asylum and thus restore order in the German state once and for all. This chapter represents the first sustained analysis of *Psichopatia criminalis*, rereading the work through the lens of genre, and with an awareness of the workings of satire. More specifically, it examines how this provocative text continually echoes the case study genre, and the medical case study compilation in particular, while also entailing a bitter polemic against members of the Munich psychiatric scene.

By definition, satire refers to the very genre it satirises; the self-reflexive nature of parodic expression is characterised by 'repetition with critical distance'.[5] It stands to reason that traditions of medical case writing can be reflected in satirical ways. In his bold game of make-believe, Panizza presents the reader with a work that closely imitates the generic characteristics of the psychiatric case study compilation in the manner of Richard von Krafft-Ebing. Accordingly, *Psichopatia criminalis* consists of a short preface and introduction that establish a framing narrative, followed by four 'diagnostic chapters' on the phenomena of: softening of the brain; mania; melancholy; and paranoia. In turn, these are followed by five sets of case notes about intellectuals afflicted with the frightful condition. The threefold structure of *Psichopatia criminalis* is a most peculiar form that contributes both to the satirical character of the work and to its subversion. Preface and introduction establish the framework of reference and entail a hefty satire against members of the Munich psychiatric scene; the four main chapters constitute Panizza's 'psychiatric' examination of the German state, while the case vignettes present the reader with an anti-utopian genealogy of oppositional and persecuted pre-socialist thinkers.

In short, this chapter answers the question: was *Psichopatia criminalis* a satire? It does so with reference to writings on parody by scholars such as Linda Hutcheon and discourse analyst Paul Simpson. The latter argues that for a text to function as satire, a prime element (or 'discoursal prime') serves as an echoic frame which draws intersemiotically on 'real discourses'.[6] Panizza's direct reference to the psychiatric case study compilation is easily identified as such a 'real discourse'. As per Simpson's schema, this prime element needs to be supplemented by a text-internal device called a dialectic, which forms the antithesis to the prime, and 'induces a collision of ideas or appeals to a line of reasoning that falls outside the straightforward'. Panizza does this by exaggerating the German state's supposed willingness to prescribe psychiatric treatment for all citizens ever guilty of a dissident thought. This second step is followed by a satirical uptake that places the reader on a 'satirical footing' and requires 'a special configuration of the three principal claims of sincerity, appropriateness and truth' – categories Simpson borrows from German philosopher Jürgen Habermas.[7] In this context, the dystopian and oxymoronic character of Panizza's work becomes obvious.

Panizza's choice of the psychiatric case study compilation as a prime can be traced back to the intimate knowledge he had of this case modality, as a former psychiatrist. Already the choice of title expresses his intention to problematise the forensic imbrication of legal and medical discourse. '*Psichopatia criminalis*' – in Panizza's phonetic spelling – obviously references Krafft-Ebing's influential *Psychopathia Sexualis* (1886), as well as the groundbreaking *Kriminalpsychologie* (*Criminal Psychology*, 1898) by Hans Gross (1847–1915), although the latter did not contain any case studies. Panizza's detailed knowledge of the field of psychiatry and its practices, as well as his critical stance towards his former colleagues, function to characterise him as an expert. In the Preface to *Psichopatia criminalis*, Panizza shows himself to be very familiar with the names and works of present and past psychiatric experts when he mentions German psychiatrist Heinrich Schüle (1840–1916) and influential French psychiatrist Valentin Magnan (1835–1916), a prominent representative of degeneration theory.[8] Panizza knew many such men well, whether as former fellow students or as colleagues. He had studied medicine in Munich and in the same city he had begun an estimable medical career as a psychiatrist, starting out as an assistant doctor for prominent

Munich-based psychiatrist Bernhard von Gudden (1824–86), who was formerly a director of the Zurich Burghölzli clinic (1870–72) and then of the Oberbayrische Kreisirrenanstalt (1872–86).[9] Gudden died in 1886, under mysterious circumstances: shortly after being appointed personal physician to Bavaria's King Ludwig II, and declaring the latter mentally incompetent to rule, both Gudden and the King were found dead in Lake Starhemberg; it is possible that Gudden was drowned by Ludwig II.[10] In a bitter twist of fate, just a few years after the publication of *Psichopatia criminalis*, Gudden's son was responsible for judging the state of Panizza's deteriorating mental health.

From the opening of *Psichopatia criminalis*, Panizza creates the dialectic in his framing narrative by representing the voice of the first-person narrator as that of the chief psychiatrist for the German nation. This practitioner holds the view that German revolutionaries should be incarcerated and undergo psychiatric treatment as a new way to prevent civil unrest. Panizza describes the narrator's fictitious psychiatric clinic as a 'moderately sized mental asylum built between the rivers Nekar [*sic*] and Rhine, the size of a palatinate and on the grounds of Rhineland-Palatineon, the very ground on which have flourished the most tumultuous intellects'.[11] This asylum can be identified by means of geographical proximity as Illenau, the model German mental hospital founded in 1842, at which Krafft-Ebing, Schüle and Panizza's former employer Gudden had worked. The Illenau clinic was defined by a humanitarian outlook, yet its clinicians were proponents of degeneration theory.

In *Psichopatia criminalis* Panizza evokes the humanitarian psychiatric language of his contemporaries, and then slowly undermines it over the course of his intellectual game. He comments that 'the principle of humanity … is at the fore in our generally upset times', and elaborates:

> The lenient treatment, fully tempered baths, the quiet, the remoteness, the song of the nightingale beyond the bars, the physician's benevolent words of comfort – a little bit of hyoscamine and potassium bromide – and the political insight of all these internees would have grown considerably.[12]

The idyllic picture is further underlined through an auditory evocation, the song of the nightingale, a symbol of paradise in European literature, which, however, draws attention to the patients' situation of confinement. The reader questions the psychiatrists' compassion, particularly on reading about their prescription of hyoscamine and potassium bromide. These sedatives produced considerable side-effects – they were used in very high dosage, due to the limited pharmaceutical means of intervention available at the time. Hyoscamine is a belladonna derivative and was widely used to treat schizophrenia; Krafft-Ebing suggested it was temporarily highly effective for 'motorically highly agitated patients and such, who soil themselves on purpose or are destructive'.[13] Potassium bromide was used for sedation and to treat epilepsy. Its poisonous side-effects were well known and included excessive sedation, migraines, memory loss, hallucinations, as well as mucous hypersecretion of the lungs (called *Bromschnupfen*) and acne. Krafft-Ebing writes about the abatement of bromide poisoning in several of his case studies, which indicates the medical profession's awareness of such side-effects, as well as their justification as a 'necessary evil'.[14]

At this point in the text Panizza reiterates the ostensible addressees of his volume, that is, fellow psychiatrists, although the subtitle of *Psichopatia criminalis* also mentions physicians, laypersons, jurists, legal guardians, administrators and ministers – *Anleitung um die vom Gericht für notwendig erkanten Geisteskrankheiten psichjatrisch zu eruiren und wissenschaftlich festzustellen; für Ärzte, Laien, Juristen, Vormünder, Verwaltungsbeamte, Minister etc.* Panizza seemingly softens his tone and acknowledges that 'some attentive readers, especially those belonging to the psychiatric profession, might interject that what is stated here is history, political history, literary history, reformation history, but not actually psychiatric casuistry, and not a discussion of psychopathologies'.[15] To make his point, Panizza takes as an example the first German psychiatric textbook, a work published by Rudolf Arndt in 1883. With irony Panizza adds in a footnote that this book 'has not been appreciated enough by far, and can still be purchased in its first edition'.[16] Panizza argues that Arndt

> divided human cultural history and the history of ideas into hyper- and paraesthesias [overt sensitivity to stimuli of the senses and the skin], and in this way included in his wonderful textbook the complete historical development of the Christian West, all revolutions and Schiller's *The Robbers*, all political contracts and Metternich, with the exception of rulers and princes.[17]

Indeed, like other psychiatrists of this era whose theories were heavily grounded in biological reasoning, Arndt also referenced writers and other 'greats' of intellectual history. And like the psychiatrists investigated in Chapters 1 and 2 of the present volume, Arndt used biographies of important figures in German intellectual history to illustrate certain phenomena. For instance, he referenced Martin Luther's vision of the devil on the Wartburg to illustrate the phenomenon of hallucination.[18] Yet Arndt had recourse to this strategy in only a handful of instances. Highlighted by Panizza, the terms 'hyperaesthesia' and 'paraesthesia' appear just once in Arndt's textbook of over 600 pages, namely in his two-page discussion of genius. Here Arndt summarises relatively commonplace medical and popular notions of 'genius' and outlines that highly gifted individuals suffer from 'all sorts of pathological conditions, with peculiarities, idiosyncrasies and even perversions'.[19] In this context, Arndt provides a long list of names of 'great minds' who contributed to society through their ideas but died 'psychologically clouded and broken'.[20]

In *Psichopatia criminalis*, Panizza shifts Arndt's meaning for his own satirical purposes, by misquoting Arndt and by slipping text fragments into his account of the disregarded psychiatrist. A reference to Luther now becomes the alliterative 'Luther or Lafayette, Lincoln or Lucian', and the inflated corresponding claims relating to these names wrongly attest the psychiatric pathologisation of the Reformation, the utilisation of steam, the concept of 'human rights' and sheep shearing. This exaggerating literary technique presents Arndt's work as nonsensical. The same holds true for Arndt's alleged denouncement all of human cultural and intellectual history.

Thus Panizza attacks the first German psychiatric textbook and also his former Munich teachers and colleagues. By explicitly referencing what he calls 'older psychiatric textbooks [... by] Arndt, Krafft-Ebing, Schüle, Griesinger, Esquirol, Gudden, Kräpelin, Ganser und Bumm', he discredits as outdated the relevance of a range of contemporary psychiatrists.[21] This holds particularly true for representatives of the Illenau school as well as Panizza's contemporaries in Munich: Sigbert Ganser (1853–1931), assistant psychiatrist to Gudden between 1877 and 1884; Munich professor of psychiatry Anton Bumm (1849–1903), appointed head of the Munich mental asylum (Kreisirrenanstalt) in 1897; and, most importantly, Emil Kraepelin (1856–1926), who became the pre-eminent psychiatrist in Munich, and in whose defence Paul Julius Möbius wrote his modern pathographies a few years after the publication of *Psichopatia criminalis*. In later years Kraepelin turned the critique around: in his lectures and textbooks he presented the case of Panizza – made anonymous – as an example of paraphrenia, or the organised system of paranoid delusions.[22]

After establishing an 'anti-psychiatrist' framework, Panizza presents the four symptoms of 'psichopatia criminalis' and expands his satire from the realm of the clinic to include that of the German state. As mentioned, the four antiquated diagnostic concepts that Panizza invokes in his satire are: softening of the brain; mania; melancholy; and paranoia. There is no reference to recent progress within psychiatric thinking, there is no acknowledgement of Krafft-Ebing's new intellectual adventures in the world of sexual perversion, nor of the explorations of hysteria undertaken respectively by Ganser, Sigmund Freud and Josef Breuer. The dialectic in *Psichopatia criminalis* is the exaggeration that any thought directed against authority both undermines the order of the German state and constitutes the symptom of a psychiatric illness that requires institutionalisation. Ultimately, of course, this implies that all human beings need to be committed to a mental asylum.[23]

Panizza's technique of negation is repeated in the main text of *Psichopatia criminalis*. 'Softening of the brain' queries how human beings come to have dissident thoughts. Panizza scoffs delightedly at the infectious and hereditary nature of dissident ideas. With satirical intent he states how many political opponents of 'the powers that be' come from 'inverted-democratic' families and can be found to have a history of opposition to politico-religious authority. They include: descendants of 'Salzburger Émigrés' (the protestant refugees who were expelled from Salzburg by decree in 1731); Anabaptists of the sixteenth-century Radical Reformation; and Huguenots, the members of the Protestant Reformed Church of France, many of whom established themselves in Germany in the late seventeenth century (among them the family of Panizza's mother). 'Mania' explores the 'silent rage, the secret and calm conspiracy, the inner insolent thoughts that characterise such [manic] people'.[24] Panizza explores these anti-governmental attitudes in a language characterised by oral imagery, in which German burghers are literally sick of their state (the German *den Staat gefressen haben* literally means 'to have gorged on the state'). Although they do not necessarily speak, Panizza suggests that their every thought needs to be presided over. After this vision of absolute control, 'melancholy' turns to the temporality of power and dissidence, with a particular emphasis on the failed revolutions of 1848. Panizza declares the longing for different political conditions as a German illness, and skilfully uses the distorted notion of time that characterises melancholia to criticise contemporary political discourses of legitimacy. He ironically classifies the revolutionary folk song of 1848 'Fürsten zum Land hinaus' ('Out With the Princes') as 'asylum poetry as recently defined by Lombroso'; indeed, a third of the study *The Man of Genius* (1891) by the Italian criminal anthropologist was devoted to the creative production of the mentally ill in the asylum.[25] In the section of *Psichopatia criminalis* devoted to 'paranoia', Panizza argues that 'we stand at the pinnacle of humanity' because the accused are not treated as criminals but suffer from 'psichopatia criminalis'.[26] This statement can be considered of utmost polemical importance, since it questions the humanitarian nature of the insanity defence, and with it the reason for the existence of the interdisciplinary field of forensics in the first place.

Another important parallel to the medical case study compilation is the use of casuistry in *Psichopatia criminalis*. Panizza uses this feature to create a genealogy of oppositional pre-socialist thinkers, thus inserting a more overtly political dimension. He names Roman senator and land reformer Tiberius Sempronius Gracchus (*circa* 169–33 BC); German poet Christian Friedrich Daniel Schubart (1739–91); utopian socialist Wilhelm Weitling (1808–71); German democratic politician Robert Blum (1807–48); and the early nihilistic German philosopher Max Stirner (1806–56).[27] These case vignettes are described by the narrator in a clinical and unsympathetic manner that classifies the subjects' sense of injustice and rebellious behaviour as signs of the eponymous psychiatric illness. Panizza ends his treatise with an appeal to all rulers of Europe, warning them of the impending mass epidemic of dissident thought. Similar to Krafft-Ebing's case compilations, Panizza's biographical case vignettes become a place within the larger work where readers can much more easily identify with the subject and narrative mode, as an analysis of the reception of *Psichopatia criminalis* reveals.

A dystopian satire and its reception

For a satire to be successful, Simpson contends, it needs to be comprehensible, and eventually suspend its truth, retract the claim of appropriateness and rescind the underlying claim of sincerity. *Psichopatia criminalis* challenges its readers in two respects: firstly, through the choice of the psychiatric case compilation as the satirical prime; and secondly, through its refusal to suspend the truth or rescind its sincerity.

From Simpson's standpoint, the role of the prime in satire is to provide an echoic frame which draws intersemiotically on 'real discourses', and is interpreted through a frame of general knowledge.[28] Yet the psychiatric case compilation was a very specific genre to choose for such a frame, conventionally written for and best understood at this period only by members of the medical profession. Lay people engaged with this genre when motivated by palpable interest – such as readers who self-identified as masochists – and often in an eclectic manner. Yet when compared with other contemporary attempts at anti-psychiatric satire, *Psichopatia criminalis* was the only work to satirise such an expert case modality. To the former psychiatrist Panizza, however, this choice made complete sense from a personal perspective, and from the perspectives of familiarity and authorial mastery. For the reader who did not share Panizza's erudition, his choice led to a limited comprehension and appreciation of the text. This is set forth in a review of *Psichopatia criminalis* from 1895, by an unnamed but sympathetic reviewer who writes in a journal targeted at socialist academics: 'yet the reader has to do a lot. Already the complex knowledge and the rare German words require the reader to play an active role; a Panizza encyclopaedia is asked for'.[29] Even so, for this socialist-leaning reviewer, such frustrations were presumably buffered by the chapters, with their clearly satirical description of symptomatology, and by the case notes, with their focus on dissident thinkers.

The second point of contention with regard to the question of whether *Psichopatia criminalis* is indeed a satire concerns a more fundamental aspect of the genre. Panizza's volume projects its truthfulness to the reader through the skilful recreation of psychiatric discourse, which involves the narrator taking the position of chief psychiatrist of the German nation state. Yet the satirical model is pushed to its limits, since *Psichopatia criminalis* never suspends the truth or rescinds its sincerity. Hence the work allows its readers no relief from its claustrophobic imagery. Furthermore, the continuous negation that characterises Panizza's writing pushes the text 'more into line with the various "straight" [psychiatric] anteriors', creating a dystopian anti-truth rather than a suspension of truth.[30] Readers come to occupy an uncomfortable position: they are refused the pleasure of relief from aggression, and here not even the genealogy of oppositional persecuted pre-socialist thinkers contains much relief, since the dissidents are described in a clinical manner and all suffer a pitiful fate. Readers find themselves, in other words, trapped in a negative utopia; if they are brought to laugh, they laugh on the other side of their faces.

The particular nature of Panizza's text raises questions around whether and how this work can be, and has been, adequately understood. The reception of Panizza's oeuvre has always been controversial, dominated by the clichés 'martyr' and 'madman'. These terms implicitly describe the two most important identifiable audiences for his works: a socialist, left-leaning, 'revolutionary' readership that empathised with Panizza on the basis of his anti-authoritarian sentiment, the discussion of pre-socialist thinkers and his persecution by the German state and psychiatry; a liberal discourse that was sympathetic towards Panizza but also re-evaluated his oeuvre on the basis of his biography and his mental health. These publics tended to relate to *Psichopatia criminalis* in quite different ways, the former identifying it as a satire, the latter often bypassing its significance in Panizza's oeuvre – presumably because of the struggle to combine Panizza's radical decline in mental health towards the end of his literary career with the notion of satire as a genre that requires intent.[31]

According to Robert Phiddian, the success of satire is always dependent on a consenting audience which has a vested interest in seeing its own opinions reflected.[32] By intellectuals of the left, Panizza the political 'martyr' was seen as mercilessly persecuted by state authorities after the publication of his church drama *Das Liebeskonzil*; after all, the persecution resulted in Panizza's incarceration in Amberg prison during 1895–96.[33] Creating an instant literary scandal, this court conviction attracted comments from prominent German writers such as Theodor Fontane, Thomas Mann and, later, Kurt Tucholsky.[34] After the Second World War, a critical leftist public dubbed Panizza the greatest German satirist since Luther.[35] Panizza's unremitting resistance to excessive persecution by state authorities led playwright Heiner Müller to affirm the earlier writer as a 'terrorist: those who do not want to become German should read him'.[36] For Müller, Panizza's fate represented no less than 'the misfortune of the prophet who prognosticated too early'; he sees Panizza as a victim of German unification, rejected by the German state, and an enemy of the state 'in the tradition of the counterculture of half-mad heretics'.[37] Dramaturg and film-maker Knut Boeser, in his carefully arranged collection of documents concerning Panizza's imprisonment, underlines the strict morality of the late Wilhelmine era as a factor in Panizza's demise, and compares Panizza's case with that of twentieth-century British Indian writer Salman Rushdie.[38] Indeed, from 1895 onwards Panizza's main works underwent various forms of censorship imposed by the German authorities during the Wilhelmine period and beyond, and by Panizza's family. Active steps were taken to suppress the ongoing circulation of his works and, as a consequence, his historical sacrilegious play *Das Liebeskonzil* (1894) was first produced in Paris only in 1969.

Throughout the twentieth century, reviewers observed the ideological, individualist and socialist underpinnings of Panizza's work, reading him in a manner similar to that in which Krafft-Ebing's readers read *Psychopathia Sexualis* – that is, highly selectively. Thus Fritz Brügel, socialist writer and later Czech post-war ambassador to Berlin, underlined Panizza's reputation as a satirist, noting in 1926 that *Psichopatia criminalis* represented a 'political satire about the persecution mania of German state prosecutors'. Brügel went so far as to claim that the authorities suspected Panizza of socialist leanings (other members of the same literary circle in which Panizza moved suffered this fate); he even argued – wrongly – that Panizza had been sacked from his post as a psychiatrist for this reason.[39] For Tucholsky, 'the unhappy Panizza stood out by far among Munich writers', since their political will – which was supposedly typical for the period – was too narrow, and failed to establish a 'connection with the working social democracy, which could have intellectually stimulated these writers, and rather subsided into a middle-class bohemia'.[40] This view of Panizza was rekindled by the German political left throughout the twentieth century, which considered Panizza a political forebear.

While the Weimar critics focused on Panizza's attempt to create a genealogy of German dissidents, from the 1960s onwards, and due to anti-psychiatric leanings, the new left was able to embrace Panizza's conflation of psychiatry and state politics more thoroughly than any previous readership. This becomes apparent when literary critic Jörg Drews (1938–2009) emphasises the 'exciting political reflections of the great satire *Psichopatia criminalis*' and he compares Panizza's text, with anti-authoritarian sentiment, to 'a handbook for the Verfassungsschutz [the Federal Office for the Protection of the Constitution]'.[41] For Drews, Panizza 'transforms political into psychiatric categories and – as a devil's advocate and with rapidly sustained irony – advises that all critical, that is, anti-authoritarian and specifically anti-monarchist sentiment be understood as mental illness'.[42]

The shortcomings of such forms of reception become obvious, however, in the reviewers' limited engagement with the 'uncomfortable' Panizza as conveyed in his work; his anti-Semitism, homophobia and misogyny. Perhaps more importantly, the new left's problematic embrace of Panizza is seen in the limited reflection on troublesome parallels between Panizza's delusional logic (which effectively prohibited him for taking responsibility for his own actions) and the politics of the new left, which also considered 'the system' the enemy. At the same time, such unconscious parallels may be considered responsible for much of the left's efforts to engage with Panizza and *Psichopatia criminalis* in the twentieth century. The myth of the degenerate genius is reinforced by the fact that Panizza, who was formerly a psychiatrist, eventually succumbed to his schizophrenic illness. The same myth is transformed later into that of the anti-psychiatrist becoming 'prey' to mental illness and psychiatry.

The image of the 'psychiatrist who went in his own manner towards his own madness', as Michel Foucault remarked, although contributing to an understanding of Panizza's personality, also clouds the reception of Panizza's works.[43] The context and meaning of his psychological slippage into a psychotic world have been vigorously debated among scholars, who have presented three narratives concerning the life of the modernist writer. In the first book-length study on the subject, American scholar Peter D. G. Brown considers Panizza 'the first German author to explode the taboos surrounding sex and religion'.[44] With the exception of Rolf Düsterberg, German scholarship continues to debate Panizza's status as victim of state prosecution and psychiatry or rightful patient. By contrast, Brown underlines Panizza's detrimental self-perception as a failure and the complete isolation Panizza experienced through most of his life, except in the early 1890s, when he participated in the social circles around the avant-garde association Gesellschaft für modernes Leben (Society for Modern Life).[45] Michael Bauer's comprehensive and thorough study is based on Panizza's diaries and archival materials concerning the relevant court cases. Bauer foregrounds the author's placement under guardianship and considers this a politically motivated process against an oppositional writer, a process enabled by psychiatry.[46] Conversely, German psychiatrist Jürgen Müller examines Panizza's vicissitudes from a medical perspective, and after a careful reading of the psychiatric reports reaffirms Panizza's (self-)diagnosis. For Müller, Panizza's life history remains remarkable because, as a psychiatrist, Panizza was able to and sought to assess his own pathological symptoms; Panizza's insight into his condition was unprecedented.[47]

Writing for the *Neue Deutsche Biographie*, Bauer has lamented that Panizza's psychiatric case has remained better known than his works.[48] Indeed, all scholarly studies, Bauer's included, reread Panizza's life story at least partly through the archive of his oeuvre, discussing the author's deteriorating mental health and its causes. Nor have twentieth-century feuilleton writers managed to resolve the question of whether a mentally unstable writer can produce literary works of a high quality. On the occasion of the reissue of *Das Liebenskonzil* in 1966, a writer for the German national weekly *Die Zeit* stated in agreement that 'even the editor [of *Das Liebeskonzil*, Hans Prescher] distances himself from the artistic merit and stresses the documentary value of the phenomenon Panizza for the medical history of the German empire'.[49] Another review conceded that Panizza was not a writer of significance, since 'his relationship to language was too erratic'.[50]

Scholarship has only rarely touched upon *Psichopatia criminalis* in the context of Panizza's decline in mental health during his self-exile and after his forced return to Munich. On this theme, Bauer, Panizza's literary biographer, remarks that *Psichopatia criminalis* is often directly polemical rather than satirical.[51] Düsterberg is the only scholar who has investigated Panizza's late works; he steers clear of *Psichopatia criminalis*, even as, with reference to Panizza's journal *Zürcher Diskußjonen* (*Zurich Discussions*), he highlights at great length Panizza's productivity during the Zurich period.[52] Düsterberg also concedes that from about 1895 onwards Panizza developed a pronounced paranoia centred on German Emperor Wilhelm II, whom Panizza held responsible for his persecution. Nonetheless, in his defence of Panizza, Düsterberg does not find a way to correlate Panizza's inner life and his writing as part of a productive discussion of Panizza's claustrophobic and increasingly repetitive imagery. Especially in his late oeuvre, this closed aesthetic comes to visibly parallel Panizza's delusional ideas concerning the Church, the state and psychiatry. Scholars have thus struggled with deciphering the precision and depth of *Psichopatia criminalis* – or failed to find it sufficiently compelling.

In the paucity of discussion about *Psichopatia criminalis* there hovers a rarely articulated yet persuasive assumption that Panizza the satirist was not the master of his own writings. Apparently, the unease discernible in secondary literature arises from queries about whether a delusional writer can be credited with deliberately suspending the truth in his work, as the genre commands. With this in mind, Bauer, Müller, Brown and Düsterberg would appear to conspicuously avoid discussing *Psichopatia criminalis* – which makes for a very different crisis of reception.[53]

A new interpretation of *Psichopatia criminalis*

Panizza's varied literary oeuvre includes prose poems, fictionalisations of medical case studies, short fiction with a fantastic streak, and satirical plays, as well as works of non-fiction focused on historical investigations of political persecutions, and discussion of the role of prostitution. Panizza's literary beginnings manifested as poems and songs; his narrative explorations of the early 1890s – some of which were fictionalisations of medical case studies – were later superseded by dramatic ventures. These he developed into the peculiar form of the dialogue in verse, only to return to the case study genre as satire and as cultural histories for his late works.

While the most recent interest in Panizza focuses on his early works, I argue that *Psichopatia criminalis* for Panizza indicates a new way to relate to the case study genre.[54] That volume stands at a crossroads between Panizza's literary and his cultural-historical non-fiction case writings, marking a discernible turning point in his oeuvre. It also represents, I submit, a psychological and intellectual defence against the forensic imbrication of the legal and psychiatric domains, triggered in all likelihood by an application for pardon on grounds of insanity made by his friends and supporters after his imprisonment.

Throughout his literary career, Panizza referenced medical case study traditions, not always with satirical intent. The first reference to this genre can be found in his story 'Der Corsetten-Fritz' ('The Orange Corset') (1893), in which the main character eventually enters a psychiatric ward and – on the request of its director – writes his life story.[55] From the same year, 'Ein skandalöser Fall', or 'A Scandal at the Convent' (the German title literally means 'a scandalous case') fictionalises a medical case study of the life of Herculine Barbin. This story represents Panizza's most widely known literary piece in the English-speaking world, since it was published in English and German as part of Foucault's edited volume *Herculine Barbin*. Although Foucault included 'Ein skandalöser Fall' in his own case compilation, he was disconcerted by it, since Panizza's fictionalisation of Barbin's case notes resisted his own understanding of the workings of medical power. After all, Panizza saw the religious framework of the convent as the greater contributor to Barbin's decline, rather than psychiatry.[56] Panizza critically depicts the psychiatrist in this story as a detached participant invested in a process of painful physical assessment. While the doctor's voice is described as 'gentle, compassionate', the outcome 'sad' – emotions are lacking in his clinical report.[57] In the cursory and playful introduction to the compilation, Foucault rehearsed, albeit in a self-reflexive manner, what many literary commentators had done before him: he made Panizza into 'a case' for his own argument, at the expense of exploring the 'anti-archaeology' of Panizza's text, and listening to its echoes of insanity, sex and subversion.[58]

Psichopatia criminalis was published three years after the famous 1895 court case concerning Panizza's play *Das Liebeskonzil*, and the satire represents an attempt by Panizza to come to terms with these earlier events and their consequences. The dramatic investigation was set in the late fifteenth-century papal court of Alexander VI, and became a veritable literary scandal, since the biting portrayal of the papal church depicted the rise of syphilis as God's punishment for a lewd Vatican. At the subsequent trial the Bavarian authorities convicted Panizza of blasphemy and he was sentenced to one year's imprisonment in Amberg. Certainly, in many ways the verdict prompted by *Das Liebeskonzil* represented a significant juncture in Panizza's life. Following his imprisonment he moved to Zurich (1896–98) and after his expulsion from there he relocated to Paris (1898–1901). State authorities used legally questionable methods to force his return to Munich. After they managed to acquire a copy of *Psichopatia criminalis* (with great effort), and through the help of a local bookseller from Paris, they froze his assets in Bavaria and ordered the temporarily destitute Panizza to return.[59]

In his second trial (1901) Panizza was accused of lese majesty in his works *Parisjana* (1899) and *Psichopatia criminalis* (1898). In the context of an assessment of Panizza's soundness of mind, the 1905 psychiatric report by Dr Fritz Ungemach stated that Panizza believed the German Emperor to have passed a law against prostitution in Switzerland to revenge the publication of *Psichopatia criminalis*.[60] During this second trial (and in contrast to 1895), the court no longer held Panizza accountable for his actions, and his literary peers remained distant. After his acquittal, Panizza returned to Paris, where, towards the end of his stay in 1904, the former psychiatrist diagnosed himself as suffering from 'personality dissociation'.[61] By 1905, having returned to Munich, he wished to be admitted to the public psychiatric clinic where he had once worked, but was refused because he had previously renounced his German citizenship. He later attempted to commit suicide and, after denuding himself in public, was eventually committed to the private asylum of St Gilgenberg, close to Bayreuth. In 1907 he was transferred to a nearby luxury sanatorium, the castle Herzoghöhe, where he died in 1921. One of his last literary utterances was a poem titled 'Umsonst gelebt', or 'Lived in Vain'.

The persecution of Panizza by state authorities was exemplary in its harshness and lack of mercy, and represented the greatest literary scandal of the 1890s in Germany. His contemporary Frank Wedekind (1864–1918) was sentenced to six months in Amberg jail for lese majesty in 1898 because of a poem directed at Emperor Wilhelm II. A similar fate was suffered by Hanns von Gumppenberg (1866–1928), who was convicted of lese majesty after he delivered a lecture on the socialist lyrics of German author Karl Friedrich Henckell (1864–1929) to workers and modernist writers; Gumppenberg was imprisoned for two months.[62] Thus writers in the satirical scene in Munich feared the censorship authorities for good reason, yet, unlike Panizza, both Gumppenberg and Wedekind were able to carve out an existence as creative writers, and later worked for the first political German cabaret as one of *Die Elf Scharfrichter*. Wedekind also became established as a widely successful playwright in his own right.

As a fellow writer, Gumppenberg characterised Panizza's literary method as 'historical-theological-critical'.[63] Panizza's imprisonment for a work that had not been staged – a work published across the border in Switzerland, and one that had reached a comparatively small readership – seems outstanding, even given the rule of the censor in Bavaria at the time. Like the hatred Panizza attracted from authorities and the jury, this fact is only explained by the way in which the content of *Das Liebeskonzil* targeted the Catholic Church rather than the Emperor, and by Panizza's open defiance in court. His reckoning with the Church was rooted in his childhood. Born in 1853 in the Bavarian spa resort of Bad Kissingen, he was the son of a well-to-do hotelier, and grew up in the midst of religious scandal. After the death of Panizza's Catholic father Karl, his Huguenot wife, Mathilde Panizza, insisted on a Protestant upbringing for her five children. Her husband had signed a declaration to this effect on the latter's deathbed. When the local Catholic priest challenged the attestation, arguing that Karl had not been of legally sane mind, the court found in favour of the priest in all instances.

Despite being threatened with imprisonment and monetary fines, Mathilde brought up her children in strict pietistic ways. To escape the state authorities, the children were sent to live with relatives in Swabia and Hesse. Oskar was eventually placed in a boarding school in Wurttemberg, then in different Bavarian schools in Schweinfurt and Munich, where he lived with his uncle, who was a city pastor, a profession his mother wished Oskar to occupy as well. Instead, Panizza eventually became a psychiatrist and assistant to Gudden between 1880 and 1884. He left the clinic behind when his mother made the inheritance of his father available to the children, and Panizza now devoted his energies solely to his literary career. He had found the work with patients demanding and the research – largely based on the dissection of human brains – detrimental to his mental health, and he had come to appreciate the curative and therapeutic value of writing.[64] The welcoming writerly scene in Munich gave him a sense of belonging for the first time. While critical of psychiatry as an institution, Panizza appreciated the avenues of thought his studies had opened up to him. His fictional case writings are testimony to this fact, as is the medical and historical understanding of disease that informed his attack on the papal church in *Das Liebeskonzil*. Yet at court his standing as a former psychiatrist and holder of expert medical knowledge might have actually increased the bias against him.

When *Das Liebeskonzil* was first confiscated in early 1895, Panizza had decided to remain in Munich. He did so although he had the financial means to take up residence abroad. In retrospect he acknowledged that this decision proved detrimental, but he ascribed his insistence to await trial in Munich in 1895 to his 'Hugenot lust for opposition'.[65] Despite warnings from different sides, Panizza must have envisaged it possible to instrumentalise the court as a stage for his critique of the Church, and to take a stance for the freedom of the arts. Had he succeeded, not only would this have been a considerable affirmation for the autonomy of the arts and of literature, but also he would have symbolically repealed the much older sentence against his father, whose decision to allow his children to be raised in the Protestant faith was revoked by the court. In his own court case, Panizza insisted on defending himself, and called as an expert witness the founder of the modernist Munich journal *Die Gesellschaft* (*Society*), Michael Georg Conrad, to which Panizza contributed regularly.[66] For his defence Panizza prepared a lengthy speech in which he intellectually justified his literary project and defended the freedom of the arts, but in the actual trial his speech was cut short. After admitting that as a creative writer he wished readers in Germany to engage with *Das Liebeskonzil*, the verdict was given – and the author was sentenced to immediate detention.

While his conduct raised concern among his friends, at no point in the trial was a plea on the grounds of insanity entered, although there are indications that Panizza's mental state had been of concern to him since at least the early 1880s. In 1882 he advised his mother to have his sister treated psychiatrically after she had made a suicide attempt. The death of his uncle Ferdinand in a psychiatric hospital in 1884 must have increased Panizza's fears for himself – Panizza attended his relative's post-mortem examination and wrote an extensive report.[67] In 'Genie und Wahnsinn' ('Genius and Insanity'), his first talk on the topic of genius to the bohemian and writerly audience of the modernist association Die Gesellschaft in Munich in 1891, he elaborated that 'however much the genius amazes and admires in his milieu and in history, he never is completely content. He lives alone and in continuous struggle with himself.'[68] At this point in time Panizza discussed the psychiatric discourse of genius critically, but also agreed with much of what was said. Like Arndt, Panizza contended that cases in which a genius experiences hallucinations are relatively rare, albeit with known exceptions such as Luther. 'More often', Panizza asserts, 'a condition exists by which the rising fantastical images might be strange, but are perceived as part of one's own mind'.[69] It is worth recollecting Panizza's later appropriative critique of Arndt's psychiatric textbook in *Psichopatia criminalis*.

Close study of the court files reveals that the reason why an insanity plea was not considered at trial lay with Panizza himself. As Panizza's lawyer, Dr Kugelmann, claimed, 'he had not dared to raise the question [of unsoundness of the mind] because the accused with his whole persona would have rejected in the most utmost manner such a presumption'.[70] Yet within the first month of serving his sentence, on 30 August 1895 and without Panizza's consent, Kugelmann applied for pardon for his client on these very grounds. In his petition Kugelmann wrote to Prince Regent Luitpold and argued that the content of *Das Liebeskonzil* 'immediately raises doubts as to the intellectual freedom of its author'. (This might have been a strategic means to sway the Prince Regent's favour; Luitpold was well aware of the consequences of insanity. In 1886 he had been instrumental in having King Ludwig II declared mentally incompetent. After King Ludwig's death, Luitpold remained Prince Regent in the name of Ludwig's younger brother, Otto, who had shown first signs of a mental disorder in 1865, and had been declared mentally ill in 1872.) As supporting evidence Kugelmann also provided two references: one by a Dr Nobiling and the other by Panizza's friend from university and personal physician Dr Paul Ostermaier. Both expressed the fear that solitary confinement would worsen Panizza's condition.[71] Ostermaier further elaborated that he had been in regular contact with Panizza both socially and scientifically, and had been for many years of the belief that his friend 'is to a high degree pathologically disposed and cannot be held responsible for any of his speeches and deeds'.[72]

Panizza had found the *Liebeskonzil* trial and the concomitant imprisonment on remand highly stressful. Before Kugelmann applied for his pardon, Drs Nobiling and Ostermaier had both supported an application for a two-month delay of Panizza's term of imprisonment because of anxiety attacks and nervous stomach cramps; this might have triggered Kugelmann's application for a pardon as well as Nobiling's and Ostermaier's support. Yet a month later, if prison physician Dr Schmelcher was right in his assessment, Panizza felt physically and mentally healthy, he slept well and his nervous stomach cramps had altogether disappeared.[73] It was in this somewhat stabilised situation that Panizza was called to meet with the director of the prison, who informed him of the application for pardon and the reasoning behind it. Panizza apologised profusely for having upset religious sentiments but argued that, to his knowledge, *Das Liebeskonzil* had not reached anyone in whom such upset could be fostered. As to his former state of mental health, he detailed the detrimental influence of his incarceration, yet decidedly declared that he was of sound mind, even though, 'like all intellectuals [he] suffered from mood anomalies, mental fluctuation, depression, yet [...] he had experienced such states since his earliest youth'.[74]

The application for pardon was subsequently rejected, yet it brought to the fore a central issue for Panizza. He knew that if he was to be declared legally insane, the literary value and standing of his work would be tarnished; presumably this proposition also insulted his professional pride as a psychiatrist. On a more personal level, to be classified as insane confronted him with fears he had harboured for over a decade – in a situation where he was not free to react: in order for the application to be considered, Panizza needed to present to the prison director his support for Kugelmann's application and its claim. Instead, this well-meant act forced to a head a crisis that already been at the heart of Panizza's court trial: was it more important to be right or to be free? Five years before he was acquitted on grounds of insanity in his second trial in 1901, Panizza chose the former solution.

It is in *Psichopatia criminalis* that Panizza comes to terms with the consequences of his trial, and problematises the forensic imbrication of legal and medical discourse for the first time in his wide-ranging career. Having effected a radical displacement of authority as an imaginative foundation for his project, Panizza creates a satire utilising his profound knowledge of the psychiatric case study genre to attack his former profession, the German state, and even his supporters and friends. Yet if, for the sake of argument, we read the plot of *Psichopatia criminalis* literally, a new interpretation arises. To recall, the prime of *Psichopatia criminalis* installs the author as the chief psychiatrist of Germany. In it, Panizza for the first time attacks the psychiatric profession, both from his imagined position as the German chief psychiatrist and from his position as a creative writer; moreover, this omnipotent figure holds accountable for their thoughts all citizens who had ever conceived of resistance, and commits them to a mental asylum. 'All citizens' included, surely, his lawyer and supporters Ostermaier and Nobiling, who – although with Panizza's best interests at heart – brought the eccentric and self-destructive wordsmith into a situation in which he needed to confront his innermost fears.

In the voice of the chief psychiatrist of the German state, he addresses his psychiatrist colleagues, the nominal addressees of *Psichopatia criminalis*, and highlights their lack of understanding of the poor prognosis of the disease 'psichopatia criminalis'. By offering his superior insights to the German Emperor, the chief psychiatrist insinuates the professional incompetence of his colleagues and assumes an omnipotent position; in collaboration with the Emperor he creates a system of total control from which none can escape. This reasoning had an evident underlying logic. Before the introduction of the insanity defence in the nineteenth century, the court could only convict culprits and punish them according to the law, or acquit them, which indicated their complete innocence.[75] This polarised model of condemnation or redemption was now undermined, since being held in a clinic or prison on the grounds of legal insanity did not actually resolve the underlying question of guilt. Rather, if a person was declared temporarily insane, their accountability was fundamentally undermined and they relied on the judgement of psychiatrists to be released. Consequently, the public perception of their persona might remain tainted. Panizza was the first German writer to formulate this critique at the very point at which, historically, this legal defence strategy became widely accepted. He did so – at least in the instance of his own life – with prophetic clarity.

The creative experimentalism of Panizza's achievement in *Psichopatia Criminalis* has a darker underbelly. The strategy of displacement can be understood as the creative reformulation of a painful situation which was beyond Panizza's control. This analysis agrees with Henry Lothane when he claims – attempting to buffer an overtly deterministic interpretation of Panizza's biography – that 'Panizza was not just paranoid, he was also persecuted'. Similarly, it is possible to accept as readers that Panizza was not only persecuted but also paranoid, and unwilling and unable to perceive the ways in which he contributed to his own suffering.[76] *Psichopatia criminalis* enabled Panizza to express his deep-seated frustration with the uninvited application for pardon made by friends and supporters, but the relief he must have gained from writing his satire stood in the way of re-establishing a positive relationship with his peers. A year before the publication of *Psichipatia criminalis* Panizza published his grumbling literary farewell note, *Abschied von München* (*Farewell from Munich*, 1897), in which he accused all inhabitants of Munich of being 'vassals of Rome' and the Catholic Church; *Psichopatia criminalis* expressed his increasing alienation from his Munich friends.[77]

With respect to the development of Panizza's psychosis, arguably the *Liebeskonzil* trial contains the moment of Panizza's psychological decompensation. In his discussion of Freudian concepts, Bernd Nitzschke expounds how neurosis suppresses the unwanted reality, while psychosis reformulates it.[78] Both the description of the mechanism of this loss as well as its traces can be found in *Psichopatia criminalis*. For instance, where Panizza describes paranoia as one of the four characteristics of the symptomatology of 'psichopatia criminalis', he argues that it is not easy to convict people of this disease, since they are erudite, and believe that 'because Schiller has written "The Robbers" they are allowed to think anything'.[79]

This statement can also be interpreted as a retrospective aggrandisement of Panizza's defence strategy in court. Like the characters of his case vignettes, Panizza flooded the president of the court with erudite quotes, yet, in stark contrast to *Psichopatia criminalis*, Panizza was cut short in his own defence. Moreover, a passage of his satire against Arndt directly relates to Panizza's *idée fixe* of later years, that of rulers and princes. Panizza attests that Arndt did not include the ruling classes in his critique. Yet although it is only in the context of already marginal comments on genius, Arndt's textbook does mention 'the genius of statesmen and military commanders, the Duke of Marlborough and [Roman] commander Tiberius'.[80] The textbook also notes that sufferers of 'raving madness' (*Tobsucht*) often identify themselves with great figures of history, including kings and emperors.[81] Again, Panizza does not cite this reference; rather, his writings idealise a range of prominent historical figures in the case vignettes. Panizza's own world-view was one of extreme individualism and he was carried by a belief that world history is written by singular outstanding individuals; as he confessed to his mother, he too wanted to be a 'great man'.[82] Yet another figure looms large for the first time in his writing, that of German Emperor Wilhelm II. Accordingly Panizza dedicated the manuscript of *Psichopatia criminalis* to the German Emperor: 'The Great Megalomaniac/In Deepest Dedication/The Psychiatrist'.[83] While this inscription was present only in the manuscript and not the printed version of *Psichopatia criminalis*, just a year later, in *Parisjana* (1899), Wilhelm II became the delusional metaphor within Panizza's psychosis. Panizza remained haunted by Wilhelm II – as any psychotic subject is fixated – and the German Emperor now became the only image through which Panizza could integrate his reality.

Panizza's creation of a delusional metaphor and a conformist imaginary may be read in psychoanalytic terms as an attempt by the author to repair the psyche through writing, although at the cost of the loss of a sense of reality.[84] Symbolically, the Emperor belongs to the realm of the state and stands as a punitive father figure. In this sense, the trial surrounding the anti-Catholic play *Das Liebeskonzil* represented a refusal and an inability to connect to the symbolic order of social interchange bound by the name of the father, as Jacques Lacan has argued in his essay on psychosis.[85] This tendency was already present in the play itself, as Freud observes in his *Interpretation of Dreams*. Here the reflections on Panizza's play become part of Freud's chain of associations in which he reflects on the rebellion against his own father in his dreams:

> This recalled a strongly revolutionary literary play by Oskar Panizza [*Das Liebeskonzil* (1895)], in which God the Father is ignominiously treated as a paralytic old man. In his case will and deed were represented as one and the same thing, and he had to be restrained from cursing and swearing by one of his archangels, a kind of Ganymede, because his imprecations would be promptly fulfilled.[86]

Panizza's Catholic father died when his son was only two years old. The ensuing religious conflict between his mother and the Catholic Church concerning the religious affiliation of Panizza and his siblings dominated

Panizza's childhood, and *Das Liebeskonzil* presented a literary means of siding with his mother against the persecution of the Catholic Church, and a means to carve out a troubled symbolic space for himself. Once the state impeded his freedom of movement and, as in his childhood, intervened on behalf of the Catholic Church – this is at least how the situation must have seemed to him – his defences broke down. The trial became the moment that determined his psychosis, since it revealed to him 'his own insufficiency, humiliating him at the ethical level'.[87]

With reference to this background, it can be shown that in *Psichopatia criminalis* Panizza lampoons the case study genre while also reinterpreting it. Thus *Psichopatia criminalis* can be read simultaneously as, firstly, incisive satire; secondly, Panizza's psychological defence against his own trial, and the question of unsoundness of mind that it raised for him; and thirdly, the first iteration of his persecutory doppelgänger. Moreover, it is possible to draw parallels between Panizza's shift to a satirical mode, with its attempt to reduce complexity, and his withdrawal from the social sphere. Both appear to be attempts 'to compensate for the lack of the ability to synchronise, by avoiding overcharging interactions', as philosopher and psychiatrist Thomas Fuchs outlines in his study of temporality and psychopathology.[88]

Panizza's later cultural historical case writings present a perpetuation of his genealogy of dissidents. Having started to present such case studies in *Psichopatia criminalis*, Panizza continued this work in his journal *Zürcher Diskußjonen*. While leading an isolated life, symbolically Panizza surrounded himself with a host of dissident thinkers, all of whom were martyrs for their cause. Yet his fixation with the German Emperor also remained, as his verses *Parisjana* and the unpublished 'Casus conscientiae' (1903), one of the very last texts Panizza composed, reveal. The latter piece, a short dialogue between a layperson and a priest, makes mixed reference to religious as well as medical case writing traditions, and exploits the forgotten religious case modality of the case of conscience – a form of religious reasoning used to resolve hypothetical or apparent instances of wrongdoing by analysing whether the protagonist has acted wrongly. 'Casus conscientiae' possibly restages a dialogue between Panizza and Friedrich Lippert, the chaplain at the Amberg prison who had befriended Panizza during his imprisonment, and who in 1908 became his legal custodian. In the dialogue, the figure of the layperson asks the priest if sex murder should ever receive a sentence from the courts on grounds of the diminished insanity of the accused murderer, as occurs in the context of worldly penal law. With reference to the fifth biblical commandment, the priest first denies, then follows the layperson's catch question: 'what if the prince, the margrave, the king, [or] the emperor is the sex murderer?'[89]

Had 'Casus conscientiae' been published, it would have held a notable challenge for Panizza's contemporary German readers: it illuminated the limitations of the Church's moral power in the real world and also noted the limits of German civil law. Based on positive law, the German legal system has historically relied on the understanding that the state protects its citizens and, in turn, expects its citizens to respect its laws. The only scenario in which breaking the law can be ethically justified is under a rogue regime – in this instance, a rogue emperor. Panizza in this *casus* points to the limits not only of religious reality but also of political reality, and does so from a standpoint of moral superiority. As his final negotiation with the case study genre, 'Casus conscientiae' closely resembles Panizza's own delusional system, detailing its three 'fates', Church, state and psychiatry. It also raises pertinent questions concerning the powers of these institutions and the accountability of the ruling classes.

***

'[Parody] stresses difference and through the inscription of difference in a literary or artistic tradition masters it. Its assumption is imperial.'[90] This verdict stands with reference to *Psichopatia criminalis*, in which Panizza ingeniously interweaves the reductionist nature of case writing with that of satire, while his late case writings similarly serve as sites of radical reinterpretation. Depending on the reader's frame of reference, *Psichopatia criminalis* has been received as an extravagant *pièce de résistance*, as a means of overcoming aggression, and as the author's conscious rendering of his emerging system of delusion. This chapter has aimed to show that these multiple interpretations need not be at odds with one another, but that their divergent momentum has engendered different reader responses. *Psichopatia criminalis* has suffered from limited availability and circulation, and poor critical engagement, understanding and appreciation, because it pushes satire to its very limits, while the choice of the psychiatric case study genre as a prime was not without complications. Yet this daring and distinctive project also allowed Panizza to portray the limits of forensic discourse. His interpretation was in many ways the consequence of his upbringing and medical education, combined with modernist phantasies about insanity, played within a context of Bavaria's repressive rule of law.

As Phiddian points out, satirists often claim to be prophets in the name of truth.[91] This holds true for Panizza. Panizza's decision to await his trial in Munich, his subsequent conviction for blasphemy and the harsh sentence – a year's imprisonment – undoubtedly constituted a heavy psychological burden on a man who, by his own admission, had suffered from depression since his childhood. The conviction also created a marked, ongoing interest among the Bavarian authorities in persecuting Panizza in a merciless manner. As part of this destructive situation, the Bavarian authorities confiscated Panizza's German assets – his main income – and forced him to return to stand trial for lese majesty in 1901, even though he had renounced his German citizenship and emigrated to Zurich, and then Paris. During the same years, Panizza was busy constructing, with increasing intensity, German Emperor Wilhelm II as a persecutory doppelgänger, both in his interior symbolic world and in his publications. Acquitted on grounds of insanity, later he admitted himself to the same clinic where he had once worked as a psychiatrist. Finally, he was declared incompetent in 1905. At once because of and in spite of these biographical vicissitudes, his exploration of the psychiatric case study genre in *Psichopatia criminalis* remains unprecedented.

The scandal surrounding Panizza the man has had profound consequences for the reception of his oeuvre. Panizza was demonstrably both a revolutionary *enfant terrible* and a man struggling to maintain his sharp mental faculties. Given the deeply oxymoronic nature of much of Panizza's life and oeuvre, it is not surprising there has been a divided reception of his work. His readers either sympathise with this anti-clerical, anti-monarchist and antipsychiatric author and idealise his stance against authority, sometimes at the cost of understanding the rhetorical projects tackled in his written works, or they medicalise the author, and by extension the content of his writing, challenging Panizza's status and significance as a satirist. Originally, his books were difficult to come by, because they were published by obscure publishers, often confiscated rather quickly, and subsequently published abroad in small editions. At best, the resultant rarity of copies of Panizza's publications fostered a fetishisation of his works, which gained value as collectors' items, and promoted the adulation of Panizza as a cultural-political dissenter. The accumulation since the 1980s of biographical insights into Panizza's suffering has changed readers' expectations of the satire *Psichopatia criminalis* by suspending the truth of the satire in a particular way. While, overall, the socialist reception clung to the satire's most comprehensible elements, the newer idea of Panizza's limited artistic accountability denies the writer agency over his text, and fails to provide a model for, or a clear explanation of, the impact of Panizza's mental health on his writing. This is partly a result of the incomprehensibility of certain aspects of Panizza's text, and partly follows from the specificity of his thinking, some of which, as evidenced above, can be contextualised biographically.

Both strands of reception intuitively grasp the fact that in Panizza's writing there exists a concurrence of art and mental illness, and each defends against one particular aspect of Panizza's unique system of thought, whether by means of idealisation or repression. Each of these divergent interpretations reflects characteristics inherent to Panizza's text. Prodded by generic means and inner defences, readers either idealise Panizza's dissident thought or avoid the question of whether a writer suffering from pronounced mental health problems can compose a literary text. This question is propelled by the satirical nature of *Psichopatia criminalis*, since, as Phiddian contends, satire requires intent: 'it is necessary to ascribe a rhetorical purpose to it, even if others see the purpose differently, and even if you then go on to criticise how coherent or consistently pursued that purpose may be'.[92]

This raises the much bigger question of the role and function of literature and creativity in the context of the mental health of authors. These questions are not new, and were particularly pertinent in the late nineteenth and early twentieth centuries. As discussed in Chapter 2, psychiatry assumed creative writers to be degenerate, while later psychoanalysts such as Wilhelm Stekel and Isidor Sadger tended to categorise at least some writers as neurotics. For psychoanalysts who stood in a psychiatric tradition, the creative act represented an expression of narcissism, and hence they did not pay any attention to literary texts, while Freud and his supporters championed the view that writing was a means to overcome or at least ease inner conflicts, both for writers and for their audience. Then there was contemporary criminal psychologist Erich Wulffen, a prolific writer and a master of case writing – presented in Chapter 4 – who argued that in the specific instance of criminals such as con man Georges Manolescu, writing functioned on a symbolic level as a repeat offence. Apparently Panizza was not privy to Freud's early writings, and he was already institutionalised in a psychiatric clinic when Freud elaborated on creative artists' ability to overcome their psychological impediments and resolve their inner conflicts. Nevertheless, it is possible to read *Psichopatia criminalis* for the ways in which it allowed Panizza to satirically transform his aggression against his lawyer, his supporters and psychiatry more generally into a work of literature. Simultaneously – to reference the criminal psychological discourse of Wulffen – Panizza also committed a 'crime' against himself. His retreat into language at the cost of experience was instrumental in his decline. This becomes most obvious in Panizza's focus on Emperor Wilhelm II, who came to assume the role of Panizza's eerie doppelgänger. As for the case study genre, like Alfred Döblin in the inter-war period, Panizza was one of the key German writers of the fin de siècle with an expert knowledge of a range of case modalities. He skilfully fashioned the psychiatric case study genre to invert its logic and to create a dystopian satire that challenged the institutions which traditionally had been the site of case knowledge: the Church, the court and psychiatry. His critique of psychiatric discourse as the basis of a new forensic legal mode was at the same time deeply personal and political.

Notes

1 For example, Jörg Drews, 'Aus Anlaß von Oskar Panizza. Bemerkungen zu zwei Schriften des großen Satirikers', *Süddeutsche Zeitung*, 28 October 1978; Ernst Stein, 'Ein grandioses Greuel. Scheiterhaufen oder Denkmal für Oskar Panizza', *Die Zeit*, 25 March 1966; Klaus Wagner, 'Franz Marijnens große Wut. Panizzas Liebeskonzil in Hamburg', *Frankfurter Allgemeine Zeitung*, 21 July 1977.

2 John Forrester, 'Foreword', in Joy Damousi, Birgit Lang and Katie Sutton (eds), *Case Studies and the Dissemination of Knowledge* (New York: Routledge, 2015), pp. ix–xi, p. ix.

3 'Nicht immer gelang es Panizza, die Grenzen der Satire zu wahren und nicht zur direkten Polemik gegen die Politik jener überzugehen, an die sich seine Schrift

angeblich wandte.' Michael Bauer, *Oskar Panizza. Ein literarisches Portrait* (Munich: Hanser, 1984), p. 202.

4 Bauer mentions *Psichopatia criminalis* only in passing. Despite his great interest in Panizza's Zurich writings Rolf Düsterberg does not engage with *Psichopatia criminalis*. Rolf Düsterberg, *'Die gedrukte Freiheit'. Oskar Panizza und die Zürcher Diskussionen* (Frankfurt: Peter Lang, 1984).

5 Linda Hutcheon, *A Theory of Parody: The Teachings of Twentieth-Century Art Forms* (New York: Methuen, 1985), p. 6.

6 Hutcheon, *A Theory of Parody*, p. 6; Paul Simpson, *On the Discourse of Satire: Towards a Stylistic Model of Satirical Humour* (Amsterdam: John Benjamins, 2003), pp. 8–9.

7 See Jürgen Habermas, 'What Is Universal Pragmatics?', in Thomas McCarthy (ed.) *Communication and the Evolution of Society* (London: Heinemann, 1979), pp. 1–68.

8 Oskar Panizza, *Psichopatia criminalis: Anleitung um die vom Gericht für notwendig erkanten Geisteskrankheiten psichjatrisch zu eruiren und wissenschaftlich festzustellen; für Ärzte, Laien, Juristen, Vormünder, Verwaltungsbeamte, Minister etc.* (Zurich: Zürcher Diskußionen, 1898), p. v.

9 Hanns Hippius, Hans-Jürgen Möller, Norbert Müller and Gabriele Neundörfer, *Die psychiatrische Klinik der Universität München, 1904–2004* (Heidelberg: Springer, 2005), pp. 37–8.

10 A rich corpus of literature is available concerning the life of Ludwig II, for instance: Wilfrid Blunt, *The Dream King: Ludwig II of Bavaria* (Harmondsworth: Penguin, 1973); Oliver Hilmes, *Ludwig II. Der unzeitgemäße König* (Munich: Siedler, 2013); Christopher McIntosh, *The Swan King: Ludwig II of Bavaria* (London: Lane, 1982); Hans Rall, *King Ludwig II: Reality and Mystery* (Regensburg: Schnell & Steiner, 2001). On the role of Bernhard von Gudden see: Ian Freckelton, 'Deaths of King Ludwig II of Bavaria and of His Psychiatrist, Professor von Gudden: Warnings from the Nineteenth Century', *Psychiatry, Psychology and Law*, 19:1 (2012), pp. 1–10; Heinz Häfner, 'War das psychiatrische Gutachten B. von Guddens über König Ludwig II. von Bayern korrekt?', *Der Nervenarzt*, 82:5 (2011), pp. 611–16; Wilhelm Kaltenstadler, 'Was Ludwig II Mentally Ill? Critical Remarks on the Estimate of Professor Dr med. von Gudden', *Deutsche medizinische Wochenschrift*, 136:51/52 (2011), pp. 2684–91; Jürgen L. Müller, 'Johan Bernhard Aloys von Gudden (1824–1886): Not Only the King of Bavaria's Psychiatrist', *International Journal of Psychiatry in Clinical Practice*, 5:2 (2001), pp. 135–9.

11 In Panizza's characteristic spelling: 'Ein mässig grosses Irrenhaus zwischen Nekar und Rhein, etwa von der Grösse der Pfalz, und auf eben diesem Boden, wo die turbulentesten Köpfe gediehen, errichtet'. Panizza, *Psichopatia criminalis*, pp. vi–vii.

12 '[D]as Prinzip der Humanität, welches bei unseren heutigen, auf allen Seiten aufgeregeten Zeiten, besonders auch immer an die Spitze gestellt wird.' 'Die milde Behandlung, richtig temperirte Wannenbäder, die Ruhe, die Abgeschlossenheit, Nachtigallenschlag jenseits der Gitter, der gütige Zuspruch des Arztes – ein Bischen Hyoscamin, und ein Bischen Bromkali – und die politsche Einsicht all dieser Internirter wäre bedeutend gewachsen.' Panizza, *Psichopatia criminalis*, pp. v, viii.

13 Hans C. Bangen, *Geschichte der medikamentösen Therapie der Schizophrenie* (Berlin: VWB, 1992), p. 23; Richard von Krafft-Ebing, *Lehrbuch der Psychiatrie auf klinischer Grundlage für Ärzte und Studierende*, 3rd new edition (Stuttgart: Enke, 1888), p. 298.

14 For instance, Richard von Krafft-Ebing, *Psychosis Menstrualis. Eine klinisch-forensische Studie* (Stuttgart: Enke, 1902), p. 58.

15 The German original reads: 'Mancher der aufmerksamen Leser, besonders solcher,

die Psichjater von Fach sind, möchte vielleicht hier den Einwurf wagen, dass das hier Vorgetragene ja Geschichte, politische Geschichte, Literatur-Geschichte, ReformazjonsGeschichte, aber keine eigentliche psichjatrische Kasuistik, keine Darstellung von Psichopatieen seien'. Panizza, *Psichopatia criminalis*, p. 9.

16 'Das bewundernswerte Lehrbuch ist bei weitem nicht genügend gewürdigt und noch immer in der ersten Auflage zu haben'. Panizza, *Psichopatia criminalis*, p. 9.

17 The German original reads: 'Hat doch der trefliche Forscher *Rudolf Arndt* in seinem "Lehrbuch der Psichjatrie fur Ärzte und Studirende" die ganze Kultur- und Geistesgeschichte der Menschheit in *Oxy-* und *Par-ästesieen* eingeteilt, und auf diese Weise die gesamte Entwiklungsgeschichte des Abendlandes, alle Revoluzjonen und die "Räuber" von *Schiller*, alle politischen Verträge und *Metternich* – mit alleiniger Ausnahme der Fürsten – in seinem hervorragenden Lehrbuche untergebracht!' Panizza, *Psichopatia criminalis*, p. 9.

18 Rudolf Arndt, *Lehrbuch der Psychiatrie für Ärzte und Studirende* (Vienna: Urban & Schwarzenberg, 1883), pp. 110–11.

19 '[A]llerhand krankhaften Zuständen, mit allerhand Eigenthümlichkeiten, Idyosynkrasien und selbst Perversitäten.' Arndt, *Lehrbuch der Psychiatrie*, p. 296.

20 '[P]sychisch verdüstert und gebrochen.' Arndt, *Lehrbuch der Psychiatrie*, p. 297. These elaborations are part of the fourteenth chapter (forty-eight pages long), which deals with the origins of psychosis.

21 Panizza, *Psichopatia criminalis*, p. 10. Yet in *Psichopatia criminalis* six of the nine psychiatrists that Panizza listed were his contemporaries, and only Arndt, Wilhelm Griesinger (1817–68) and French psychiatrist Jean-Étienne Esquirol (1772–1840) could be counted as 'old'.

22 See Jürgen Müller, 'Oskar Panizza: Psychiatrist, Antipsychiatrist, Patient. The Man Behind Emil Kraepelin's Case Report on "Paraphrenias"', *International Journal of Psychiatry in Clinical Practice*, 4:4 (2000), pp. 335–8.

23 Simpson, *On the Discourse of Satire*, p. 9. In Simpson's terms, while the prime is interpreted through a frame of general knowledge, the dialectic is accessed through the text, 'such that a schism or fracture occurs between these two frameworks'.

24 'Es ist die stille Wut, das geheime, ruhige Konspiriren, das innere freche Denken was diese Leute auszeichnet; es ist die mania anti-govermentalis.' Panizza, *Psichopatia criminalis*, p. 18.

25 Panizza, *Psichopatia criminalis*, p. 30; Cesare Lombroso, *The Man of Genius*, trans. H. Havelock Ellis (London: Walter Scott, 1891). The Italian original of Lombroso's study was published in 1886, the German translation in 1890.

26 Panizza, *Psichopatia criminalis*, p. 39.

27 In comparison to Panizza, Austro-Marxist Max Adler mentions as socialist forebears and relevant thinkers: Rousseau, Schiller, Kant, Fichte, Saint-Simon, Owen, Weitling, Feuerbach, Stirner, Lasalle, Engels, Marx and Hegel. See Max Adler, *Wegweiser. Studien zur Geistesgeschichte des Sozialismus* (Stuttgart: Dietz, 1914).

28 Simpson, *On the Discourse of Satire*, pp. 8–9.

29 'Man kann sie in höchster Empörung als Attentate gegen Sitte und Schönheit und dann wieder als kindlich harmlose Launenspielereien auffassen. Allein selber dazu thun muss man jedenfalls nicht wenig. Schon die vielen Gelehrsamkeiten und seltenen deutschen Wörter stellen an den Leser die Anforderung des Mitarbeitens; ein Panizza-Lexikon wäre sehr erwünscht.' 'Vatikanische Satiren', *Der sozialistische Akademiker*, 10 (15 May 1895), pp. 178–82, p. 182.

30 Simpson, *On the Discourse of Satire*, p. 136.

31 Robert Phiddian, 'Satire and the Limits of Literary Theory', *Critical Theory*, 55:3 (2003), pp. 44–58, p. 49.

32 Phiddian, 'Satire and the Limits of Literary Theory', pp. 54, 49.

33 *Das Liebeskonzil* (1894) represented a veritable literary and judicial scandal, and created religious controversy long after its creation; it was censored the

last time in Austrian Tyrol in 1983. See Peter D. G. Brown, 'The Continuing Trials of Oskar Panizza: A Century of Artistic Censorship in Germany, Austria, and Beyond', *German Studies Review*, 24:3 (2001), pp. 533–56; Gary D. Stark, 'Trials and Tribulations: Authors' Responses to Censorship in Imperial Germany, 1885–1914', *German Studies Review*, 12:3 (1989), pp. 447–68.

34 Peter D. G. Brown, *Oskar Panizza: His Life and Works* (New York: Peter Lang, 1983), pp. 36–9.

35 'Ganz ohne Frage ist der schludrige Stilist und miserable Orthograph Panizza der seit Luther derbste, deftigste, polterndste und zugleich genialistische Polemiker deutscher Sprache gewesen.' Hans J. Fröhlich, 'Der deftigste und genialischste Polemiker deutscher Sprache. Eine Neuausgabe von Oskar Panizzas "Dialoge im Geiste Huttens", *Frankfurter Allgemeine Zeitung*, 7 February 1980.

36 'Panizza ist ein Terrorist: wer kein Deutscher werden will, sollte ihn lesen.' Heiner Müller, 'Panizza oder Einheit Deutschlands', *Frankfurter Rundschau*, 4 August 1979.

37 The German original reads (with original emphasis): 'Panizzas Unglück ist das des Propheten, der zu früh vorausgesagt hat', and, further, 'Oskar Panizza ist ein Opfer der deutschen Einheit, kein REICH wollte ihn haben. Einigung ist Ausschließung, Panizza gehört zu den Ausgeschlossenen, ein Spaltpilz und Nestbeschmutzer, Gotteslästerer und Staatsfeind in der Tradition einer Gegenkultur der HALBVERRÜCKTEN Ketzer'. Müller, 'Panizza oder Einheit Deutschlands'.

38 Knut Boeser, 'Panizza und Rushdie. Vom gefährlichen Leben der Schriftsteller in moralischen Zeiten', in Knut Boeser (ed.), *Der Fall Oskar Panizza: ein deutscher Dichter im Gefängnis; eine Dokumentation* (Berlin: Hentrich, 1989), pp. 220–9, p. 220.

39 '[P]olitische Satire über die Verfolgungswut der deutschen Staatsanwälte.' Fritz Brügel, 'Der kaiserliche Wahnsinn', *Arbeiterzeitung*, 2 August 1926.

40 'Der politische Wille dieser Münchner war – wie hätte es in dem Wilhelminischen Deutschland auch anders sein können! – viel zu eingeengt, und eine Verbindung mit der praktisch arbeitenden Sozialdemokratie, die die Literaten wieder geistig hätte befruchten können, und verebbte schließlich in Bürgerbohème.' '[S]o ragte über die Münchner der unglückliche Oskar Panizza weit hervor.... [Oskar Panizza] hat noch hassen können, wie heute nur Heinrich Mann haßt. Er hat sein Land geliebt und Die verabscheut, die es zu einem Kasernenhof und zu einer Tretmühle gemacht haben, derweil sie selbst nicht mitzutun brauchten: denn für galten keine Gesetze. Vorschriften gelten nur für *die*, die sie gemacht haben.' Kurt Tucholsky (writing as Ignaz Wrobel), 'Panizza', *Die Weltbühne*, 38 (11 September 1919), p. 321.

41 'Große Satire aber und geradezu aufregende politische Reflexionen allerdings bietet die "Psichopatia criminalis".... Bei der Lektüre braucht man bisweilen nur einige wenige Adjektive zu ändern, um Panizzas Anweisungen brauchbar zu machen als Handbuch für den zeitgenössischen Verfassungsschutz.' Drews, 'Aus Anlaß von Oskar Panizza'.

42 'Panizza verwandelt die politischen Kategorien in psychiatrische und rät als Teufels Advokat, mit einer rasant durchgehaltenen Ironie dazu, alle kritische, sprich: antiobrigkeitliche und speziell antimonarchistische Gesinnung als Geisteskrankheit, nämlich als verbrecherische Psychopathie zu verstehen.' Drews, 'Aus Anlaß von Oskar Panizza'. A similar sentiment is expressed by Klaus Völker, 'Phantast und Gelehrsamkeitspedant. Oskar Panizza: Auf dem Weg zu einer Wiederentdeckung des Verfemten', *Frankfurter Rundschau*, 19 January 1980.

43 Michel Foucault, *Herculine Barbin: Being the Recently Discovered Memoirs of a Nineteenth-Century French Hermaphrodite*, trans. Richard McDougall (Brighton: Harvester Press, 1980), p. xvii.

44 Brown, *Oskar Panizza*, p. 183.

45 Brown, *Oskar Panizza*, p. 182.

46 Bauer, *Oskar Panizza*, p. 219.
47 Jürgen Müller, *Der Pazjent als Psychiater: Oskar Panizzas Weg vom Irrenarzt zum Insassen* (Bonn: Narrenschiff, 1999), pp. 197–8.
48 Michael Bauer, 'Panizza, Leopold Hermann Oskar', *Neue Deutsche Biographie*, 20 (2001), pp. 30–2, www.deutsche-biographie.de/pnd118739131.html, accessed 13 August 2015.
49 '[S]elbst der Herausgeber ... rückt von einem künstlerischen Anspruch ab und betont den dokumentarischen Wert seiner Erscheinung für die Krankengeschichte des Kaiserreichs.' Ernst Stein, 'Ein grandioses Greuel. Scheiterhaufen oder Denkmal für Oskar Panizza', *Die Zeit*, 25 March 1966.
50 'Ein bedeutender Dichter war er nicht; dazu war sein Verhältnis zur Sprache zu unkontrolliert.' Fröhlich, 'Der deftigste und genialischste Polemiker deutscher Sprache'.
51 'Nicht immer gelang es Panizza, die Grenzen der Satire zu wahren und nicht zur direkten Polemik gegen die Politik jener überzugehen, an die sich seine Schrift angeblich wandte.' Bauer, *Oskar Panizza*, p. 202.
52 Düsterberg, '*Die gedrukte Freiheit*', pp. 138–9.
53 Bauer, *Oskar Panizza*, p. 202; Müller, *Der Pazjent als Psychiater*, pp. 95–7. Brown carefully separates biography and literary works, and while Panizza's works underpin his biography, he simply neglects Panizza's late oeuvre. Brown, *Oskar Panizza*, pp. 55–6. As for Bauer, Panizza's case writings play a minor role in his analysis, whereas, ironically, the psychiatrist Müller presents them – like his medical predecessors – both as a means of exoneration and as an expression of Panizza's delusion, without, however, considering their literary merit, or presenting the reader with a language-based understanding of psychosis.
54 See Joela Jacobs, '*Verbrechen wider die Natur*. Oskar Panizza's First Encounter with Censorship', in Godela Weiss-Sussex and Charlotte Woodford (eds), *Protest and Reform in German Literature and Visual Culture, 1871–1918* (Munich: Iudicium, 2015), pp. 125–38; Sophia Könemann, 'Von "Menschen-Bälgen", "kostbaren Rassen" und "Canarienvögeln": Fetischismus in Oskar Panizzas Erzählung "Der Corsetten-Fritz"', in Sophia Könemann and Anne Stähr (eds), *Das Geschlecht der Anderen. Figuren der Alterität: Kriminologie, Psychiatrie, Ethnologie und Zoologie* (Bielefeld: Transcript, 2011), pp. 171–86. Jacobs discusses *Das Verbrechen in Tavistock-Square* (1891) and Könemann 'Der Corsetten-Fritz' (1893).
55 Panizza also references psychiatry in his poetry; see the edited collection Oskar Panizza, *Das Rothe Haus. Lesebuch zu Religion, Sexus und Wahn*, ed. Michael Bauer (Munich: Allitera, 2003).
56 A detailed reception history of the English, French and German editions can be found in Birgit Lang, 'Michel Foucault, Herculine Barbin, and the Case Study Genre', in Tess Do, Véronique Duché and Andrea Rizzi (eds), *Mélanges. Festschrift for Anne Freadman* (Paris: Classiques Garnier, 2015), pp. 243–57.
57 Oskar Panizza, 'A Scandal at the Convent', in Foucault (ed.), *Herculine Barbin*, pp. 155–99, p. 193.
58 The original context of publication was Panizza's 1893 collection of short stories titled *Visionen. Skizzen und Erzählungen* (*Visions, Sketches and Stories*) – after *Dämmerungsstücke* (*Twilight Stories*) of 1890 and *Aus dem Tagebuch eines Hundes* (*Dog Diaries*) of 1892, his third and last extensive work of literary prose.
59 Staatsarchiv München (State Archives, Munich), Prosecution File 7122 (*Parisjana*).
60 Staatsarchiv München (State Archives, Munich), Prosecution File 7122 (*Parisjana*), Report Dr Ungemach, dated 10 March 1905, p. 11.
61 Müller, *Der Pazjent als Psychiater*, p. 212.
62 Hanns von Gumppenberg, *Lebenserinnerungen. Aus dem Nachlass des Dichters* (Berlin: Eigenbrödler Verlag, 1929), pp. 174–9.
63 Gumppenberg, *Lebenserinnerungen*, p. 173.
64 Bauer, *Oskar Panizza*, p. 99; Brown, *Oskar Panizza*, p. 83.

65 Quoted in Müller, *Der Pazjent als Psychiater*, p. 89.
66 Oskar Panizza, *Meine Verteidigung in Sachen 'Das Liebeskonzil': nebst dem Sachverständigen-Gutachten des Dr. M. G. Conrad und dem Urteil des k. Landgerichts München I* (Zurich: Schabelitz, 1895).
67 Bauer, *Oskar Panizza*, pp. 98–9.
68 'Wie sehr auch das Genie von der Mit- und mehr noch von der Nach-Welt angestaunt und bewundert wird, es selbst ist nicht glücklich. Es lebt vereinsamt und im steten Kampfe mit sich selbst.' Oskar Panizza, 'Genie und Wahnsinn, Vortrag', *Münchner Flugschriften*, 1:4/5 (1891), reprinted in Oskar Panizza, *Die kriminelle Psychose, genannt Psichopatia criminalis* (Munich: Matthes & Seitz, 1978), pp. 85–117, p. 117.
69 'Häufiger besteht jener Zustand, wo die aufsteigenden Bilder der Phantasie zwar als fremd, aber doch im eigenen Kopfe vorgehend, erkannt warden.' Panizza, 'Genie und Wahnsinn', p. 107.
70 Staatsarchiv München (State Archives, Munich), Prosecution File 7119 (*Liebeskonzil*): Petition for pardon dated 30 August 1895 submitted by defence lawyer Dr Kugelmann to His Most Serene Highness Prince and Ruler. (This was Luitpold Karl Joseph Wilhelm of Bavaria, Prince Regent for Otto I, who had been declared mentally incompetent on 10 June 1886; he died on 11 October 1916.) The German original reads: 'Ich habe als Verteidiger desselben die Frage indessen nicht anzuregen gewagt, weil der Angeklagte eine derartige Unterstellung nach seinem ganzen Temperament sehr schwerst zurückgewiesen haben würde'. The doctors who attested that Panizza was not of sound mind were Panizza's physician and friend Dr Paul Ostermaier (report dated 24 August 1895) and Dr Nobiling (report dated 21 August 1895). Dr Schmelcher, the resident physician of the prison in Amberg, disagreed (report dated 15 September 1895).
71 Staatsarchiv München (State Archives, Munich), Prosecution File 7119 (*Liebeskonzil*): Medical certificate, Dr Nobiling, dated 21 August 1895; medical certificate, Dr Ostermaier.
72 Staatsarchiv München (State Archives, Munich), Prosecution File 7119 (*Liebeskonzil*). The relevant passage from Ostermaier's report states: 'Herr Dr Oskar Panizza ist dem Unterfertigten seit nunmehr 19 Jahren genau bekannt. Der Unterfertigte hat seit dieser Zeit viel mit dem Rubrikaten sowohl gesellschaftlich als wissenschaftlich verkehrt und ist seit vielen Jahren zur Überzeugung gekommen, daß derselbe psychisch hochgradig krankhaft veranlagt ist und für alle seine Reden und Handlungen nicht zur Verantwortung gezogen werden kann'. Brown, *Oskar Panizza*, p. 46, summarises the above. Bauer, *Oskar Panizza*, p. 186, suggests that Kugelmann's plea contributed to Panizza's legal incapacitation later on.
73 Staatsarchiv München (State Archives, Munich), Prosecution File 7119 (*Liebeskonzil*), Report concerning Panizza by Dr Schmelcher, Amberg Prison, dated 15 September 1895.
74 Staatsarchiv München (State Archives, Munich), Prosecution File 7119 (*Liebeskonzil*), Report by Head of Amberg Prison Eiger, Amberg Prison, dated 20 November 1895. The German original reads: 'Bezüglich seines dermaligen geistigen Zustandes erklärt Panizza, daß er sich zwar noch als vollkommen zurechnungsfähig erachten zu denken glaube, jedoch zeitweilig wie alle verschiedenen geistig Arbeitenden an Stimmungsanomalien, geistigen Schwankungen, Depressionen leide, daß aber derlei Zustand bei ihm schon seit seiner frühesten Jugend bestanden hätte und sich auch naturgemäß unter dem Einfluss der Zellhaft und bei dem durch die Anstaltsverhältnisse bedingten, für ihn persönlich nicht ausreichenden freien Bewegung in frischer Luft ungünstig fortentwickeln müßte, daß er daher wiederholt inständig um Begnadigung oder doch eine Umwandlung seiner Haft in Festungshaft bitte'.
75 See Ylva Greve, *Verbrechen und Krankheit: Die Entdeckung der 'Criminalpsychologie' im 19. Jahrhundert* (Cologne: Böhlau, 2004).

76 Henry Zvi Lothane, 'Romancing Psychiatry: Paul Schreber, Otto Gross, Oskar Panizza – Personal, Social and Forensic Aspects', in Werber Felber, Albrecht Götz von Olenhusen, Gottfried Maria Heuer and Bernd Nitzschke (eds), *Psychoanalyse und Expressionismus. 7. Internationaler Otto-Gross-Kongress, Dresden* (Marburg: LiteraturWissenschaft.de, 2010), pp. 461–93.
77 Oskar Panizza, *Abschied von München. Ein Handschlag* (Zurich: Schabelitz, 1897), p. 15.
78 Bernd Nitzschke, *Die Psychoanalyse Sigmund Freuds: Konzepte und Begriffe* (Wiesbaden: VS Verlag, 2011), p. 165.
79 'Diese Leute glauben wahrhaftig, ... oder weil *Schiller* die "Räuber" geschrieben hat, sei ihnen Alles zu denken erlaubt.' Panizza, *Psichopatia criminalis*, p. 40.
80 Arndt, *Lehrbuch der Psychiatrie*, p. 297.
81 Arndt, *Lehrbuch der Psychiatrie*, pp. 486–7. Panizza never succumbed to such ideas. He was not deluded that he was the Emperor, but was deluded that the Emperor was persecuting him, and was deluded that Nietzsche did not exist.
82 Panizza, *Psichopatia criminalis*, p. 203.
83 'Dem Großen Megalomanen/In tiefster Ehrfurcht dargebracht/Der Psichjater.' Quoted in Düsterberg, '*Die gedrukte Freiheit*', p. 64.
84 Stijn Vanheule, *Subject of Psychosis: A Lacanian Perspective* (Basingstoke: Palgrave Macmillan, 2011), p. 73.
85 Jacques Lacan, *The Psychoses. The Seminar of Jacques Lacan. Book III 1955–1956*, ed. Jacques-Alain Müller (New York: Routledge, 1993), p. 193.
86 Sigmund Freud, 'The Interpretation of Dreams', in *The Standard Edition of the Complete Psychological Works of Sigmund Freud*, ed. James Strachey, with Anna Freud, Alix Strachey and Alan Tyson, vol. IV (London: Hogarth Press and Institute for Psychoanalysis, 1953), pp. ix–627, p. 217. The German original reads: '[Es] erinnert an ein stark revolutionäres Buchdrama von Oskar Panizza, in dem Gottvater als paralytischer Greis schmählich genug behandelt wird, dort heißt es: Wille und Tat sind bei ihm eines, und er muß von seinem Erzengel, einer Art Ganymed, abgehalten werden zu schimpfen und zu fluchen, weil diese Verwünschungen sich sofort erfüllen würden'. Sigmund Freud, 'V: Das Traummaterial und die Traumquellen', in Sigmund Freud, *Gesammelte Werke, chronologisch geordnet*, ed. Anna Freud, in collaboration with M. Bonaparte, E. Bibring, W. Hoffer, E. Kris and O. Isakower, vol. II/III (London: Imago, 1948), pp. 169–282, p. 222.
87 Jacques Lacan, *Paranoid Psychosis and Its Relation to the Personality* (1932), quoted in Vanheule, *Subject of Psychosis*, pp. 10–11.
88 Thomas Fuchs, 'Temporality and Psychopathology', *Phenomenology and the Cognitive Sciences*, 12:1 (2013), pp. 75–104, p. 93.
89 Monacensia, Literary Archive of the City of Munich, Oskar Panizza Papers, Oskar Panizza, 'Casus Conscientiae novissimorum temporum vom Pfaffen Panitius', unpublished manuscript of twenty-four pages dated 21 March 1903, p. 3, where the German original reads 'Wenn der Landesfürst, der Markgraf, der König, der Kaiser der Lustmörder ist?'
90 Vincent Crapanzano, 'The Postmodern Crisis: Discourse, Parody, Memory', in Amy Mandelker (ed.), *Bakthin in Contexts: Across the Disciplines* (Evanston: Northwestern University Press, 1995), pp. 137–50, p. 138.
91 Phiddian, 'Satire and the Limits of Literary Theory', p. 53.
92 Phiddian, 'Satire and the Limits of Literary Theory', p. 49.

4

Erich Wulffen and the case of the criminal

Birgit Lang

In 1927, the leading illustrated weekly *Berliner Illustrirte Zeitung* (*BIZ*) introduced its readers to the twenty-one most influential German criminologists of the day. Each was represented by a portrait photograph and a caption. The result was an iconography of experts in the burgeoning fields of studying, solving and writing about crime and criminals. Among the select group was Dr Erich Wulffen (1862–1936), Head of Department in the Saxon Ministry of Justice.[1] The photo essay describes Wulffen as the author of several criminological works on sex crime. Actually, the former state prosecutor can be considered Wilhelmine Germany's first legal expert; with reference to Reiner Grundmann and Nico Stehr's definition of such an expert, Wulffen was undoubtedly a broker of knowledge between specialist discourse and the wider public in modern society.[2] In addition, Wulffen wrote creative fiction on criminal psychology and legal reform.

During Wulffen's lifetime his published oeuvre included an unprecedentedly wide range of interdisciplinary cases: his case study compilations integrated sexological, psychiatric, psychoanalytic and anthropological insights to broaden the legal understanding of criminality. Through these compilations, Wulffen targeted the milieus of the court, the university and professionals within the penal system, but also the educated public. As a broker of knowledge between the law and the German people in the Wilhelmine and Weimar periods, Wulffen deserves special credit for shaping two new case modalities: the expert case and the case story. Wulffen's expert case studies relied on his privileged position and expertise to communicate new academic insights to the reading public. Wulffen's case stories were conceived as creative works of fiction with the purpose of illustrating certain criminal psychological insights gained in his academic work.

This chapter represents the most in-depth scholarly engagement with the breadth and nuance of Wulffen's case writings, and explores the intellectual contexts and case writing traditions that influenced Wulffen's use of case modalities: his humanist education, the cases and case writing traditions of the legal profession and forensics, and, most importantly, the role of the legal reform movement. Further, this chapter contextualises Wulffen's case writings in relation to his wider emancipatory project of educating a range of publics about the psychology of criminals – part of his attempt to further society's understanding of the criminal mind. Wulffen cleaved to his pedagogical project across the divide of the First World War, his sustained use of the case study genre defined by an ability to adapt case writings to particular audiences in Wilhelmine Germany. The period of the Weimar Republic proved more challenging to his larger project and to preserving the authority of what turned out to be a genre in crisis.

Like the fellow experts featured in the news magazine, Wulffen was a *modern* German mandarin. Fritz Ringer originally used the term 'mandarin' to reference the conservative nature of Germany's academic and legal elite, yet Wulffen was part of an overlooked group of legal reformers who sought to change the legal system from within.[3] This progressive German intellectual elite aimed to close the ever widening gap between intellectuals and the German public and – during the Weimar era – stood in support of the Republic. If Wulffen's efforts on behalf of legal reform in the Wilhelmine era had entailed a range of professional and political difficulties, after the war the tables turned. He returned from exile in Zwickau to his home town of Dresden, where he began a stellar career, soon becoming the first Director of the Saxon State Court; in 1923 he was appointed Head of Department in the Saxon Ministry of Justice. English-language secondary literature in particular tends to emphasise Wulffen's political engagement as a member of the German Democratic Party, and his sustained interest in legal reform, thus situating him at the (albeit crumbling) liberal hub of Weimar Germany.[4] He is overwhelmingly viewed as one of the early twentieth century's discerning observers of the psychological effects of war, who was also able to present 'a multifaceted picture of members of the criminal class'.[5]

Such a portrayal contrasts with German historiography, where Wulffen is considered to have perpetuated Cesare Lombroso's biological theories, and to have disseminated stereotypes about criminals, furthering the dreaded biologisation (*Biologisierung des Sozialen*) which culminated in discriminatory and calamitous National Socialist policies.[6] Yet, with the exception of female felons, Wulffen assumed criminality to be the result of three key factors: nature, nurture and fate. Accordingly, he took a sophisticated stance towards the Italian criminal anthropologist. That is, he summarised critical discourse concerning the reception of Lombroso in Germany and directly questioned Lombroso's theories.[7] It is notable that Berlin psychiatrist, psychoanalyst and social reformer Otto Juliusburger (1867–1952) called Wulffen 'the ingenious successor of Lombroso, and the destined reformer of the brittle, doomed old penal system'. This genealogy did not contradict Wulffen's acknowledged distance from Lombroso, nor the interdisciplinarity of Wulffen's approach – Juliusburger was well aware of Wulffen's psychoanalytic leanings.[8] Rather, Wulffen's works promised a new understanding of criminality and the criminal that transcended criminal anthropological insights. The pronounced differences between Lombroso and Wulffen were remarked upon by another contemporary, in a newspaper article which asserted one of the pillars of legal reform, namely that 'in contradiction to Lombroso's theories of the born criminal, Wulffen vindicates the point of view that criminality is latently present in every human being'.[9]

The most satisfying way to describe Wulffen's position during the Weimar period is as a mediator between the opposing discourses of nature and nurture in Weimar criminology, which, as Richard F. Wetzell has noted, became increasingly dominated by biological explanatory models.[10] Psychoanalysts and criminal psychologists focused their attention on criminality's effects on society, while criminal biology increasingly favoured biological explanations of crime. The criminal psychologist Wulffen sympathised with the former position – although he became disgruntled by psychoanalysis – while insisting on the relevance of biological factors, and adhering to a medical framework that he had referenced from the very beginning of his explorations of crime. The partial judgement of Wulffen as an adherent to notions of degeneration originates in Wulffen's post-war works on female criminality, in which he did revive some of Lombroso's theories. The fact that against the zeitgeist Wulffen viewed female felons as more degenerate than their male counterparts can be partly explained by his methodology. For better and for worse, Wulffen's empiricist framework and case-based methodology were not amenable to drastic paradigm shifts, since change could be accommodated only through the integration of new case material. Consequently, he was unable to integrate the paradigm shift represented by the emancipation of women in the Weimar era.

In addition, Wulffen's position as a writer of case studies became increasingly complicated due to the criminological fantasies of German society. The depiction of crime in Weimar popular culture, its 'dominance and prevalence as a cultural symbol' for the Weimar era, have long been noted in secondary literature.[11] Todd Herzog has skilfully elaborated how, in the face of rising crime statistics, discourse about crime became all-encompassing and remained so even after 1924, once criminality declined.[12] For Weimar journalists and many of their readers, criminals became a central symbol for the disrupted social order of the time.[13] Correspondingly, the pervasiveness of criminality as a metaphor becomes obvious in the works of key Weimar intellectuals such as Walter Benjamin and Carl Schmitt.[14] Herzog shows how the complex interweaving of documentary evidence with sensationalist cases, as seen, for instance, in Fritz Lang's cinematic oeuvre, led to a collapse of boundaries between fact and fiction.[15] Such new developments brought into question Wulffen's educational project, in which fiction was put to serve criminology, although with a keen awareness of the limitations of conflating fact with fiction. In

Wulffen's eyes this could only further the negative romanticising of crime and sexuality in contemporary society. Thus, during the Weimar era, this unorthodox thinker and practitioner of the case became a somewhat conflicted proponent of sexual modernity.

Indeed, the five-part definition of sexual modernity put forth by Harry Oosterhuis is particularly applicable to a study of Wulffen's ideas.[16] Firstly, Wulffen believed sexuality to be an inevitable, natural force and one that greatly influenced criminality. Secondly, Wulffen's understanding of the effects of criminality and sexuality was psychological. Thirdly, as a criminal psychologist, Wulffen both classified and subverted the normal and abnormal, always assuming that anyone had the potential to become a criminal. He did, however, incontrovertibly favour the procreative norm over the pleasure and relational dimensions of sexuality. He believed the latter to be an important factor in the development of female criminality in particular, a topic that became central to Wulffen's late oeuvre. Despite the great success of his academic case compilations on criminal psychology and sex offenders, his views on female felons proved controversial among colleagues and his wider readership. Wulffen's views of sexual identity – the fifth criterion in Oosterhuis's definition – also grew increasingly conflicted with regard to the nexus between sexuality and criminality. This conservatism represented an 'occupational hazard' of sorts. Yet it is also expresses the dilemma of seeking to retain a balanced position in political and academic milieus that became increasingly radicalised on the one hand and biologised on the other.

Embracing the case

Wulffen's adoption of the case study genre in Wilhelmine Germany was extraordinarily successful. Above all, his academic case compilations hit a nerve and were well received in psychiatric, legal and progressive circles. *Psychologie des Verbrechers* (*The Psychology of Criminals*), first published in 1906 and reissued in 1908, was reviewed in all the major German newspapers.[17] Similarly, *Der Sexualverbrecher* (*Sex Offender*) was reprinted three times in three months following its first publication in 1910. Hailed as the new Lombroso by Juliusburger, even reviews that were critical of some aspects of the work welcomed the new turn to casuistry. In his review of *Der Sexualverbrecher*, Carl Gustav Jung (1875–1961), founder of analytic psychology and at that time still a robust ally of Sigmund Freud, noted that the criminalistic casuistry presented by Wulffen, and the investigation of crime's psychological and sociological foundations, made the volume 'a valuable source' ('eine schätzenswerte Quelle') for future psychoanalytic enquiries in the field.[18]

The inspiration for embracing a genre that by the mid-nineteenth century had been pushed out of the realm of legal instruction at university originated from a desire to understand the driving forces behind criminality and to gain insight into the psyche of the criminal. In German legal history, such a way of thinking is inextricably linked with legal reformer Franz von Liszt (1851–1919), a younger cousin of the famous composer. Liszt had founded the Internationale Kriminalistische Vereinigung (or IKV, the International Criminological Association) in 1889, together with Belgian criminologist Adolphe Prins, Professor at Brussels University (later Vice Chancellor), and Dutch law professor Joost Adrian van Hamel. Liszt's scholarship in criminal law – widely disseminated through his 1881 textbook *Das deutsche Reichsstrafrecht* (*German Imperial Criminal Law*) – had already managed to shift the prevailing perspective from the authority of the law to that of the criminal act and its perpetrators. It opened positive law to a key new thought, namely that anyone could become a criminal given the chance: hence the degree of criminality should be judged by the perpetrator's potential for reform. Liszt consequently argued that opportunistic criminals should receive suspended sentences; reformable perpetrators should receive custodial sentences, with special measures taken for their resocialisation; repeat offenders should be held permanently in custody. In all, Liszt spearheaded the modern school of criminology and, as remarked by American legal scholar Arthur J. Todd in 1914–15, Germany's new penal code rested 'to no small extent upon the work of the I.K.V.'[19]

Wulffen's encounter with Liszt's modern school of criminology in 1903 had a palpable effect on his writings, and forms the beginning of Wulffen's new appreciation of the case study genre, a genre which had already defined his everyday work as a state prosecutor for several years. The passion and playfulness that Wulffen displayed in his engagement with this genre were mediated through forensic medicine and shaped by his humanistic education as well as his literary ambitions. Case writing gave voice to a crisis of expression that had accompanied Wulffen through his legal studies, glimpses of which are expressed in his 1913 roman-à-clef *Frau Justitias Walpurgisnacht* (*The Walpurgis Night of Mrs Justice*). Publication of this novel saw Wulffen demoted from his post as State Prosecutor for Criminal Affairs in Dresden to the status of Councillor for Civil Affairs at the Magistrate's Court in provincial Zwickau.[20] An unpublished autobiographical sketch dating to 1932 likewise reveals that Wulffen's first inclination had been to study not law, but literature.[21] However, a fatherly intervention and the son's orientation towards the goals of his fellow high school students resulted in a decision to study law.[22] In Wulffen's roman-à-clef the main character, Wartenberg, is easily identifiable as the author; for instance, Wartenberg – just like Wulffen in 1908 – delivers a lecture titled 'Der Strafprozeß – ein Kunstwerk der Zukunft' ('The Criminal Trial as a Future Work of Art'). Wartenberg 'went with a full, warm heart into [the] unknown academic field [of law]', only to realise that 'matters of the heart were of no relevance'.[23] The novel criticises the 'stuffy' court systems of the time, as well as German legalese, renowned for its impenetrability. When Wartenberg seeks to challenge legal writing conventions he is rebuffed:

> Now he had to hear that he had no clue about legal writing style. From the corrections of the local judge he saw what was needed. He had stressed the emotional and lively side of the criminal event. That was not allowed.[24]

Likewise, the autobiographical sketch reports how, during his time as an assessor, Wulffen was criticised for his ornate writing style, which not did not seem austere enough.[25]

According to Wulffen, his literary and theatrical ambitions subsided only after his encounter with representatives of the German division of the IKV, an occasion he describes as a 'decisive turning point' ('entscheidende Wendung') in his life, at age forty-one. In 1903, Wulffen had been invited to the association's ninth German gathering, in Dresden, and he reported on the event for the scientific supplement of the most important local daily newspaper, the *Dresdner Anzeiger*.[26] In the modern school of criminology Wulffen found the answer to his question of whether law and art could complement one another. Apparently, the insight that criminal proceedings could and should utilise analysis of the 'interior life and character, motif and environment of the perpetrator' meant that Wulffen could invest his imaginative powers in his work, rather than into separate creative ventures.[27] The same insight enabled him to reframe works of German and world literature as 'textbook examples of criminal psychological literature'.[28] Friedrich Schiller and Johann Wolfgang von Goethe and their engagement with criminality held a special fascination for Wulffen throughout his career, and in time he put these figures into the service of criminology.[29]

Two years after his first encounter with the modern school of criminology, Wulffen's first published discussion of a legal case (1905), 'Ein kriminalpsychologisches Experiment' ('A Criminal Psychological Experiment'), highlighted the shift in his understanding of crime and his new affiliation with the burgeoning field of criminal psychology. Published in Gustav Aschaffenburg's well respected journal *Monatsschrift für Kriminalpsychologie und Strafrechtsreform* (*Monthly Journal for Criminal Psychology and Legal Reform*), the case history essays the possibilities for ethically influencing the life of a 'criminal character'. Wulffen presents the example of twenty-six-year-old 'Arthur Br.', who had been wrongly convicted of theft as a repeat offender. Under Wulffen's administration the case had gone to retrial and the accused was acquitted, but Arthur Br. approached Wulffen, seeking to regain his status as a prisoner, because life in prison had provided him with 'food, work and order'.[30] Wulffen was eventually able to place Arthur Br. with a Dresden welfare association and even invited Arthur Br. to his own home for the Christmas celebrations. Nonetheless, when the court financially compensated Arthur Br. for his wrongful imprisonment, he quit his job, paid his debts and left for

Berlin, only to return once depleted of his funds. By way of a conclusion, Wulffen states that 'ethical interference' ('ethische Beeinflussung') might bring temporary relief, thus exerting some positive influence. Yet his verdict is unambiguous:

> Disposition, education and fate have made him [Arthur Br.] what he is, and what he is destined to be. There is no escape from these three sisters of fate. Weakness of the will is his allotted part, as other people suffer from different organic failures. So help him God![31]

Wulffen's first case history written for an educated and professional public exemplifies the conflation of scientific and moral categories of analysis that Silviana Galassi considers typical for Wilhelmine criminology.[32] It also discloses the empathy of a state prosecutor and – in this case at least – Wulffen's exceptional goodwill. The same article underlines contemporary prejudice towards former convicts, and presents a 'best practice' case: Wulffen outlines how he arranges for Arthur Br.'s wages to be paid daily, and advises him to open a savings account, presenting his subject in a likeable light. He also emphasises that, based on aspects of the circumstantial evidence, and other details of the case, any other court would have convicted Arthur Br., since errors of justice are inherent to the justice system. Wulffen's stern assessment of the inevitable fate of Arthur Br. could be rendered more generously: the facts that Arthur Br. paid off his debt with the compensation monies, and did not commit another criminal offence, might be interpreted together as an indication of reasonable success.

Wulffen's turn to the case study genre was unusual for someone in his profession. This seems surprising, considering that legal cases and related case studies represented an integral part of judicial life. As a state prosecutor in the German legal system, Wulffen came into contact with a whole range of case files; he was responsible for the preparation of a great variety of such files in connection with the three-stage German court process. To this day, the process comprises an initial investigatory phase (*Vorverfahren*), the decision-making process if the case should proceed to trial (*Beschlusskammer*) and the trial itself (*Hauptverfahren*).[33] In the role of state prosecutor, Wulffen was actively involved in all three stages, collecting, examining and partly composing or supervising the composition of relevant materials and organising these neatly into a court file register, where the various entries were made chronologically: the record of interrogation of the accused; witness statements; on-site inspections; the results of the *Beschlusskammer*; as well as contributions from court-appointed experts, and from forensic, psychiatric and police reports; and any other significant incriminating materials, such as letters or diaries.

Despite the prevalence of case studies in the everyday professional life of the court, legal journals refrained from publishing casuistry. As a consequence, journals important to the German legal profession, such as the generalist *Deutsche Juristen-Zeitung* (1896–1919) (*Organ of German*

Jurists), in which Wulffen published his views on legal reform, were not publishing casuistry. *Der Gerichtssaal* (1849–1919) (*The Courtroom*), a progressive journal dedicated to popular law and scientific practices, presented case writings only rarely. Until Wulffen's arrival in criminal psychological circles, even Gustav Aschaffenburg's influential journal *Monatsschrift für Kriminalpsychologie und Strafrechtsreform* (*Monthly Journal for Criminal Psychology and Penal Reform*) presented case studies in a designated section titled 'Sprechsaal', a 'speakers' corner' concerned with day-to-day judicial business. Earlier criminal psychological works such as Hans Gross's *Kriminalpsychologie* (1898) remained widely discursive and did not include case materials. This lack was a direct consequence of the fact that the German legal system was (and is) not case-based like the common law, but was defined through abstract and conceptual reasoning. While legal change in a common law system is driven by precedent, and thus makes casuistry highly relevant to legal professionals, civil law negotiates changes through federal parliament. Within the German legal system, judges have traditionally had greater influence than those in common law legal systems.

When Wulffen himself set about writing academic case compilations, he used the generic frame provided by forensic medicine. Richard F. Wetzell has helpfully outlined the mutual benefits arising from the medicalisation of penal reform and sees 'the penal reform agenda ... significantly influenced by medical theories and practices'.[34] The combination of discourse and casuistry that defined forensic textbooks became determinative for Wulffen's academic case studies as well. The first reference to forensic psychiatry in Wulffen's oeuvre can be found in an eleven-page discussion of the treatment of legal issues in the play *Rose Bernd*, a 1903 drama by naturalist German writer Gerhart Hauptmann (1862–1946), inspired by Hauptmann's jury service on the case of child murderer Hedwig Otte. Wulffen's discussion explains the legal context of the drama and elaborates on Hauptmann's inclusion of psychiatric knowledge of female hysteria.[35] In this context, Wulffen quotes leading psychiatrist August Cramer (1860–1912), then director of the psychiatric clinic in Göttingen, and his work *Gerichtliche Psychiatrie* (*Forensic Psychiatry*), which was written for physicians and lawyers, and contained a range of case studies. Thereafter, all of Wulffen's criminal psychological textbooks followed the forensic model.

Criminal psychological case compilations differed from medical case studies through the evidence provided, which, as expected, originated from medical and legal discourse but also included expertise from fields such as criminal statistics, criminal anthropology, psychoanalysis and literature. A review of *Der Sexualverbrecher* by Dresden lawyer Dr Glaser underlines, for instance, the value of the new psychoanalytic aetiology that was championed by Wulffen for the world of law. To conceptualise crime and criminality through the lens of sadism, masochism, fetishism and homosexuality, in combination with social factors, had the advantage of pointing out phenomena which, 'especially for the judge, were not considered enough, if at all. And it sheds light into the gaping abyss of criminal souls, that even today remain murky and incomprehensible to many'.[36]

In twenty-first-century secondary literature, this medley of knowledge is usually ignored, or criticised. Well known historian of sexuality Volkmar Sigusch considers Wulffen's works unscientific, while Sace Elder calls Wulffen 'an indefatigable synthesizer and popularizer of criminal science (often at the expense at scientific rigor)'.[37] Galassi has argued more generally that the insufficient academic professionalisation opened the door to the political appropriation of criminology by National Socialism.[38] Yet such criticism does not explain the appeal of Wulffen's compilations for his contemporaries, which lies in the interdisciplinary method now disparaged. Reviewers of Wulffen's works were most impressed by his ability to synthesise several discourses from a range of monographs and professional journals, and to provide much-needed reference works.[39] Thus, the overall goal of these case compilations was to educate readers and to sharpen expert eyes by making available comparable casuistry and new explanatory frameworks. They provided professional and educated readers with an archive of casuistry, allowing them to make more informed judgements about criminals and their crimes.

Like medicine, criminal psychology needed to find laws for irregular phenomena that were embodied by a specific group of people.[40] Such an undertaking required a range of theories; in the case study compilation these were represented through broad discursive-scientific narratives. The individual cases then provided evidence for these theories, while also serving as illustrations. Neither doctors nor criminal psychologists assumed that any single individual would fit their categories perfectly. As Wulffen outlines in his contested *Das Weib als Sexualverbrecherin* (*Female Sex Offenders*), 'the individuals questioned are never typical men or women, but – according to biological knowledge – can only ever be individuals with a greater or lesser element of the characteristics of the opposite sex'.[41] This also implies that a range of theories could coexist, although they did not always seamlessly integrate.

Yet Wulffen did not stop at the creation of case study compilations. Against the backdrop of the crisis of legitimacy surrounding the German legal system in the late nineteenth and twentieth centuries, accused of class bias (*Klassenjustiz*) and of being disconnected from 'the real world' (*Weltfremdheit*), Wulffen also developed the case study genre beyond criminal psychological case compilations.[42] His choice of register for these more unusual case modalities – that is, his expert legal commentaries and crime novels – were informed by case knowledge he had acquired during his education in a humanist gymnasium. Wulffen attended the renowned Dresden Kreuzgymnasium (literally, 'High School of the Cross'), one of the oldest German schools, dating to the fourteenth century. Like all graduates from Wilhelmine gymnasia, he was familiar with the case as a rhetorical device through the study of classical literature. As a gymnasium student he would have learned about the necessity of aligning an illustrative case with his main argument in order to remain convincing; from Cicero in particular he learned to address his audiences in different registers, whether to inform, to move or to delight.[43] As a writer, Wulffen made a precise and deliberate appeal to his readership. Through his criminal psychological case compilations he aimed to inform; readers were delighted by his expert case studies of criminals, as well as his literary and cultural histories of the representation of sexuality in art and literature. His case stories aimed to move the wider general public and to illustrate criminal psychological knowledge. In all three case modalities he aimed to convey the insights of criminal psychology.

Wulffen's key concerns are easily discernible and shaped by his legal reform background and his close affinity to the modern school of criminology. While Wulffen might appear a 'Jack of all trades', if he did include a wide range of evidence in his case studies he did so with the self-confidence of a legal professional. Unlike the common law system, where evidence must conform to a number of rules to be admissible, the legal system in Germany accepts as evidence whatever the judge sees fit to admit. Wulffen differed from fellow members of the judiciary in that he showed a genuine preoccupation with the emotional and interior life of criminals. This could not be expressed in his legal studies until his encounter with the modern school of criminology, and subsequently with the case study genre, which made it possible for Wulffen to explore a legal language that he felt comfortable to speak.

Exceptional criminals: con men

Throughout his career, Wulffen retained a deep concern with exceptionally intelligent criminals, especially con men. Analysis of Wulffen's case writings on the topic brings to light ways in which he fashioned different case modalities. The profile of the con man as a type of criminal seemed to Wulffen different from that of other offenders: criminals were usually considered to be below average in intelligence, already facing learning problems while in the educational system, and liable to experience difficulties in logical thinking. Con men operated in a different league.[44] Their deceptive nature, their theatrical talents and their methods for seducing their victims, while loved by the public, made them an especially pertinent subject of investigation for criminal psychology. Imposture was the topic that inspired Wulffen to write his first book-length expert case study – on Georges Manolescu (1871–1908), con man and hotel thief extraordinaire – as well as several fictionalised case stories inspired by the Manolescu case. The most successful of these was Wulffen's 1917 best-selling crime novel *Der Mann mit den sieben Masken* (*The Man with the Seven Masks*), which was made into a film in 1918.

A comparison of expert case study and case story showcases Wulffen's ability to adapt case writings to particular audiences in an attempt to educate them, as well as to communicate criminal psychological insights to a wide readership. Wulffen's pioneering work on con men represents the earliest academic investigations of this phenomenon in the German-speaking world and it preceded relevant psychoanalytic investigations by nearly two decades. If psychoanalysis has contributed most to the psychological understanding of imposture, it was also instrumental in sidelining Wulffen's earlier insights, as the following explorations show.

By the early twentieth century, Wulffen's interest in legal reform, and his attempt to close the communication gap between the court and the public, had led him to deliver public lectures, write contributions to academic and legal journals, and write to newspapers on the topic of criminality.[45] Wulffen's first extensive expert case study, *Georges Manolescu und seine Memoiren. Kriminalpsychologische Studie* (*Georges Manolescu and His Memoirs: A Criminal Psychological Study*) was published in 1907, following the publication of Manolescu's memoirs in 1905 and 1907.[46] The media hype surrounding these memoirs represented an ethical challenge, due to the romanticisation of criminality, but also an opportunity. The memoirs allowed Wulffen to develop new insights into the workings of a fascinating criminal mind, to build his profile as an expert in legal matters, and to promote the criminal psychological cause beyond the academic sphere. They also permitted Wulffen to remind the German public of the detrimental consequences of Manolescu's actions, and of the unstable source of their excitement. After all, Wulffen believed that those members of the German public who so feverishly consumed the works of the suave Romanian hotel thief were also easily victimised. It was Wulffen's view that, due to their love of everything foreign, Germans were especially credulous and susceptible to imposture.[47]

Manolescu was one of the first convicted criminals in Germany to publish his memoirs with a reputable and entrepreneurial publisher, Paul Langenscheidt. This made the memoirs accessible not only to a specialised readership but, simultaneously, to a general audience. Up to this point, case studies by convicted criminals had been published in academic contexts, notably in Lombroso's *Archivio di Psichiatria* (1880–1909), which contained a series of autobiographical texts by psychiatric patients, together with Lombroso's extensive commentary – sometimes without the patient's awareness of the publication. A more religious framework of penance was the context for publications edited by prison chaplains, such as Johannes Jaeger's *Hinter Kerkermauern* (1906). In British autobiographies of convicted criminals, the theme of redemption played an important role until the 1930s, when a shift occurred towards a more psychological interpretation, though it still included the notion of redemptive suffering.[48] The more psychological narratives helped to curb the potential hype surrounding these works and gave them an aura of respectability. In the German context, a shift to a psychologising framework took place much earlier.

In retrospect, such publication practices certainly appear ethically questionable, and represent key examples of the control wielded by clinics and prisons over their subjects, as emphasised by Michel Foucault. Yet Manolescu's publication of his memoirs for a general readership through Langenscheidt involved its own ethical challenges, including the romanticising and trivialisation of crime in general, and secondary trauma caused to victims. It also yielded financial and potential emotional benefits to a convicted criminal who had escaped from psychiatric institutionalisation in Germany, and who eventually settled as a free man in France, where he died in 1908.[49]

Wulffen's study of Manolescu negotiated in new ways the worlds of law and the public sphere and made Langenscheidt the publisher of the first legal expert case study. Wulffen set forth a new kind of in-depth analysis of the character of a con man in German criminology. Written in a measured tone, and in a language that was free from legal jargon, this expert case study presented a thoroughgoing character analysis of Manolescu himself, and explained the impact of Manolescu's deeds on his victims (including Manolescu's wife and daughter). Wulffen brought to this analysis more than just an inquisitive mind and a deep understanding of the German legal system. As a state prosecutor, he was a respectable public figure. Through his professional role he enjoyed privileged access to a wide range of police and court files often unavailable to other contemporary writers and crime reporters such as Paul Lindau (1839–1919), Hans Hyan (1868–1941) or Paul Schlesinger (1878–1928).[50] These well known crime writers were obliged to request permission from the local court for access to court files and they were unable to order files from other jurisdictions, while Wulffen consulted relevant judicial and police records from other European countries.[51] Wulffen's high standing might explain also why the megalomaniac Manolescu agreed to correspond with him. In his memoirs Manolescu acknowledged his attraction to the 'cat and mouse' game he played with judicial and penal authorities as well as the police; according to Wulffen, Manolescu even offered his own remains to Lombroso, revealing his enthralment with the word of criminology.[52]

By today's standards, Manolescu fulfils all assessment criteria of the Hare Psychopathy Checklist – Revised (PCL-R); since the 1990s this psychological diagnostic tool has been commonly used to assess the presence of psychopathy in individuals. Judging from Manolescu's autobiography and Wulffen's study, Manolescu was superficially charming, possessed a grandiose sense of self-worth, lied pathologically and was cunning and manipulative. His affective capacities were limited and he lacked remorse; he was emotionally shallow, lacked empathy and failed to accept responsibility for his actions. His lifestyle was parasitic and revealed a need for stimulation. He lacked realistic long-term goals (apart from becoming rich), was impulsive and irresponsible. In all, he demonstrated a range of antisocial behaviours, as well as promiscuous sexual behaviour.

Aspects of Wulffen's criminal psychological language for describing Manolescu's behaviour prefigure this current vocabulary of psychopathology; he includes biological and environmental explanations. To Wulffen, Manolescu unambiguously presented as a degenerate maniac, that is, a person whose mental illness is marked by periods of great excitement, delusions and over-activity, and who is missing the physical, mental or moral qualities considered normal and desirable. Manolescu's Romanian origins and his southern race played a key role in Wulffen's profiling of the con man, and was used to explain the degree of his mania, factors that helped Wulffen to situate Manolescu's crimes in line with contemporary forensic notions of criminality. Yet to Wulffen the most important reason why Manolescu was 'in reality even more interesting and of greater significance than the memoirs reveal him to be' lay in the psychological make-up of Manolescu's personality.[53]

Wulffen's expert case study includes a detailed reconstruction of Manolescu's life history, based on police and judicial files, the original French manuscripts of the memoirs, newspaper articles and other materials, which are compared in detail with statements made by Manolescu in his autobiography. Wulffen verifies Manolescu's statements where possible, unveils his lies, describes Manolescu's omissions in his memoirs and corrects his exaggerations.[54] In addition, Wulffen questions Manolescu's self-image as energetic, disciplined, self-controlled and determined. These were largely figments of Manolescu's imagination – so Wulffen argues – with Manolescu's character defined by an 'instinctual primordialism' that led Manolescu to reinterpret his actions retrospectively, and to embellish his explication with grandiose notions of self.[55]

Wulffen's psychological insights into Manolescu's psyche seem considerable. They pre-empt and parallel psychoanalytic insights on imposture that to this day dominate in the relevant specialist literature. For example, his insights parallel Helene Deutsch's 1955 case study of imposture, in which she states:

> Reading his [the patient Jimmy's] life history, one sees that he was perpetually in pursuit of an identity which would do justice to his narcissistic conception of himself in terms of 'I am a genius,' and which at the same time would serve to deny his own identity. This denial of his own identity appears to me to be the chief motive for his actions, as is true in the case of other impostors.[56]

Similarly, Wulffen convincingly argues that Manolescu fails to take responsibility for his actions, and lacks ethical feelings for victims of his crimes.[57] Two years before Freud described the 'family romances' of neurotics, and half a century before Phyllis Greenacre identified the compulsive pressure to live out the 'dominant and dynamically active family romance' as one of three constitutive factors in the personality of impostors, Wulffen describes Manolescu's fixation on his family romance, repeated in his relationships with his wife and daughter.[58]

The difference between the criminal psychological analysis and psychoanalytic analysis of imposture is important to discern, because it helps to explain the ways these two fields of knowledge developed. Specifically, a comparison between Wulffen's works and the first exploratory case study of the phenomenon by German psychoanalyst Karl Abraham in 1925, 'Die Geschichte eines Hochstaplers im Lichte psychoanalytischer Erkenntnis' ('The History of an Impostor in the Light of Psychoanalytical Knowledge'), sheds light on the differences in methodology and the mutual reception of criminal psychology and of psychoanalysis.[59] As mentioned, Wulffen's aetiology was based on psychoanalytic categories. Indeed, the minutes of the Vienna Psychoanalytic Society, or WPV, reveal that his reception of psychoanalytic theories was noted in psychoanalytic circles.[60] However, in the mid-1920s, when psychoanalysts turned their investigations towards the area of the law and criminality, considerable tension arose between criminal psychologists like Wulffen and psychoanalysts like Abraham. Abraham sidelined Wulffen's body of work, and yet the insights developed in the two fields of knowledge are complementary.[61]

Abraham's 1925 case study describes the fate of a con man who overcame his condition–through a marriage that represented the 'complete psychological fulfilment of an infantile wish-situation'.[62] Wulffen also contemplates the reasons behind Manolescu's marriage, but does not focus on the positive influence of this marriage, which seems to have enabled Manolescu to abstain from committing criminal acts for almost a year. Rather – and here lies a key difference in approach – Wulffen describes the detrimental effects of the marriage on Manolescu's wife and daughter. While Abraham focuses on the childhood fantasies of his subject of study, Wulffen engages with Manolescu's adult fantasies. According to Wulffen, Manolescu remained fixated on his family (his marriage to a German countess can be interpreted as wish fulfilment) but the 'affect for his daughter remains phantasmatic, in that it is not directed in a real, practical, and caring manner towards his daughter'.[63] Instead, Manolescu 'torments his family and then cries about the fact like a child'.[64]

The respective case studies authored by Wulffen and Abraham lie nearly twenty years apart, and their contrasting focus can be explained in part by the severity of symptoms presented by the two criminal subjects in question, and partly by the different methodology the intellectuals used. Wulffen explains Manolescu's disposition with considerable psychological insight, and underlines the impacts of Manolescu's behaviour on his family and society in general. He develops the language of criminal psychology further through a contemporary medical framework that identifies Manolescu as an incorrigible criminal. Abraham steers his argument in another direction. Although he states that his article represents a bridge between psychoanalysis and criminology, he takes a decided stance in relation to degeneration, arguing that 'we should not overestimate heredity, "degeneration" in its role in the genesis of asocial and criminal behaviour'.[65] Rather, concludes Abraham, his case represents another instance that strongly suggests a fundamental role played by early childhood, while the phenomenon of the con man is usually explained through the degeneration model.[66]

Abraham's comment on the prevalence of the degeneration model in criminology might be read as an allusion to Wulffen's Manolescu study, or to his 1923 study *Die Psychologie des Hochstaplers* (*The Psychology of the Con Man*), which again contained biological but predominantly psychological insights, and was published two years before Abraham's article. Otherwise Abraham chose to sideline Wulffen altogether. There would have been ample opportunity to relate Wulffen's psychological insights in his own study, but Abraham's article constitutes a notable occasion on which a psychoanalytic thinker skated over a body of knowledge first explored through criminal psychology. Abraham preferred to reference the work of Austrian school teacher and psychoanalyst August Aichhorn (1878–1949), who was at the time working with troubled youth. Thereby Abraham constructed a narrative of hope and change, rather than what he perceived to be a narrative of stigmatisation. As discussed below, this strategy might have contributed to Wulffen's alienation from the formerly revered Viennese school of thought.

Wulffen did not yet have at his disposal the psychoanalytic vocabulary for analysis of imposture, but his description of Manolescu seems closer to later psychoanalytic explanations of the phenomenon than to the biological framework otherwise employed in *Georges Manolescu und seine Memoiren*. He foreshadowed a relational approach, which emerged predominantly in American psychoanalytic thought, first through psychiatrist Harry Stack Sullivan (1892–1949) and then through the relational turn of the 1980s. Conversely, Abraham focused solely on the subject of his case, gave informed speculations about the latter's childhood fantasies – he had not able to conduct psychoanalysis – but did not consider the implications of the marriage for the spouse and her family. His sidelining of Wulffen might have been a reaction to the shift towards the biological model in psychiatry, but also an attempt to claim new psychoanalytic territory, at the cost of a loss of knowledge.

Der Mann mit den sieben Masken as a case story

Wulffen's expert case studies and academic case compilations aimed to convince an educated public through insightful observation and by means of argumentation. His case *stories*, on the other hand, illustrated the criminal psychological arguments developed in his analytical work, educating the wider public through their recreational reading and by means of catharsis. Poetic licence also allowed Wulffen to explore case materials that were inappropriate in his academic and expert case studies:

he could write so as not to reveal personal details and further stigmatise the victims of impostors.

Wulffen's case stories of imposture comprise a range of works, the most important of which is his 1917 crime novel *Der Mann mit den sieben Masken*. Wulffen wrote his crime novels during his period 'in exile', after his transfer to Zwickau between 1914 and 1919, following publication of his roman-à-clef. Each novel represents a mixture of legal thriller and police procedural, mostly featuring as the main investigator a state prosecutor who is interested in criminal psychology.[67] Three works stand out for their success: *Der Mann mit den sieben Masken* focuses on imposture; *Die Kraft des Michael Arbogast* (*The Powers of Michael Arbogast*), published in the same year, describes the fate of a former criminal who fails once his previous conviction becomes known; and *Die geschlossene Kette* (*The Closed Chain*) (1919) problematises conviction for murder where the evidence is only circumstantial. Each of these works illustrates insights that Wulffen had gained in his academic case studies, and makes them palpable to a reading audience beyond the educated middle class.

Der Mann mit den sieben Masken became Wulffen's greatest success as a writer of fiction. The work was first printed as a serialised novel in 1916 in the *Berliner Tageblatt*, which together with the *Vossische Zeitung* was the most influential Berlin newspaper at the time.[68] *Der Mann mit den sieben Masken* then reached four reprintings with publisher Reissner in the first year of its publication in 1917, and was reprinted as a serialised novel in the Protestant nationalist *München-Augsburger Abendzeitung*.[69] In August 1918, Wulffen was approached by Messter Film Berlin concerning the film rights to the story. Within five weeks the film was adapted for the screen by Danish film actor, director, producer, silent-movie pioneer and creator of a Sherlock Holmes series Viggo Larsen (1880–1957); Wulffen provided the film script.[70] Lastly, in 1922 and 1928, renowned publisher Ullstein, one of the most active and successful German publishers of popular literature, included *Der Mann mit den sieben Masken* in the first and second incarnation of the Yellow Series, which focused on crime, adventure and society novels, and targeted a mass audience.

Der Mann mit den sieben Masken was well received in legal as well as progressive liberal circles, and more generally by the wider German public. In an essay on the nature of imposture the then Director of the Brandenburg State Court Albert Hellwig (1880–1950) stressed the importance of Wulffen's achievement.

> I do not feel the urge to comment on the literary value of [t]his work. From the perspective of criminal psychology, however, without doubt we are dealing with an extraordinarily instructive book, which nonetheless forms a compelling and good read [*Unterhaltungslektüre*] as well. The expert will recognise the original material from which the poet-criminologist draws [i.e. the Manolescu case]. It is remarkable how Wulffen has utilised his academic sources, how he created poetically from reality, without negating the criminal psychological meaning of his account.[71]

Other reviews focus on the story-line in greater detail, especially on the most evocative protagonist of the crime novel, state prosecutor Dr Sperl, who, like other characters in the book, falls victim to the charms of con man Niklas Györki. While at least partly conscious of his fascination with Györki, through a mixture of epistemophilia and insecurity, the all-too-human Sperl becomes deeply involved in the con man's psychological game, ultimately compromising Sperl's own ethical boundaries. Sperl's complicity in this relationship makes him vulnerable, and leads him to commit suicide.

All reviews comment on the scene in which Györki 'reels in' the enthusiastic criminal psychologist who believes himself capable of analysing and convicting the con man. The *Dresdner Volkszeitung* attests to the importance of this incident, while Helene Stöcker's progressive feminist journal *Die neue Generation* concedes as weaker those scenes in which Wulffen introduces his criminological knowledge: 'it seems unrealistic that a state prosecutor will engage so deeply and intimately in conversation with a convicted criminal that the latter is allowed to declaim scenes from Richard III or Hamlet in order to explain his psychological considerations, and that in turn the accuser feels so defeated that he commits suicide'.[72] Austrian botanist and local historian Dr Friedrich Morton (1890–1969) came to a different conclusion in his enthusiastic and thoughtful evaluation of the work, having found the portrayal of Sperl convincing. He opines that the state prosecutor's weakness brings about his demise, and he underlines Györki's poetic and acting skills, his knowledge of languages and his forces of fantasy in general.[73]

Sperl's character caught the imagination of reviewers most likely because they could identify with the erudite state prosecutor. Yet Wulffen shows over and over again how imposters intuitively and ruthlessly honed in on the wishes and desires of their victims, as well as their feelings of guilt; thus the victims frequently enabled the offences in the first place. This feature of the victim profile of impostors was discussed by American psychoanalyst and psychiatrist Phyllis Greenacre, who argued in 1958 that

> in some of the most celebrated instances of imposture, it indeed appears that the fraud was successful only because many others as well as the perpetrator had a hunger to believe in the fraud, and that any success of such fraudulence depended in fact on strong social as well as individual factors and a special receptivity to the trickery. To this extent those on whom the fraudulence is imposed are not only victims but unconscious conspirators.[74]

Wulffen illustrates this propensity in all the characters of *Der Mann mit den sieben Masken*. However, he portrays the con man's impact on female victims as graver than that on the male victims involved: most male victims are defrauded of money that they give willingly in attempts to compensate for past failures, or for career advancement. Sometimes they lose wives, lovers and daughters to the ingenious trickster. Women, by contrast, bear a greater emotional cost: divorce, suicide, being committed to a mental asylum or becoming complicit to the extent of manslaughter and murder. Wulffen makes clear in other contexts that he considers women more vulnerable than men, due to the 'female fate' to love just one man (men in turn were perceived as 'physiologically different, less favourably organised [polygamous]', than women).[75] He promoted the increased participation of women in society, publicly supported the admission of female lay assessors (*Schöffen*) for juvenile courts, preferred female prison officers over their male counterparts. Nonetheless, Wulffen was convinced that women's only concept of honour and morality was defined by 'sexual honour' ('Geschlechtsehre'), their respectability, that is, pride in her virginity, and later in being a faithful wife.[76] At the same time, he did not consider social factors, and held responsible the parent generation in their duty of care towards young women.

This stance towards women is best illustrated in Wulffen's description of the character Klarika in *Der Mann mit den sieben Masken*. Klarika is seduced by Györki as an under-aged girl and remains under his spell until the end of their lives. Wulffen's description of Klarika is based on qualities entirely different from those of Sperl, and is phrased in the language of sexual pathology. Klarika first met Györki and fell in love with him aged fifteen in Baden, where he was involved in an affair with Mrs Ferenczi. Klarika's seduction at an early age represents her downfall. Her love – as Wulffen writes about female criminals in his academic case compilation *Der Sexualverbrecher* – represents 'the absolute, sometimes slavish complaisance to the man of her choice [that] leads her on a criminal path'.[77] In the novel, this is exemplified through Klarika's criminal negligence of a patient she is nursing, who dies because, yet again, Klarika pursues her lover and leaves behind a life she has built for herself. Other characteristics also portray her in a language of sexual pathology. She is unable to recognise him after she has broken away from him, and afterwards enters a kind of 'waking state' in which she leads a respectable life. Klarika certainly seems somnambulistic in a close-up through the eyes of Sperl when he interviews her for the court case, and after that in the meeting with Györki; then again as the nun who leaves behind her sick patient and departs with Györki for the USA; and finally, on her last journey back to European shores. Wulffen's vocabulary for the encounter with Sperl is distinct – his narrative voice describes Klarika speaking slowly and monotonously, hardly looking at Sperl, her facial expression 'faraway', and never calling Györki by his real name, but only by his false names. Overall, 'she seemed to take this opportunity to live through the lost dream again'.[78] Upon meeting Györki she is paralysed, unable to move, and begins shaking; her look becomes veiled. The description of this physical reaction does not offer insight into her feelings, just as readers do not gain direct insight into Györki's emotional life; however, Klarika's dependence is vividly portrayed.

Wulffen's multifaceted explorations of imposture pre-empt later psychoanalytic insights about con men, and more generally about narcissistic behaviour. He presents relevant case materials in a range of publications and case modalities, yet these do not so much represent different insights as reveal how Wulffen targeted both expert and lay audiences in his case compilations, expert case studies and case stories. The key difference between Wulffen's expert case study of Manolescu and his most famous case story of imposture lies in the factual specificity and formal register of the former, and in the general claims and entertaining descriptions of the latter. While the expert case study was based on discursive arguments and logic, the case story illustrated in detail how characters were made fools of, and how they suffered as a consequence, topics Wulffen was able to discuss only briefly in his expert case study.

The representation of a con man in his novel *Der Mann mit den sieben Masken* is notable as a detailed illustration of Wulffen's psychological insights, as well as his biological explanatory framework concerning imposture. While he holds a certain admiration for con men, and expresses pity for their victims, Wulffen outlines the real distinction between criminals and their victims through the powers of biology. For Wulffen, Klarika represents the 'downright marked female fate, to love only one man, [which] became true for her in a tremendous and harrowing way'.[79] Sperl and Klarika epitomise Wulffen's gendered criminal psychological theories: Sperl as the example of the guardian of the law who is fooled by his desire for knowledge; Klarika as the example of a prematurely sexually active teenager whose sex makes her vulnerable. This is what Sperl does not understand, and what causes or at least hastens Klarika's downfall. Tensions between psychological explanations of criminality and notions of biological determinism in Wulffen's thinking became more marked over time. During the Weimar period these tensions opened his work to critique from various factions.

Female felons and the crisis of the expert case study

If imposture was the favourite topic of Wulffen's exploration of criminality during the late Wilhelmine era, female felons became his subject of choice during the Weimar Republic. As established elsewhere in discussion of the Grete Beier case, Wulffen's concern with changing female gender roles and the perceived dangers were linked with societal change, and placed the stern democrat on an awkward footing with progressive forces in Weimar Germany.[80] This argumentative shift seems somewhat surprising, since Wulffen's framework for understanding male criminality had always been more complex, and had developed greatly since his first explorations in *Psychologie des Verbrechers* (1908). He reworked this study for publication 1926, with the new title *Kriminalpysychologie. Psychologie des Täters* (*Criminal Psychology. Psychology of the Perpetrator*). In this version, Wulffen left behind the pre-war focus on physiology and biology; he had developed a new criminal psychology that none less than Bernhard

Weiß, Vice President of the Berlin Police Force, described as '*the* key work of contemporary criminal psychology ... an apex not only of German criminalistic literature, but of criminalistic world literature'.[81] The volume encompassed a range of new case studies as well as insights into a variety of crimes, from imposture to theft and murder; it included considerations of wider crime-related phenomena, such as affective states after a crime and false confessions.

With such rich materials and methodologies to hand, the reasons for Wulffen's comparatively simplistic exploration of female felons are more complex than have been perceived in scholarly discourse so far. They are an expression of a confluence of factors: an increasing 'nature–nurture' divide between psychiatry and criminal psychology on one side and psychoanalysis on the other – neither of which Wulffen found convincing; a perceived rise in criminality; his increasingly troubled relationship with the explicit nature of public discourse about sex; and, importantly, the decline of Wilhelmine notions of respectability and morality in a traumatised post-war society, which was tending to romanticise sexual crime. All these factors helped to undermine the standing of the case study genre as a site of academic discourse, and as a site of respectable and empirical discourse about sexuality.

Wulffen's increased interest in female criminality after 1919 was influenced by his stellar rise in the Weimar Republic, to the position of a chief public servant in the Saxon Ministry of Justice, and his election to the Saxon parliament as a member of the socially liberal German Democratic Party (DDP). As a member of the DDP he sat at the disintegrating centre of Germany's increasingly polarised political landscape. Like no other party, the DDP aimed to represent a balanced position on many questions of post-war life, and did so as a government party. From its foundation in 1919 to 1932 the DDP was nearly continuously part of Weimar coalition governments, although its influence declined steadily.[82] In a climate of rapidly changing social attitudes and moral values, the DDP sought to represent the middle ground. It supported progressive social reform-oriented legislation, but also – to the great dissatisfaction of German left-wing writer Kurt Tucholsky – the 1926 Schund und Schmutz (filth and trash) paragraph, instating the first Weimar-era censorship, mainly aimed at the protection of youth.[83]

With his undiminished sense of mission when it came to legal reform, Wulffen throughout his career successfully identified new criminological trends. When crime statistics showed a spike in female criminality, he reacted with characteristic vigour and wrote the first and only book-length German specialist volume on the topic in the 1920s, titled *Das Weib als Sexualverbrecherin* (1923). This work has been widely quoted in studies of Weimar gender relations and criminality, either because of its perceived tendentious outlook, or because of the rich casuistry it provides.[84] As in Wulffen's other case compilations, the case studies collected here offer examples for a range of discourses. They include contributions to the three argumentative strands that defined debate about female criminality in the new Republic. In the Weimar Republic gender difference helped to explain both why women committed fewer crimes overall, and the existence of specific 'female' felonies such as murder by poisoning, or procuring (prostitution) among female criminals. The rise of female criminality was more broadly explained by the perceived masculinisation of women that followed from the First World War and the post-war brutalisation of society – further explored in Chapter 5 of this volume.[85]

As when writing about imposture, Wulffen assumed the German people, including German academics and writers, to be naive in their understanding of female criminality; evidence for such naivety could be seen, for instance, in a new leniency in juries' sentencing of female offenders.[86] Indeed, criminological fantasies in Weimar Germany predominantly portrayed women as victims rather than perpetrators. Wulffen challenged this bias in particular because the new Republic provided 'the weaker sex' with new rights and opportunities, but also with a range of 'temptations'. According to Wulffen, the lost war, revolution and female suffrage – which to him represented women's unconditional emancipation – created a materialistic ethos among male and female youth that diminished differences between the sexes, a view widely shared by twenty-first-century scholars of Weimar Germany. However, Wulffen insisted on the gender difference between men and women, and that young women, as exemplified in Klarika in *Der Mann mit den sieben Masken*, were more vulnerable than men. This position shows parallels with the stance of the DPP on Schmutz und Schund literature, a debate that, in Luke Springman's words, 'provided a thoroughly structured sentimental archetype of youth threatened by decadent society'.[87] Such debates can be interpreted as evidence of cultural anxiety in the face of radical change, couched typically for the period in terms of concern for the next generation.

Wulffen most decisively expressed this sentiment in his introductory essay to the collection of expert case studies *Irrwege des Eros* (*Aberrations of Eros*) of 1928, a volume that showcases the downfall of fourteen female criminals. Because Wulffen perceived crimes to be the result of misdirected sexual urges, and Weimar's sexualisation was beyond the control of the law ('since too many old and young people live on such things'), in *Irrwege des Eros* he appealed to the intellectual and spiritual ideals of the previous generations as a guiding light.[88] In the context of this moralistic plea Wulffen contended that mothers did not appreciate how vastly gender roles had changed, and that their daughters needed guidance, particularly since the relationship between mothers and daughters presented a lacuna in the German imagination – in fiction as well as in reality.[89]

While *Irrwege des Eros* parades its female criminals as a deterrent for its female readers, and appeals to mothers to bridge a generational divide that shaped the Weimar era, in *Das Weib als Sexualverbrecherin* Wulffen addressed his professional audience to consider – against the criminological fantasies of the time – the possibility of female felony.[90] Wulffen expresses the belief that his work will further the understanding of female criminality for science, judicial practice and the arts; that the casuistry would stand independently and be self-explanatory.[91] The introduction to *Das Weib als Sexualverbrecherin* elaborates most succinctly Wulffen's theoretical stance. Firstly, Wulffen observes that a lack of systematic exploration of female sex offenders has created the need to showcase female criminality, since previous works in the field provide no or at least insufficient casuistry.[92] Secondly, he stresses the criminal psychologist's assumption that criminality is innate to human existence and not solely a reflection of the social ills of society. At the same time, he rejects the experimental culture of knowledge that had begun to dominate German psychology, biological criminology and forensic psychiatry. Wulffen perceived this approach as remote from legal practice, confined to its psychiatric ivory tower.[93] To Wulffen such a retreat from the case study genre also represented a move away from an empiricism that refused both a purely sociological framework and a purely biological framework for explaining female criminality.

At the same time – and seemingly in a contradictory manner – Wulffen reiterated the argument that heredity or degeneration contributed to female criminality. He did so to explain why a minority of women committed crimes in the first place, and thus to take a stance against an exclusively social constructionist approach that, in his view, furthered the sexualisation of society. The combination of these arguments shaped much of the reception of *Das Weib als Sexualverbrecherin* and caused considerable antagonism. Colleagues such as fellow sexologist Juliusburger backed a more liberal and emancipated view and, like other reformers, worked towards the normalisation of female sexuality. He had sympathetically reviewed many of Wulffen's works in the past, but now declared incomprehensible the argument that 'female criminality less than its male counterpart is caused by social conditions'.[94] Similar critique was voiced behind the scenes. In 1931, just before *Das Weib als Sexualverbrecherin* was to be published in a third edition by HRW publishers, the editor formulated his critique along comparable lines. HRW had recently purchased the copyright for the series 'Encyklopädie der modernen Kriminalistik' ('Encyclopaedia of Modern Criminology') from Langenscheidt, the company that had published most of Wulffen's academic works.[95] To update *Das Weib als Sexualverbrecherin*, the new editor suggested a range of changes, most importantly a revision of what he perceived to be the 'at some points too pessimistic' view of women.[96] In light of new publications on the topic, the publisher suggested adaptations and revisions on a range of issues (from female procuring to prostitution) and championed the 'modern' view of crime as solely explained by social factors.[97]

Such critique of Wulffen's perception of women coincided with a crisis in the book market and with a decline in sales numbers, as outlined elsewhere.[98] As documented in his correspondence with his publishers, Wulffen found himself in a marketplace where book titles were used to 'lure' readers, as were photographs and suggestive advertisements for sexological works. This only reinforced his view that 'our complete intellectual world has become impregnated [*sic*] by sexuality' and did nothing to ease his concerns about the vulnerability of women.[99] Wulffen's struggle to retain agency over the presentation and wording of his own works becomes obvious in a number of ways. For instance, Julius Brüll, the publisher of *Irrwege des Eros*, suggested changing the title of the volume to the more titillating and ambiguous *Erotische Verbrecherinnen* (*Erotic Female Felons*); Wulffen refused.[100] In preliminary discussions about a third edition of *Das Weib als Sexualverbrecherin*, HRW pushed Wulffen to include more of the graphic photographs that had undoubtedly attracted a wider readership. The publisher found the photographs duly submitted by Wulffen 'excellent', but argued that 'the number of images can easily be doubled without undermining the scientific character of the publication'.[101] Emphasising that selling books had become 'a hundredfold harder in these hard times', HRW also suggested that Wulffen increase his publicity by launching articles in illustrated newspapers and high-circulation magazines, and by using 'lively and striking images' for advertising the book.[102]

Wulffen's dispute with HRW about images lasted over nine months, during which time he remained adamant about the academic respectability and appropriateness of the materials. He favoured images from official sources, such as the criminal museum in Hamburg or the police.[103] HRW highlighted a concern with sales numbers and suggested that images would also be much valued by the police and other readers with a professional interest in the material, but Wulffen remained unconvinced.[104] When HRW pointed out to Wulffen that he had published a chapter in the sexological cultural studies series 'Die Erotik in der Photographie' ('The Erotics of Photography'), which had also produced a supplementary volume of photographs, Wulffen disputed having ever seen these images; this seems plausible, given the publishing history of the supplementary volume.[105] He argued that 'while recently sadistic-masochistic and fetishist images have become so common, this constitutes nonsense that we absolutely should not take part in'.[106] Upholding his pre-war assumption about his different target audiences, he further suggested that while such images might have their place in an academic volume about erotic photography, and even in a literary or artistic context, they were of no relevance to a volume on sex crime, which would be concerned with reality and not staged masochistic and other scenarios.[107]

Libel presented another problem. In a later letter to HRW, Wulffen complained of market competition from books by non-academic authors.[108] Specifically, Wulffen complained about Robert Heymann (1879–1946), film director and writer of popular fiction and popular cultural histories, whose volume *Der Sexualverbrecher* (*The Sex Offender*) was published in 1931 by Lykeion.[109] Wulffen raised the issue of title copyright with his own publisher and a compromise was negotiated with Lykeion. New imprints of Heymann's book showed a title change to *Das Verbrechen. Eine Sittengeschichte menschlicher Entartung* (*Crime. A History of Human Aberration*) and those copies already printed received a paper jacket printed with the new title.[110] The ambiguous sales strategy adopted by Lykeion represents an excellent example of the practices employed by many publishers in the Weimar Republic. Like other publishers of cultural studies, Lykeion stretched the boundaries of sexological respectability on the way to sexual modernity. Many new titles referenced sexological discourse; however, it was often difficult to identify whether they foregrounded academic or expert knowledge, represented a further popularisation or eroticisation of these discourses, or were merely a means to avoid censorship. For instance, Lykeion printed works of respected academic authors like literary historian Paul Englisch, as well as more provocative series such as Heymann's 'Sexuelle Hörigkeit. Sittengeschichte der Erotomanie' ('Sexual Enslavement. A History of Erotomania'), which included titillating titles such as *Der masochistische Mann* (*Masochist Man*) and *Die hörige Frau* (*The Sexually Enslaved Woman*), both published in 1931.[111]

This increasing willingness to explore sensationalist and erotic literature was partly due to economic necessity. The courts' inability to contain such publications was concurrent with the Weimar public's potent fascination with criminality. Such 'criminalistic fantasy' – a term recently revived by Todd Herzog but first coined in 1927 by Bernhard Weiß of the Berlin police – threatened Wulffen's reform project and the legitimacy of his reliance on the case study genre. The new ubiquitous presence and commercialisation of confessional and autobiographical writing during the Weimar period exerted an influence on the case study genre, challenging traditional boundaries between academic discourse and popular fiction. Where Wulffen had carefully crafted a space for his expert case studies and case stories, new autobiographical case studies began to appear. Such personal narratives were infused with the respectable language of sexological or psychoanalytic discourse and also romanticised criminal acts. As Wulffen all too clearly realised, this 'lay' use of specialist terminology affected the popularisation and diffusion of the meaning of such discourses.

There is no better way to portray the ambiguous shift in sexual modernity from the respectable norm to the agency of the 'perverse' individual than through Wulffen's exchange with Edith Cadivec. Cadivec was a private language teacher, a convicted paedophile and a writer of erotic literature. In 1924 she was convicted of having sadistically abused her protégé and four pupils in her care; the court case revealed that a range of respectable Viennese burghers had paid to watch this punishment for their own sexual gratification. As a consequence, Cadivec was sentenced to seven years in jail – of which she served less than four years – while just two of the co-defendants were placed on probation. Austrian feuilletonist and writer Alfred Polgar criticised the double standards of this court ruling, but wrote that Cadivec 'was not really entitled to claim any sympathies'.[112]

On 2 June 1932, Cadivec wrote a letter to Wulffen, a document that has not been studied before. In the letter she demanded an apology from Wulffen for purportedly denying the truthfulness of her statements, while having previously complimented her on her willingness to confess. By way of defending her position to Wulffen, Cadivec curtly argued, 'knowledge deceives and betrays. Truth is what we experience.'[113] From Wulffen's perspective, Cadivec's attempt at agency was ill conceived. His 1928 *Irrwege des Eros*, produced by the publishing house Avalun, contains an expert case study of Cadivec as a self-proclaimed sadist. It must have been troubling to Wulffen that, after publication of *Irrwege des Eros*, his publisher, Julius Brüll, the owner of Avalun, approached Cadivec and published her volume *Bekenntnisse und Erlebnisse* (*Confessions and Experiences*) in 1931. Furthermore, Brüll used Wulffen's expert case study in an endorsement for Cadivec's autobiography.[114] Wulffen was not impressed, and when Cadivec's book was banned he agreed with the verdict of the court, although the volume was offered only as a subscription volume for libraries and academics; he refused to support Brüll in overturning the censorship decision.[115] This refusal was in line with the court and with the position of the DDP. It represented a small and futile attempt to suppress Cadivec's writings, which soon became classics of sadistic and paedophile literature.[116]

In the shape of a pseudo-psychoanalytic case study, Cadivec explained her life story. Her confessions in *Bekenntnisse und Erlebnisse* include erotic and pornographic passages. The book's paedophile content contrasts starkly with the explanatory psychoanalytic framework and language that Cadivec uses to account for herself.[117] She referenced psychiatric, but mostly psychoanalytic discourse, a fact that had been noted by the forensic expert in his report for her trial.[118] One of Cadivec's co-defendants, lawyer Alphons Peter Kuh-Chrobak, underwent psychoanalytic treatment with Ludwig Jekels, but Cadivec did not submit herself to psychoanalysis.[119] This might have been due to financial constraints, but her intense and eclectic engagement with psychoanalytic discourse meant that Cadivec – as stated in the psychiatric report at her trial – 'with the help of auto- and other [psychoanalytic] suggestions, had been able to develop a perception of her actions that did not contradict morality'.[120] That is, Cadivec adapted the narrative of authentic truth that underlies psychoanalysis, but, like a con artist, she was unable to take any responsibility for her actions. Her writings showed no compassion for her daughter, her protégé or the pupils whom the court found she had sadistically abused.[121] Rather, Cadivec resolutely sought new court hearings: following her conviction in September 1924, she applied for new hearings of her case eleven times (the last time in 1953), always in lengthy and well formulated submissions; all her applications were rejected.

No doubt Wulffen was not surprised by this development, nor by Cadivec's need to write. The parallels to Manolescu are telling, although Wulffen never spelled them out. As Wulffen underlines in his expert case study of the latter, Manolescu's writing career began after he was prevented from thieving 'in reality', due to the loss of his arm.[122] Cadivec commenced writing when imprisoned, and due to the loss of her reputation as a teacher. Wulffen was also familiar with the criminalistic fantasies of convicted criminals that centred on institutions of authority and their representatives. Hence Manolescu's day-dream of selling his skull to Lombroso, or the second volume of Manolescu's autobiography, which contained a plea against psychiatric containment; hence those con artists who involved Wulffen in their criminal fantasies. Two undated newspaper clippings in the archive of Wulffen's papers reveal that farmer Hermann Friedrich Karl Thürnau had posed as a baron and one of his false names was Erich von Wulffen. In another example, when accused of fraud, Margaret Engel alleged Wulffen to have wooed her, and wrote to abdicated Emperor Wilhelm II to request that he convince Wulffen to divorce his wife. After Engel was acquitted on grounds of diminished responsibility, she defrauded a range of businesses, including first-class hotels, arguing that the Saxon courts would pay the costs because Wulffen had falsely accused her.[123]

Cadivec's publications were, however, of a different nature. Wulffen saw her use of a sexualised language – in her *Bekenntnisse and Erlebnisse* and in her letter – as symptomatic of post-war German and Austrian society in general. Cadivec's use of case study fragments in her confessions must have deeply concerned him. This contributed to a remarkable development: the former supporter of psychoanalysis now took the view that psychoanalysis, far from serving as a cure, was furthering the sexualisation of society. Presumably, Wulffen's re-assessment of psychoanalysis was based at least in part on the Cadivec case. In an undated four-page manuscript titled 'Siegmund [*sic*] Freud' Wulffen elaborates:

> Especially the sexual lure that surrounds the whole theory; the assertion that all our feelings and thoughts and every interpretation of our state and behaviour has a sexual context holds an extraordinary attraction for human beings in general, and especially at this time. That it represents a crass materialism is hardly noticed. Existence and life become eroticised in the extreme, sexualised in a time where all other stimulants fail. The over-eroticisation and sexualisation from which the present suffers are due, in the main, to the Freudian teachings.[124]

In turning his back on psychoanalysis, Wulffen also distanced himself from the field of knowledge that, after the 1920s, retained the strongest connection to the case study genre. Originally, in the early twentieth century, Wulffen had responded enthusiastically to Freud's theories. In a 1910 review of *Der Sexualverbrecher*, Juliusburger pointed out that Wulffen's works were based on Freud.[125] Indeed, Wulffen accepted the fundamental impact of sexuality on human nature that Freud's theories proposed. This led to the subsequent unusual classification of a wide range of criminal offences as sex crimes (from theft to sex murder). Wulffen's embrace of psychoanalytic theories becomes very evident in his critique of William Shakespeare's *Hamlet*, published in 1913, a work that argues from sexological and psychoanalytic perspectives.[126] Nevertheless, with the benefit of hindsight, in a review of 1932 Juliusburger names Wulffen among a large number of criminologists who had come to the conclusion that the 'psychoanalytic turn' from 1913–14 was no longer scientifically responsible.[127] The mounting dissatisfaction with psychoanalysis also resulted from attempts by psychoanalysts like Abraham to establish their hold in the legal world, and their ignorance of Wulffen's writings.[128] While Wulffen granted Freud a consistency in methodology, he pointed to the danger of manipulation in the psychoanalytic process: free association permits mistakes, lack of discrimination, self-suggestion and deception, making patients susceptible to 'all kinds of interpretations'. For Wulffen this disqualified psychoanalytic methods from being used in court, either during interrogation or for witness statements.[129]

It is also possible that Wulffen held the psychoanalytic method of free association responsible for the highly problematic tone and content of *Bekenntnisse und Erlebnisse*. Cadivec's use of free association created a work of erotic literature in which conventional distinctions between reality and fantasy collapsed. (A psychoanalytic interpretation of Cadivec's case would have rejected her interpretation as an expression of narcissism.) In all, Wulffen was well aware of the attraction that Cadivec held for her readers. In 1931, a certain Friedrich Harth wrote to Wulffen seeking direct contact with Cadivec. Harth had read Wulffen's expert account of Cadivec in *Irrwege des Eros*, which quoted passages of Cadivec's self-description. After reading these passages Harth was 'moved and galvanised'; Wulffen's commentary did not have this effect. Harth hoped to read everything written by Cadivec, to help him solve his 'puzzle of his soul'.[130] Wulffen's account could not compete with the fascination exercised by Cadivec's writing.

Wulffen's expert and pedagogical use of the case study genre had insisted on an authoritative distinction between criminal fantasy and legal reality that did not prove helpful for Harth. In other words, Harth was drawn to the particular blend of reality and fantasy that Herzog describes as characteristic of Weimar's criminalistic fantasies. Harth's reading of Cadivec might point to an underlying trauma, his attraction to Cadivec based on similar desires that represented an attempt to resolve or repeat this trauma. Such ambiguity lies at the heart of the making of German sexual modernity, and in the context of criminality it raised serious ethical questions.

Whether expressed in connection with Cadivec's case conviction and censorship, or more generally in his call for chastity among young women, Wulffen's solution to the question of female criminality seems a mixture of appropriate, old-fashioned and unrealistic. Wulffen interpreted the increasingly noticeable collapse between the respectable language of sexology and the sexualisation of language as a sign of the brutalisation of post-war society. The same trends and shifts can also be interpreted as a consequence of the onset of sexual modernity – a sexual modernity to which Wulffen had made a significant contribution, notably through his popularisation of several case modalities. Sexual modernity now represented a crisis for Wulffen's reformist and pedagogical project. He distanced himself from psychiatry, with its new experimental ethos and new scientific style of writing. He blamed psychoanalysis as the cause of the sexualisation of language. These attitudes contained, furthermore, a refusal to reflect on his own role in the dissemination of sexological knowledge. After all, over a period of almost three decades Wulffen had skilfully fostered multiple reading publics for case study compilations, expert case studies and case stories. The recent and more democratic uptake of the case study genre that Wulffen witnessed with trepidation destabilised the genre's respectability. In a certain way this made the genre unviable for academic discourse; having helped to make manifest the German populace's embrace of criminalistic and sexual fantasies, the case study was revealed as deeply subjective. Wulffen's experience, then, was that of the modern mandarin more generally. The liberal hub of Weimar Germany crumbled, and Wulffen's reservations and anxieties concerning the changing respectability of the case study genre, the role of women and the romanticisation of criminality exemplify challenges faced by the old liberal elite in cleaving to their notions of propriety and related ethical standards.

Notes

1 Sächsische Landesbibliothek – Staats- und Universitätsbibliothek, Dresden (hereafter SLUB), Nachlass des Schriftstellers und Kriminalisten Min.-Direktor Dr Erich Wulffen (1862–1936): Signatur: Mscr. Dres. App. 1832, 102 (5), 'Deutsche Kriminalisten', *Berliner Illustrirte Zeitung*, 17 (1927), pp. 700–1.

2 Reiner Grundmann and Nico Stehr, *Experts: The Knowledge and Power of Expertise* (New York: Routledge, 2011), pp. 8–13.

3 Fritz Ringer, *The Decline of the German Mandarins: The German Academic Community, 1890–1933* (Hanover: University Press of New England, 1969), p. 248.

4 For the liberal leanings of criminal psychologists see Richard F. Wetzell, *Inventing the Criminal: A History of German Criminology, 1880–1945* (Chapel Hill: University of North Carolina Press, 2000), pp. 168–74; Wulffen is explicitly mentioned in Jason Crouthamel, 'Male Sexuality and Psychological Trauma: Soldiers and Sexual Disorder in World War I and Weimar Germany', *Journal of the History of Sexuality*, 17:1 (2008), pp. 60–84; Andrew Lees, *Cities, Sin, and Social Reform in Imperial Germany* (Ann Arbor: University of Michigan Press, 2002), pp. 169–70, pp. 181–4.

5 Crouthamel, 'Male Sexuality', p. 75.

6 Monika Frommel, 'Internationale Reformbewegung zwischen 1880 und 1920', in Jörg Schönert (ed.), *Erzählte Kriminalität. Zur Typologie und Funktion von narrativen Darstellungen in Strafrechtspflege, Publizistik und Literatur zwischen 1770 und 1920* (Tübingen: Niemeyer, 1991), pp. 447–96, p. 489; on Wulffen's view on prostitution see Peter Becker, 'Weak Bodies? Prostitutes and the Role of

Gender in the Criminological Writings of 19th-Century German Detectives and Magistrates', *Crime, History and Societies*, 3:1 (1999), pp. 45–70, pp. 60–1.

7 Erich Wulffen, *Psychologie des Verbrechers. Ein Handbuch für Juristen, Ärzte, Pädagogen und Gebildete aller Stände* (Groß-Lichterfelde Ost: Paul Langenscheidt, 1908), pp. 318–49; Erich Wulffen, *Kriminalpsychologie. Psychologie des Täters. Ein Handbuch für Juristen, Justiz-, Verwaltungs- und Polizeibeamte, Ärzte, Pädagogen und Gebildete aller Stände* (Berlin: Paul Langenscheidt, 1926), pp. 133–6. Even Wulffen's benevolent obituary of Lombroso contains a critical discussion of some of the latter's insights: SLUB, Nachlass des Schriftstellers und Kriminalisten Min.-Direktor Dr Erich Wulffen (1862–1936): Signatur: Mscr. Dres. App. 1832, 1383, Erich Wulffen, 'Cesare Lombrosos Lehre vom Verbrecher', *Nord Süd*, circa 1909, n.p.

8 '[D]e[n] geniale[n] Fortsetzer der Tat Lombrosos und [er] ist der berufene Reformator des morschen, dem Untergange reifen alten Strafsystems.' Otto Juliusburger, 'Der Sexualverbrecher', *Die neue Generation*, 14:7 (1910), pp. 259–64, p. 264.

9 SLUB, Nachlass des Schriftstellers und Kriminalisten Min.-Direktor Dr Erich Wulffen (1862–1936): Signatur: Mscr. Dres. App. 1832, 81. 'Im Gegensatz zu Lombrosos Theorie vom geborenen Verbrecher verficht Wulffen die Anschauung, daß in jedem Menschen Kriminalität latent vorhanden sei': 'Erich Wulffen 70 Jahre alt', *Dresdner Neueste Nachrichten*, 2 October 1932, p. 5.

10 Wetzell, *Inventing the Criminal*, pp. 125–78.

11 Udi E. Greenberg, 'Criminalization. Carl Schmitt and Walter Benjamin's Concept of Criminal Politics', *Journal of European Studies*, 39:3 (2009), pp. 305–19, p. 315. On biologisation, see Wetzell, *Inventing the Criminal*, pp. 125–78; on the depiction of crime in popular culture, see, for example, Maria Tatar, *Lustmord: Sexual Murder in Weimar Germany* (Princeton: Princeton University Press, 1995).

12 Todd Herzog, 'Crime Stories: Criminal, Society, and the Modernist Case History', *Representations*, 80 (2002), pp. 34–61, p. 35.

13 Daniel Siemens, 'Explaining Crime. Berlin Newspapers and the Construction of the Criminal in Weimar Germany', *Journal of European Studies*, 39:3 (2009), pp. 336–52, p. 337.

14 See Greenberg, 'Criminalization'.

15 Todd Herzog, *Crime Stories: Criminalistic Fantasy and the Culture of Crisis in Weimar Germany* (New York: Berghahn, 2009), p. 4.

16 Harry Oosterhuis, 'Sexual Modernity in the Works of Richard von Krafft-Ebing and Albert Moll', *Medical History*, 56:2 (2012), pp. 133–55.

17 SLUB, Nachlass des Schriftstellers und Kriminalisten Min.-Direktor Dr Erich Wulffen (1862–1936): Signatur: Mscr. Dres. App. 1832, 1477.

18 C. G. Jung, 'Besprechung von Erich Wulffen "Der Sexualverbrecher"', *Jahrbuch für psychoanalytische und psychopathologische Forschungen*, 2:2 (1910), p. 747.

19 Arthur J. Todd, 'Review of *Der Entwurf eines deutschen Strafgesetzbuches* und *Die Postulate der Internationalen Kriminalistischen Vereinigung und die Beschlüsse zweier Strafrechtskommissionen*', *Journal of the American Institute for Criminal Law and Criminology*, 5 (1914–15), pp. 789–95, p. 790. A comprehensive history of German penal reform is yet to be written; however, Wulffen's dedicated involvement in the reform process is well documented in his writings. The following references discuss the history of the International Criminological Association in some detail: Frommel, 'Internationale Reformbewegung', pp. 447–96; Elisabeth Bellmann, *Die Internationale Kriminalistische Vereinigung, 1889–1933* (Frankfurt: Lang, 1994); Sylvia Kesper-Biermann, 'Wissenschaftlicher Ideenaustausch und "kriminalpolitische Propaganda". Die Internationale Kriminalistische Vereinigung (1889–1937) und der Strafvollzug', in Desiree Schauz and Sabine Freitag (eds), *Verbrecher im Visier der Experten: Kriminalpolitik zwischen Wissenschaft und Praxis im 19. und frühen 20. Jahrhundert* (Stuttgart: Steiner, 2007), pp. 79–97.

20 Erich Wulffen, *Frau Justitias Walpurgisnacht. Roman* (Berlin: Duncker, 1913). (*Roman* means 'novel' and was often used as a subtitle at the time.) In the Weimar era some newspaper articles would later claim that publication of this novel triggered the transfer of Wulffen from Dresden to Zwickau for disciplinary reasons. Since work records for Wulffen are lost, it is possible only to speculate whether their content alone contained sufficient fuel for professional conflict, or whether Wulffen's 'exile' was due to his novel's story of love and secret engagement between the young State Prosecutor Wartenberg, and the foster daughter of a judicial great. Even if Wulffen did not court the foster daughter of his teacher at university, the eminent scholar Karl Binding, it can be assumed that the novel was understood as an attack on his former professor, who retired in the same year as the novel was published. Moreover, *Walpurgisnacht* may have upset certain influential members of the legal profession, as did Wulffen's critique of the functioning of the court.

21 SLUB, Nachlass des Schriftstellers und Kriminalisten Min.-Direktor Dr Erich Wulffen (1862–1936): Signatur: Mscr. Dres. App. 1832, 1330, Erich Wulffen, 'Mein Umweg über die Dichter', circa 1932.

22 Wulffen, *Walpurgisnacht*, pp. 34–5; Wulffen, 'Mein Umweg über die Dichter'; Hugo Dingeldey, 'Erich Wulffen', in Alexander Baumgarten and Hugo Dingeldey (eds), *Erich Wulffen. Festschrift zu seinem siebzigsten Geburtstag* (Berlin: HRW, 1932), pp. 12–40, p. 13.

23 '[M]it einem vollen warmen Herzen an dieses ihm unbekannte Studium'; 'es dabei auf das Herz gar nicht ankommen sollte'. Wulffen, *Walpurgisnacht*, p. 39.

24 'Jetzt hörte er, daß er keine Ahnung von juristischer Schreibweise hatte. Aus der Korrektur des Amtsrichters sah er, worauf es ankam. Er hatte das Gefühlsmässige und Lebendige in dem kriminellen Vorgang betont. Das sollte nicht sein.' Wulffen, *Walpurgisnacht*, p. 41.

25 Wulffen, 'Mein Umweg über die Dichter'.

26 Wulffen, 'Mein Umweg über die Dichter'.

27 'Innenleben und Charakter, Verbrechensmotive und Umwelt des Täters.' Wulffen, 'Mein Umweg über die Dichter'.

28 'Schulbeispiele der kriminalpsychologischen Analyse.' Wulffen, 'Mein Umweg über die Dichter'.

29 Herewith a chronological listing of Wulffen's writing and lecturing on Goethe and Schiller: *Kriminalpsychologie und Psychopathologie in Schillers Räubern* (Halle: Marhold, 1907) (reprinted with a biography, comments and reviews through editor Jürgen Seul, Berlin: BWV, 2007); SLUB, Nachlass des Schriftstellers und Kriminalisten Min.-Direktor Dr Erich Wulffen (1862–1936): Signatur: Mscr. Dres. App. 1832, 1478, 'Aus Schillers tiefster Seele (im Lichte einer neuen Zeit)' – announcement of a lecture in Zwickau on 29 January 1919; SLUB, Nachlass des Schriftstellers und Kriminalisten Min.-Direktor Dr Erich Wulffen (1862–1936): Signatur: Mscr. Dres. App. 1832, 1478, 'Kriminalpsychologie bei Schiller und Goethe', lecture delivered 1912–13; SLUB, Nachlass des Schriftstellers und Kriminalisten Min.-Direktor Dr Erich Wulffen (1862–1936): Signatur: Mscr. Dres. App. 1832, 1325, 'Ein hygienischer Ausspruch Schillers', radio presentation from 1931; 'Bekanntes und Unbekanntes über Goethe als Kriminalisten', in Volker Wahl (ed.), *'Das Kind in meinem Leib': Sittlichkeitsdelikte und Kindsmord in Sachsen-Weimar-Eisenach unter Carl August; eine Quellenedition; 1779–1786* (Weimar: Böhlau, 2004), pp. 232–327; SLUB, Nachlass des Schriftstellers und Kriminalisten Min.-Direktor Dr Erich Wulffen (1862–1936): Signatur: Mscr. Dres. App. 1832, 1377, 'Kriminalpsychologie in Goethes Iphigenie auf Tauris', undated.

30 '[S]ein[em] Essen, sein[er] Arbeit und sein[er] Ordnung.' Erich Wulffen, 'Ein kriminalpsychologisches Experiment', *Monatsschrift für Kriminalpsychologie und Strafreform*, 2 (1905), pp. 734–8, p. 735.

31 'Veranlagung, Erziehung und Lebensschicksale haben ihn zu dem gemacht, was er ist und zu bleiben hat. Gegenüber diesen Schicksalsschwestern gibt es kein Entrinnen. Willensschwäche ist sein beschieden Teil, wie andere Menschen an organischen Schwächen leiden. Er kann nicht anders. Gott helfe ihm!' Wulffen, 'Ein kriminalpsychologisches Experiment', p. 730.

32 Silviana Galassi, *Kriminologie im Deutschen Kaiserreich. Geschichte einer gebrochenen Verwissenschaftlichung* (Stuttgart: Franz Steiner, 2004), p. 424.

33 Benjamin Carter Hett, *Death in the Tiergarten: Murder and Criminal Justice in the Kaiser's Berlin* (Cambridge: Harvard University Press, 2004), pp. 26–7.

34 Richard F. Wetzell, 'Psychiatry and Criminal Justice in Modern Germany, 1880–1933', *Journal of European Studies*, 39 (2009), pp. 270–89, p. 285.

35 Erich Wulffen, 'Gerhart Hauptmann's "Rose Bernd" vom kriminalist. Standpunkte', *Juristisch-psychiatrische Grenzfragen. Zwanglose Abhandlungen*, 4:3 (1906), pp. 13–23, pp. 20–2. For his analysis Wulffen took inspiration from Josef Kohler (1849–1919), another jurist, and also a poet and cultural critic, whose works analysed legal questions raised in the work of William Shakespeare. Compare Josef Kohler, *Shakespeare vor dem Forum der Jurisprudenz* (Würzburg: Stahel, 1883).

36 '[I]nsbesondere vor dem Strafrichter bislang, wenn überhaupt, weit unter Gebühr gewürdigt wurden. Und sie verbreitet Licht in Abgründen von Verbrecherseelen, die bis heut weiteren Kreisen dunkel und unbegreiflich erscheinen.' Dr Glaser, '*Der Sexualverbrecher* von E. Wulffen', *Geschlecht und Gesellschaft*, 5:9 (1910), pp. 415–24, p. 416.

37 Volkmar Sigusch, 'Erich Wulffen', in Volkmar Sigusch and Günter Grau (eds), *Personenlexikon der Sexualforschung* (Frankfurt: Campus, 2009), pp. 783–8, p. 784; Sace Elder, *Murder Scenes: Normality, Deviance, and Criminal Violence in Weimar Berlin* (Ann Arbor: University of Michigan Press, 2010), p. 25.

38 Galassi, *Kriminologie im Deutschen Kaiserreich*, pp. 424–6.

39 The following are all relevant reviews, sourced as clippings at SLUB, Nachlass des Schriftstellers und Kriminalisten Min.-Direktor Dr Erich Wulffen (1862–1936): Signatur: Mscr. Dres. App. 1832, 1477: 'Ein Buch vom Kinde. Erich Wulffen: *Das Kind, sein Wesen und seine Entartung*', *Vossische Zeitung*, 4 July 1914, n.p.; 'Literaturübersicht', *Gerichtliche und Militärmedizin* (no further reference details available). A number of reviews underline the value of Wulffen's books as reference works: Dr A. Weingart, '*Psychologie des Verbrechers*', *Deutsche Juristen-Zeitung*, 14 (1909), p. 612; Heinrich Rustige, '*Psychologie des Verbrechers*', *Die Hilfe*, 27 December 1908, n.p.; 'Literaturübersicht [on *Sexualverbrecher*]', *Gerichtliche und Militärmedizin* (no further reference details available); Willy Helpbach, 'Sexualverbrechen', *Frankfurter Zeitung*, 19 March 1910, n.p.; [on *Das Kind, sein Wesen, seine Entartung und seine Erziehung*], *Vossische Zeitung*, 4 July 1914, n.p.; Max Marcuse, [on *Weib als Sexualverbrecherin*], *Zeitschrift für Sexualwissenschaft*, 19:8 (1932), n.p.

40 Ludwik Fleck, 'Some Specific Features of the Medical Way of Thinking (1927)', in Robert S. Cohen and Thomas Schnelle (eds), *Cognition and Fact: Materials on Ludwik Fleck* (Dordrecht: Springer Netherlands, 1986), pp. 39–46, p. 39.

41 'Untersuchungspersonen [können] niemals der Vollmann oder das Vollweib [sein], sondern nach biologischer Erkenntis immer Personen mit einem mehr oder minder großen Einschlage der entgegengesetzten Geschlechtlichkeit.' Erich Wulffen, *Das Weib als Sexualverbrecherin. Ein Handbuch für Juristen, Polizei- und Strafvollzugsbeamte, Ärzte und Laienrichter* (Berlin: Paul Langenscheidt, 1923), p. 6.

42 Hett, *Death in the Tiergarten*, pp. 3–4; Birgit Lang, 'Influencing Public Knowledge: Erich Wulffen and the Criminal Case of Grete Beier', in Joy Damousi, Birgit Lang and Katie Sutton (eds), *Case Studies and the Dissemination of Knowledge* (New York: Routledge, 2015), pp. 49–65, pp. 50–2.

43 Gert Üding and Bernd Steinbrink, *Grundriss der Rhetorik. Geschichte – Technik – Methode* (Stuttgart: Metzler, 2011), pp. 278–83.

44 Wulffen, *Psychologie des Verbrechers*, p. 263.
45 Lang, 'Influencing Public Knowledge', 50–1.
46 Georges Manolescu, *Ein Fürst der Diebe. Memoiren* (Groß-Lichterfelde Ost: Paul Langenscheidt, 1905); Georges Manolescu, *Gescheitert. Aus dem Seelenleben eines Verbrechers* (Groß-Lichterfelde Ost: Paul Langenscheidt, 1907); Erich Wulffen, *Manolescu und seine Memoiren. Kriminalpsychologische Studie* (Groß-Lichterfelde Ost: Paul Langenscheidt, 1907).
47 Wulffen, *Psychologie des Verbrechers*, pp. 317–18.
48 Matt Houlbrook, 'Commodifying the Self Within: Ghosts, Libels, and the Crook Life Story in Interwar Britain', *Journal of Modern History*, 85:2 (2013), pp. 321–63, pp. 331, 335.
49 On the publisher's additional strategies for counteracting such tendencies see Birgit Lang 'Verbrecher im Fokus. Zur Zirkulation verbrecherischer und kriminalpsychologischer Fallgeschichten um 1900', in Wolfgang Hackl, Kalina Kupcyznska and Wolfgang Wiesmüller (eds), *Sprache, Literatur, Erkenntnis* (Vienna: Praesens, 2014), pp. 301–13.
50 Paul Lindau was a well known German writer whose crime writings represented only one strand of his creative output. His largest contribution to crime literature was his volumc *Interessante Fälle. Criminalprocesse aus neuester Zeit* (Breslau: Schottlaender, 1888). Hans Hyan was a German cabarettist, writer and crime reporter who wrote over thirty crime-related novels in the first third of the twentieth century. Paul Schlesinger was the best-known crime reporter of the Weimar Republic.
51 Wulffen, *Manolescu*, p. 7.
52 Wulffen, *Manolescu*, p. 110.
53 '[I]n Wirklichkeit … noch interessanter und … von tieferer Bedeutung, als ihn die Memoiren geben.' Wulffen, *Manolescu*, p. 9.
54 For example, Wulffen reconstructs from the police files that Manolescu told his wife he was innocent when he had already confessed to the police. Wulffen, *Manolescu*, p. 51. Wulffen also identifies a range of omissions in the memoirs and corrects Manolescu's distortions of events. For instance, the latter underlines in his memoirs his physical resistance to the police, while in fact he was noted to have behaved very cooperatively. Wulffen, *Manolescu*, p. 49.
55 '[I]nstinktiven Naturwüchsigkeit.' Wulffen, *Manolescu*, p. 19.
56 Helene Deutsch, 'The Impostor: Contribution to Ego Psychology of a Type of Psychopath [reprint from 1955]', *Psychoanalytic Quarterly*, 80: 4 (2011), pp. 1005–24, pp. 1014–15.
57 See particularly Wulffen's analysis of Manolescu's family relations: Wulffen, *Manolescu*, pp. 38–55.
58 Sigmund Freud, 'Der Familienroman der Neurotiker (1909)', in Sigmund Freud, *Gesammelte Werke, chronologisch geordnet*, ed. Anna Freud, in collaboration with M. Bonaparte, E. Bibring, W. Hoffer, E. Kris and O. Isakower, vol. VII (London: Imago, 1952), pp. 227–31; Sigmund Freud, 'Family Romances', in *The Standard Edition of the Complete Psychological Works of Sigmund Freud*, ed. James Strachey, with Anna Freud, Alix Strachey and Alan Tyson, vol. IX (London: Hogarth Press and Institute for Psychoanalysis, 1959), pp. 235–42; Phyllis Greenacre, 'The Impostor', *Psychoanalytic Quarterly*, 27 (1958), pp. 359–82, p. 362.
59 Karl Abraham, 'Die Geschichte eines Hochstaplers im Lichte psychoanalytischer Erkenntnis', *Imago. Zeitschrift für Anwendung der Psychoanalyse auf die Geisteswissenschaften*, 9:4 (1925), pp. 355–70, p. 368; Karl Abraham, 'The History of an Impostor in the Light of Psychoanalytical Knowledge', *Psychoanalytic Quarterly*, 4 (1935), pp. 570–87.
60 Hermann Nunberg and Ernst Federn (eds), *Protokolle der Wiener Psychoanalytischen Vereinigung. Band II (1908–1910)* (Gießen: Psychosozial-Verlag, 2008), p. 67. This affinity was also noted by other reviewers, such as Alfred Adler,

who was about to be ousted as President of the Vienna Psychoanalytic Society. The protocols of the Society from 9 December 1908 further reveal the awareness of psychoanalysts of Wulffen's work, and note that, in the description of a legal case, Wulffen used psychoanalytic 'nomenclature'. Abraham's premature death in 1925 was conceived by Freud's biographer and fellow psychoanalyst Ernest Jones as 'the most cruel and severe [blow to the science of psychoanalysis]' before the rise of National Socialism. Ernest Jones, 'Introductory Memoir', in *Selected Papers of Karl Abraham, M.D.*, trans. Douglas Bryan and Alix Strachey (London: Hogarth Press, 1927), pp. 9–41, p. 9.

61 Ernest Jones, 'Introductory Memoir', in Ernest Jones, *Selected Papers of Karl Abraham*, trans. Douglas Bryan and Alix Strachey (London: Hogarth Press, 1927), pp. 9–41, p. 9.

62 '[I]m psychologischen Sinne vollkommene Erfüllung einer infantilen Wunschsituation.' Abraham, 'Geschichte eines Hochstaplers', p. 368; Abraham, 'History of an Impostor', p. 584.

63 'Empfindung [bleibt] lediglich ein Phantom und [nimmt] gar keinen realen, praktischen, auf das Wohl der Tochter gerichteten Inhalt an.' Wulffen, *Manolescu*, p. 45.

64 '[Quälte] erst die Seinen, dann weinte er darüber wie ein Kind.' Wulffen, *Manolescu*, p. 52.

65 '[W]ir die hereditäre Belastung, die "Degeneration" in ihrer Bedeutung für das Entstehen dissozialer und krimineller Antriebe nicht überschätzen sollen.' Abraham, 'Geschichte eines Hochstaplers', p. 368.

66 Abraham, 'Geschichte eines Hochstaplers', pp. xxx and 370.

67 *Die Traumtänzerin: Ein Roman* (Berlin: Duncker, 1914); *Vorgelesen, genehmigt! Roman* (Berlin: Duncker, 1915); *Die Kraft des Michael Argobast, Roman* (Dresden: Reißner, 1917); *Der Mann mit den sieben Masken, Roman* (Dresden: Reißner, 1917); *Das Haus ohne Fenster, Roman* (Berlin: Duncker, 1919); *Die geschlossene Kette: Roman* (Berlin: Mosse, 1919); *Der blaue Diamant: Roman* (Leipzig: Leipziger Zeitungsverlag Dr Wolfgang Huck, 1919). Other fictional works from this period are: *Deutsche Renaissance: Roman* (Dresden: Reißner, 1917) and *Die Frauen von Loburg, Roman* (Berlin: Uhlmann, 1921).

68 SLUB, Nachlass des Schriftstellers und Kriminalisten Min.-Direktor Dr Erich Wulffen (1862–1936): Signatur: Mscr. Dres. App. 1832, 102(3), *Der Weltspiegel. Illustr. Halb-Wochenschrift des Berliner Tageblattes*, 2 November 1916, p. 3.

69 SLUB, Nachlass des Schriftstellers und Kriminalisten Min.-Direktor Dr Erich Wulffen (1862-1936): Signatur: Mscr. Dres. App. 1832, 1478. 'Der Mann mit den sieben Masken unser neuer Roman', *Münchnon Augsburger Abendzeitung*, 23 September 1917.

70 Wulffen composed a less successful drama titled *Immakulata*, fictionalising the story of Manolescu's first marriage. Wulffen also tried a dramatisation for the stage under the title *Mehr als Proteus*. This version, however, remained unfinished. See SLUB, Nachlass des Schriftstellers und Kriminalisten Min.-Direktor Dr Erich Wulffen (1862–1936): Signatur: Mscr. Dres. App. 1832, 1044.

71 'Über den literarischen Wert seines Werks ein Urteil abzugeben, fühle ich mich nicht berufen. Vom Standpunkt der Kriminalpsychologie aber haben wir es hier zweifelsohne mit einem außerordentlich lehrreichen Buche zu tun, das zum mindesten auch eine fesselnde und gute Unterhaltungslektüre bildet. Der Kenner der Kriminal-Geschichte wird übrigens das Urmaterial, aus dem der Dichter-Kriminalist schöpft erkennen. Es ist erstaunlich, in wie seiner Weise Wulffen seine wissenschaftlichen Quellen ausgebeutet hat, wie er die Wirklichkeit dichterisch gestaltet hat, ohne doch dadurch der kriminalpsychologischen Bedeutung seiner Schilderung irgendwie Abbruch zu tun.' SLUB, Nachlass des Schriftstellers und Kriminalisten Min.-Direktor Dr Erich Wulffen (1862–1936): Signatur: Mscr. Dres. App. 1832, 1478, Albert Hellwig, 'Dichter und Hochstapler', *Universum*, undated.

72 SLUB, Nachlass des Schriftstellers und Kriminalisten Min.-Direktor Dr Erich Wulffen (1862–1936): Signatur: Mscr. Dres. App. 1832, 1478, 'Erich Wulffen: *Der Mann mit den sieben Masken*', *Dresdner Volkszeitung*, 18 July 1917; 'Erich Wulffen: Der Mann mit den sieben Masken', *Die neue Generation* (issue number unclear) (1917), pp. 160–3. The quoted text (found at p. 162) is: 'Es ist unwahrscheinlich, daß sich ein Staatsanwalt in so intime Reden mit einem überführten Verbrecher einlassen wird, daß er sich dessen psychologischen Beweggründe bis zum Vordeklamieren von Szenen aus Richard III. oder Hamlet erläutern lassen und daß er selbst so sehr in seinen Bann geraten wird, daß er schließlich, weil er sich als Ankläger besiegt fühlt, Selbstmord begeht.'

73 SLUB, Nachlass des Schriftstellers und Kriminalisten Min.-Direktor Dr Erich Wulffen (1862–1936): Signatur: Mscr. Dres. App. 1832, 1478, Dr Friedrich Morton, '*Der Mann mit den sieben Masken*', *Villacher Zeitung*, 9 November 1917.

74 Greenacre, 'The Impostor', p. 360.

75 '[P]hysiologisch ... anders, ungünstiger ... organisiert.' Erich Wulffen, *Irrwege des Eros. Mit einer Einleitung Mütter und Töchter* (Hellerau bei Dresden: Avalun, 1929), p. 12.

76 SLUB, Nachlass des Schriftstellers und Kriminalisten Min.-Direktor Dr Erich Wulffen (1862–1936): Signatur: Mscr. Dres. App. 1832, 1407, Erich Wulffen, 'Weibliche Schöffen im Jugendgericht', undated; Erich Wulffen, *Reformbestrebungen auf dem Gebiete des Strafvollzugs* (Dresden: von Zahn & Jaensch, 1905); Wulffen, *Psychologie des Verbrechers*, p. 269.

77 '[D]ie unbedingte, manchmal sklavische Hingebung an den Mann ihrer Wahl führt sie auf den verbrecherischen Weg.' Erich Wulffen, *Der Sexualverbrecher. Ein Handbuch für Juristen, Verwaltungsbeamte und Ärzte* (Groß-Lichterfelde Ost: Paul Langenscheidt, 1910), p. 362.

78 '[S]ie schien die Gelegenheit zu benutzen, den verflogenen Traum noch einmal zu durchleben.' Wulffen, *Der Mann mit den sieben Masken*, p. 147.

79 'Gerade das ausgesprochene Frauenschicksal, in Liebe nur einem einzigen Manne zu gehören, hatte sich an ihr in wunderbarer, erschütternder Weise erfüllt.' Wulffen, *Der Mann mit den sieben Masken*, p. 229.

80 See Lang, 'Influencing Public Knowledge', pp. 49–65.

81 SLUB, Nachlass des Schriftstellers und Kriminalisten Min.-Direktor Dr Erich Wulffen (1862–1936): Signatur: Mscr. Dres. App. 1832, 1477. The pronouncements 'die Kriminalpsychologie der Gegenwart..., eine Zierde nicht nur der deutschen kriminalistischen Literatur, sondern der kriminalistischen Weltliteratur' are found in Bernhard Weiß, 'Kriminalpsychologie', *Die Polizei*, no date available.

82 The DDP was founded by Parish priest and liberal politician Friedrich Naumann (1860–1919), German writer and publicist Theodor Wolff (1868–1943) and lawyer Hugo Preuss (1860–1925), the 'father of the Weimar constitution'. Prominent members constituted modern mandarins such as Bernhard Weiß, foreign minister Walther Rathenau (1867–1922) and sociologist Max Weber (1864–1920).

83 See for example Kurt Tucholsky, 'Old Bäumerhand, der Schrecken der Demokratie', in *Gesammelte Werke in zehn Bänden*, ed. Mary Gerold-Tucholsky and Fritz J. Raddatz, vol. IV (Reinbek bei Hamburg: Rowohlt Verlag, 1975), pp. 556–9.

84 Elder, *Murder Scenes*, pp. 24–5, 95, 164–88; Hania Siebenpfeiffer, *'Böse Lust': Gewaltverbrechen in Diskursen der Weimarer Republik* (Cologne: Böhlau, 2005), pp. 69–72; Karsten Uhl, *Das 'verbrecherische Weib'. Geschlecht, Verbrechen und Strafen im kriminologischen Diskurs 1800–1945* (Münster: LIT, 2003), pp. 142–5.

85 Uhl, *Das 'verbrecherische Weib'*, p. 115.

86 Elder, *Murder Scenes*, pp. 164–88.

87 Luke Springman, 'Poisoned Hearts, Diseased Minds, and American Pimps: The Language of Censorship in the *Schund und Schmutz* Debates', *German Quarterly*, 68:4 (1995), pp. 408–29, p. 408.

88 'Von all diesen Dingen nähren sich zu viele, Alte und Junge.' Wulffen, *Irrwege des Eros*, p. 18.
89 Wulffen, *Irrwege des Eros*, pp. 6–9.
90 On the generation gap see Detlev Peukert, *Weimar Germany* (New York: Hill & Wang, 1992), pp. 86–100.
91 Wulffen, *Das Weib als Sexualverbrecherin*, pp. 3–4.
92 See Wulffen, *Das Weib als Sexualverbrecherin*, pp. 10–23. Before Wulffen outlines the biological premises of criminality, his introduction surveys the attempts in Italian, French and Spanish criminological literature so far on the subject matter at hand: Lombroso's narrative of biologisation and generalisation; the French 'feminist' understanding of female criminality (exemplified through Camille Granier, born in 1858, who remains forgotten in the twenty-first century); the Spanish predominantly sociological understanding of criminality.
93 Wulffen, *Das Weib als Sexualverbrecherin*, p. 6. For the history of psychology in Germany, and the shift from empirical to experimental psychology, or from philosophy to science, see: Horst U. K. Gundlich, 'Germany', in David B. Baker, *The Oxford Handbook of the History of Psychology: Global Perspectives* (Oxford: Oxford University Press, 2012), pp. 255–88, especially pp. 267–74; Wulffen, *Das Weib als Sexualverbrecherin*, p. 8, 4.
94 SLUB, Nachlass des Schriftstellers und Kriminalisten Min.-Direktor Dr Erich Wulffen (1862-1936): Signatur: Mscr. Dres. App. 1832, Otto Juliusburger 'Das Weib als Sexualverbrecherin', *Vorwärts*, 15 February 1923, containing the phrase 'weibliche Kriminalität weniger als die männliche durch die sozialen Umstände hervorgerufen werde'.
95 SLUB, Nachlass des Schriftstellers und Kriminalisten Min.-Direktor Dr Erich Wulffen (1862–1936): Signatur: Mscr. Dres. App. 1832, 769, HRW publisher to Erich Wulffen, 12 August 1930. Wulffen eventually filed a law suit against Langenscheidt because of outstanding royalty payments, a sad end to what had been a successful partnership over more than two decades. With HRW he planned to release the third edition of *Das Weib als Sexualverbrecherin* and the twelfth edition of *Sexualverbrecher.*
96 SLUB, Nachlass des Schriftstellers und Kriminalisten Min.-Direktor Dr Erich Wulffen (1862–1936): Signatur: Mscr. Dres. App. 1832, 783, folio 1, HRW publisher to Erich Wulffen, 9 December 1930, containing the phrase 'in manchen Punkten etwas zu pessimistisch'.
97 SLUB, Nachlass des Schriftstellers und Kriminalisten Min.-Direktor Dr Erich Wulffen (1862–1936): Signatur: Mscr. Dres. App. 1832, 783, HRW publisher to Erich Wulffen, 9 December 1930, and 795, HRW publisher to Erich Wulffen, 28 April 1931. Wulffen commented in pencil on some of these suggestions. It has proved impossible to locate the third edition of *Das Weib als Sexualverbrecherin*, which is not held in any major library across the globe. As a consequence, it is impossible to check how much of this advice Wulffen and the publisher took on board for the third edition.
98 Lang, 'Influencing Public Knowledge', pp. 59–60.
99 '[U]nsere gesamte Geisteswelt sexuell geschwängert [wird] und Leser und Leserin erotisiert.' Wulffen, *Irrwege des Eros*, p. 12.
100 SLUB, Nachlass des Schriftstellers und Kriminalisten Min.-Direktor Dr Erich Wulffen (1862–1936): Signatur: Mscr. Dres. App. 1832, 456, Julius Brüll (Avalun publisher) to Erich Wulffen, 28 January 1927.
101 SLUB, Nachlass des Schriftstellers und Kriminalisten Min.-Direktor Dr Erich Wulffen (1862-1936): Signatur: Mscr. Dres. App. 1832, 783, HRW publisher to Erich Wulffen, 9 December 1930, containing the phrase 'ganz gut die doppelte Anzahl von Bildern untergebracht werden könnte, ohne dem Werk seinen wissenschaftlichen Charakter zu nehmen'.
102 SLUB, Nachlass des Schriftstellers und Kriminalisten Min.-Direktor Dr Erich

Wulffen (1862–1936): Signatur: Mscr. Dres. App. 1832, 806, HRW publisher to Erich Wulffen, 24 November 1930, containing the phrases 'hundertmal so schwer wie früher'; 'lebhafte und auffallende Bilder'.

103 SLUB, Nachlass des Schriftstellers und Kriminalisten Min.-Direktor Dr Erich Wulffen (1862–1936): Signatur: Mscr. Dres. App. 1832, 804, Erich Wulffen to HRW publisher, 18 May 1931.

104 SLUB, Nachlass des Schriftstellers und Kriminalisten Min.-Direktor Dr Erich Wulffen (1862–1936): Signatur: Mscr. Dres. App. 1832, 787, HRW publisher to Erich Wulffen, 28 February 1931.

105 SLUB, Nachlass des Schriftstellers und Kriminalisten Min.-Direktor Dr Erich Wulffen (1862–1936): Signatur: Mscr. Dres. App. 1832, 791, Erich Wulffen to HRW publisher, 12 April 1931.

106 SLUB, Nachlass des Schriftstellers und Kriminalisten Min.-Direktor Dr Erich Wulffen (1862–1936): Signatur: Mscr. Dres. App. 1832, 791, Erich Wulffen to HRW publisher, 12 April 1931.

107 SLUB, Nachlass des Schriftstellers und Kriminalisten Min.-Direktor Dr Erich Wulffen (1862–1936): Signatur: Mscr. Dres. App. 1832, 791, Erich Wulffen to HRW publisher, 12 April 1931. Wulffen contributed to academic works on the history of photography with two major contributions: *Die Erotik in der Photographie* (1931) and 'Die behördliche Verfolgung des geheimen Photohandels', *Die geschichtliche Entwicklung der Aktphotographie und des erotischen Lichtbildes und seine Beziehungen zur psychopathia sexualis* (Vienna, Berlin, Leipzig: Verlag für Kulturforschung, 1931), pp. 187–210. See also Erich Wulffen and Felix Abraham, *Fritz Ulbrichs lebender Marmor. Eine sexual-psychologische Untersuchung* (Vienna, Berlin, Leipzig: Verlag für Kulturforschung, 1931). For the analysis of the self-perception of sexologists in this context, see Birgit Lang, 'Die Erotik in der Photographie: Zum Habitus von Sexualwissenschaftern', *LiTheS. Zeitschrift für Literatur und Theatersoziologie*, 5 (2010), pp. 5–24.

108 SLUB, Nachlass des Schriftstellers und Kriminalisten Min.-Direktor Dr Erich Wulffen (1862–1936): Signatur: Mscr. Dres. App. 1832, 791, Erich Wulffen to HRW publisher, 12 April 1931.

109 SLUB, Nachlass des Schriftstellers und Kriminalisten Min.-Direktor Dr Erich Wulffen (1862–1936): Signatur: Mscr. Dres. App. 1832, 797, Erich Wulffen to HRW publisher, 18 May 1931.

110 SLUB, Nachlass des Schriftstellers und Kriminalisten Min.-Direktor Dr Erich Wulffen (1862–1936): Signatur: Mscr. Dres. App. 1832, 797, Erich Wulffen to HRW publisher, 18 May 1931; also 810, HRW publisher to Wulffen, 14 September 1931.

111 Other works include by Robert Heymann include *Sexualwahn* (with Otto Warneyer and Walter Bahn) (1928); *Sing-sang der Liebe; ein buntes Buch von Liedern, Ludern und Lastern* (1928); *Weiber, Könige, Henker. Roman* (1928); *Christinens Weg durch die Hölle. Roman* (1929); *Das Verbrechen* (1930); *Ein Weib, ein Narr, ein Mörder* (1930); *Der masochistische Mann* (1931); *Die hörige Frau* (1931); *Sexuelle Hörigkeit* (1931); *Das hemmungslose Mädchen. Roman* (1932); *Nimm mich zu dir* (1933).

112 '[H]at wenig Anspruch auf Sympathie.' Alfred Polgar, 'Ein Kriminalfall (1924)', in Edith Cadivec, *Bekenntnisse und Erlebnisse* (Munich: Belleville, 2008), pp. 357–58, p. 357.

113 SLUB, Nachlass des Schriftstellers und Kriminalisten Min.-Direktor Dr Erich Wulffen (1862–1936): Signatur: Mscr. Dres. App. 1832, 159, Edith Christally to Erich Wulffen, 2 June 1932, containing the phrase 'Wissen täuscht und betrügt. Die Wahrheit ist die, die man erlebt'. Note that Cadivec changed her second name to Christally after her conviction in 1927.

114 Cadivec, *Bekenntnisse und Erlebnisse*, p. iv.

115 SLUB, Nachlass des Schriftstellers und Kriminalisten Min.-Direktor Dr Erich

Wulffen (1862–1936): Signatur: Mscr. Dres. App. 1832, 159, Edith Christally to Erich Wulffen, 2 June 1932.
116 Armand Coppens, 'Memoiren eines Erotica-Händlers (1969)', in Cadivec, *Bekenntnisse und Erlebnisse*, pp. 443–6, p. 445; 'Bibliographische Verweise', in Cadivec, *Bekenntnisse und Erlebnisse*, pp. 447–51.
117 Cadivec, *Bekenntnisse und Erlebnisse*, p. iv.
118 Wulffen, *Irrwege des Eros*, p. 277. The psychiatric report is missing in the Viennese case files.
119 'Attest des Psychoanalytikers Ludwig Jekels für Walter Taussig', in Cadivec, *Bekenntnisse und Erlebnisse*, p. 442.
120 '[M]it Hilfe der Auto- und Fremdsuggestion sich eine Auffassung gebildet habe, die ihre Handlungsweise mit der Moral zu versöhnen suche.' Wulffen, *Irrwege des Eros*, p. 277.
121 Neda Bei, 'Zum Strafverfahren gegen Edith Cadivec im Wiener "Sadistenprozess", 1924 (2005/2007)', in Cadivec, *Bekenntnisse und Erlebnisse*, pp. 397–428, p. 414.
122 Wulffen, *Manolescu*, p. 108.
123 SLUB, Nachlass des Schriftstellers und Kriminalisten Min.-Direktor Dr Erich Wulffen (1862–1936): Signatur: Mscr. Dres. App. 1832, 1448, 'Hochstaplerrache am Staatsanwalt', *Deutsche Allgemeine Zeitung*, 30 March 1923; 'Fall Engel', undated.
124 SLUB, Nachlass des Schriftstellers und Kriminalisten Min.-Direktor Dr Erich Wulffen (1862–1936): Signatur: Mscr. Dres. App. 1832, 974, Erich Wulffen, 'Siegmund [*sic*] Freud', where the German reads: 'Vor allem ist es die sexuelle Lockung, welche die ganze Theorie umgaukelt. Die Behauptung, all unser Fühlen und Denken und jede Deutung unserer Zustände und unseres Verhaltens habe sexuellen Zusammenhang, hat für den Menschen ganz allgemein und besonders in der Gegenwart eine ausserordentliche Anziehung. Dass darin ein krasser Materialismus steckt, wird kaum bemerkt. Dasein und Leben werden im Höchstmass erotisiert, sexualisiert zu einer Zeit, da alle sonstigen Reizmittel versagen. Die Übererotisierung, die Übersexualisierung, an der die Gegenwart leidet, sind zu einem Hauptteil der Freudschen Lehre mit zuzuschreiben'.
125 Juliusburger, '*Der Sexualverbrecher*', p. 259.
126 Erich Wulffen, *Shakespeares Hamlet. Ein Sexualproblem* (Berlin: Duncker, 1913).
127 SLUB, Nachlass des Schriftstellers und Kriminalisten Min.-Direktor Dr Erich Wulffen (1862–1936): Signatur: Mscr. Dres. App. 1832, 1478, Otto Juliusburger, 'Enzyklopädie der Kriminalistik [Review of *Sexualverbrecherin*]', *Fortschritte der Medizin*, 13 May 1932, p. 419; a similar concern was raised in the forum *Psychiatrische-neurologische Wochenschrift*, 9 April 1932.
128 Erich Wulffen, 'Siegmund Freud'.
129 '[F]ür alle möglichen Auslegungen empfänglich.' Wulffen, 'Siegmund Freud'.
130 SLUB, Nachlass des Schriftstellers und Kriminalisten Min.-Direktor Dr Erich Wulffen (1862–1936): Signatur: Mscr. Dres. App. 1832, 1495, Friedrich Harth to Erich Wulffen, 19 July 1932, containing the phrase 'ergriffen und aufgerüttelt' and 'Seelenrätsel'.

5

Alfred Döblin's literary cases about women and crime in Weimar Germany

Alison Lewis

After the First World War, European writers turned increasingly to consideration of social problems in the metropolis, and the impact of the war on sexual and mental health more broadly. In particular, the topics of violence against women, and women who commit violence, which many writers began to tackle in new ways, proved popular among readers in Weimar Germany, especially in the cities of Munich and Berlin. Stories about real cases were at once frightening and titillating – and for the first time such stories were readily available, through the diversification of literary markets, and the plethora of newspaper and print media that began to report on contemporary trials and curious cases. Middle-class and petit-bourgeois publics were keen to consume thrilling and shocking stories of crime and sexuality in newspapers and novels. They did so, and as a result these publics grew more literate and discerning, which in turn compelled writers to invent novel ways of presenting the strange but real cases. On the one hand, authors whose professional lives brought them into close contact with remarkable real-life cases (of either sexual deviance or criminality, or both), found themselves uniquely placed to cater for the appetites of these publics. Through writing and publishing case studies based on their first-hand experience, they were able to capitalise on their insider knowledge of crime and the criminal mind. These writers could easily obtain graphic source material about sensational cases through their professional associations, and provide additional expert commentary on well known cases. On the other hand, doctors and judges needed to find a point of difference between their kinds of writing about the criminal mind and underworld and writing by other sources, such as first-person accounts of crime authored by con men and criminals themselves. The experienced writer of literature with additional expertise in medicine or the law was undoubtedly better placed to interpret these real-life cases and to draw general conclusions from them. Yet he or she needed to find new ways to seize and hold a reader's attention. This was the conundrum that aspiring young German writer Alfred Döblin (1878–1957), a medical practitioner working in one of Germany's most seductive and dangerous metropolises, faced at the beginning of the Weimar Republic.

Born in the seaport city of Stettin in 1878, Döblin was a resident of Berlin who trained as a medical practitioner. He had harboured literary aspirations from an early age, but suppressed them in order to pursue a passion for medicine and the natural sciences. Many novelists of the day, such as Ernest Hemingway, began their career as newspaper reporters and strove to replicate the facticity of newspaper reporting in their literature. By contrast, while concurrently pursuing a career in medicine, Döblin indulged sporadically in writing until he first met with commercial success in 1929 through the publication of his novel *Berlin Alexanderplatz*.[1] Hence, it was not to journalism and print media that he turned to articulate his views on crime and violence – although Döblin did borrow his plots from the daily press – nor to the many psychoanalytic or medical journals of the time, but to literature.[2]

Here it will be suggested that literature provided Döblin (and indeed others before him, such as Bertolt Brecht and Erich Wulffen) with a metaphorical laboratory to revel and experiment in. Döblin's literary laboratory was not sealed off from the outside world, like a rarefied scientific space, but was an open, public forum that came with an appreciative audience, and with its own enlightened, educated reading public. This public was sufficiently distinct from other competing publics represented by newspaper readers and the like, and to Döblin it must have seemed advantageous to write for a 'captive audience'. Specifically, the so-called objective, empirically based literature of New Objectivity (*Neue Sachlichkeit*) in Germany offered Döblin a welcome medium in which to explore shocking and risqué themes of the day.

Many of Döblin's contemporaries, such as Erich Kästner and Hans Fallada, sought inspiration in the plethora of dynamic new urban spaces and milieus opening up in the cities of Berlin or Munich – seedy bars, brothels and alluring cinemas. Others, like Döblin, looked further afield to underpin their irrepressible flights of creative fantasy about modern city life. Döblin valued empirical sources for his stories, but, in addition to realistic settings, he chose to draw on the empirical human or 'life' sciences for guidance. After all, Berlin was, as Andreas Killen observes, the 'breeding ground' for nervous and mental illness, and for a new discourse about nervous exhaustion, or neurasthenia.[3] With its modern medicine and unique social welfare system, Berlin provided those writers like Döblin who practised a profession such as medicine with ample material to mine. In Berlin Döblin could observe the 'hidden costs' of modern capitalism in the rise of sexually motivated crimes and modern pathologies, which were now manifesting not merely as middle-class problems but as mass social phenonema.[4]

French writers of the nineteenth century had already observed that the modern age urgently needed to anchor its literature in real life and to document modern maladies. The sickness of their era was hysteria and writers such as Gustave Flaubert plumbed this topic for a voracious readership.[5] But by the early twentieth century, bourgeois forms of cultural expression needed to adapt in order to contend with newer maladies and social ills. As the privileged cultural form of the *Bildungsbürgertum*, literature faced challenges from many quarters, challenges that an empirical turn could not adequately address without a more radical reinvention of the parameters of literature itself. In the modern metropolis, the writers of *belles-lettres* found themselves faced not only with great complexity and interconnectivity of life forms, but with competing and multiplying forms of knowledge about these life forms, which must have daunted any attempt to make sense of the many innovations in science and the arts.

In style and scope, Döblin's works have most often been compared to the high modernism of James Joyce and the American John Dos Passos.[6] A writer of remarkable diversity and inventiveness, Döblin wrote on an astonishing range of topics, including the Manchu dynasty in China, the Thirty Years' War, modern urban life in Berlin, the 1918 November Revolution and European colonialism. He penned mostly novels as well as a few dramas, radio plays and dozens of essays on politics, religion and art. Although usually grouped under the banner of modernism, his works in fact span a number of quite heterogeneous genres, from historical fiction, science fiction, travel writing to crime fiction. While such breadth is possibly less surprising when one considers that Döblin witnessed some of the most turbulent decades of twentieth-century European history, the scope of his literary output, which now fills thirty volumes of 'selected works', is by all standards impressive. He lived through the last years of the Wilhelminian era, two world wars, the Weimar Republic, National Socialism, exile in France and the USA, as well as the post-war Federal Republic of Germany.

It remains something of a mystery, therefore, that Döblin, although critically acclaimed as a writer of international stature, never achieved the popularity of other writers in the modernist canon, most of whom who were just as difficult and complex.[7] In the Weimar Republic, Döblin was certainly a prominent figure through his short stories, his journalistic writings and his many novels – in 1925 Thomas Mann already described him as 'one of our foremost novelists'.[8] Actually, few of his works were commercial successes until *Berlin Alexanderplatz* in 1929. Focused on a factory owner who loses a battle with his competitor, Döblin's second novel, *Wadzeks Kampf mit der Dampfmaschine* (*Wadzek's Battle with the Steam Turbine*), from 1918, was labelled 'cubist' and deemed a critical failure.[9] Döblin was thought to redeem himself with his next novel, *Wallenstein*, a grand anti-war epic in two volumes, which went into a second print run.[10]

To be sure, Döblin was fortunate to have secured the support of an influential publisher in Samuel Fischer, who published his first work, in 1916 – about the Wu-wei resistance movement, *Die drei Sprünge des*

Wang-Lun (*The Three Leaps of Wang-Lun*) – and subsequent novels until 1933. Döblin was in good company, since S. Fischer was also the publishing house of Germany's two other great writers of the era, Gerhart Hauptmann and Thomas Mann. But unlike Hauptmann, who had been awarded the Nobel Prize in Literature in 1912, and Mann, who was its recipient in 1929, Döblin's fame was largely limited to Germany. Throughout his career he lived very much in the shadow of his two literary forebears. When he found himself struggling to pay the rent in exile in Los Angeles as the Manns were preparing to build a palatial residence on the Riviera, he was reminded once again that he was, by comparison with Mann, only a middling writer.[11]

Alfred Döblin, realism, naturalism and modernism

Döblin's strongest literary influences were undoubtedly the great French realists of the nineteenth century, and the Berlin naturalists Hauptmann and Wedekind. And yet, in the 1930s, when Döblin was admitted into the canon of world literature, taking his place alongside Joyce and Dos Passos, it was not as a realist or naturalist but as a moderniser and modernist.[12] Hence in German literary circles Döblin is rarely compared to his French literary forebears Gustave Flaubert, Honoré de Balzac and Émile Zola. This is curious, all the more so since Döblin proclaimed once in 1924 that the modern 'European-American world' was on the cusp of a naturalist age.[13]

Among French literary historians, German naturalism is often regarded as an imitation of French naturalism, which was superseded by symbolism and a new 'nervous romanticism'. In a recent revision of this idea, Stéphane Michaud has argued in favour of seeing classical works of German modernism by Musil and Döblin as the legitimate heirs to French naturalism.[14] Alternatively, we could view expressionism, the successor to naturalism, as does Richard Heinrich, as a 'naturalism of nerves'.[15] Richard Daniel Lehan goes further, proposing that the literary modes of naturalism and realism were the crucial 'vortex through which the novel passed' across Europe and the Americas for 100 years. Both naturalism and realism represent a 'powerful way of seeing the physical world' that responded to large-scale social changes.[16] Naturalism, for instance, can be considered a response to Darwinian theories of heredity and the environment 'that would ground the literary work in a factual and scientific context'.[17] Indeed, in Germany naturalism was far from dead at the turn of the century; it was being reinvented through the discipline of psychology. Naturalism's focus on heredity and degeneration was being replaced by an intense interest in human desire and the social determinants of human actions.[18] Döblin's work demonstrates that naturalism found a new expedient ally in the medical, legal and psychoanalytic case history – that most empirical of new-found genres – thus prolonging the life of the naturalist spirit in global literature well beyond its heyday in the Second French Empire.

The diversity of Döblin's output has posed a challenge to scholarship. His oeuvre is most commonly linked to Brecht's innovations in epic theatre, especially since several of his major novels present epic treatments of grand historical themes. A feature of his approach to historical topics is, like Brecht's, his sympathy with the powerless masses of history.[19] Closely related to this is another of his major concerns, namely with the harsh realities of modern urban life as experienced through various low-life or lower-class characters – criminals, prostitutes and working-class figures. But unlike Brecht, Döblin chose the medium of the novel to develop these themes rather than drama, and in doing so was possibly overshadowed by other great masters of the modern novel of the time in Thomas Mann and Robert Musil.

Berlin Alexanderplatz, written in the middle of his career, appears to stand across both strands of his writing: it manages to bring Döblin's fascination with the anonymous masses in history together with his keen interest in exploring individual psychology. Although its title suggests an epic treatment of a contemporary theme, the novel focuses on the fortunes of a recently released criminal, Franz Biberkopf, and is set on the fringes of the underworld of Berlin's teeming metropolis of the 1920s, with which Döblin was only too familiar from working with social welfare patients. Döblin develops a distinctive aesthetics of empathy for the 'small man' in this work, which was to augur well for the novel's positive critical reception at the time and in later years. A pivotal stage in the development of the writer's avowed sympathies for the lower middle classes – which he shared with contemporaries like Kästner and Brecht but not with Musil or Mann – is a far less well known work, from 1924, *Die beiden Freundinnen und ihr Giftmord* (*Two Girlfriends Commit Murder by Poison*).[20] This earlier work, so modest that it is often omitted from surveys of Döblin's oeuvre, is a case study that combines medical and legal traditions of case writing. It is this work, it will be argued, that plays a crucial role in the development of Döblin's specific brand of literary modernism.

These two literary works, which are both indebted to the case study genre, stand in a complex dialogic relationship to the newer styles of modernism and the older modes of naturalism and realism. In many ways, Döblin's works from this period of transition deserve Heinrich's epithet of a sort of 'naturalism of the nerves'. Döblin is often thought to belong to the camp of left-leaning modernist writers, such as Brecht, who responded to the crisis of individualism by advocating a revival of epic traditions in prose and drama.[21] Scholarship has tended to stress Döblin's break with nineteenth-century realism and present his later works as a modernist breakthrough to a new anti-realist style. These classifications capture part of the story of Döblin's massive oeuvre; however, they fail to account adequately for the innovations Döblin made in documentary realism, or, more accurately, in criminal or medical realism.

The case study genre can be shown leading the charge in innovating around the conventions associated with realism and naturalism. Rather than abandoning the realist traditions of the nineteenth century, through his case studies of ordinary working-class men and women situated on the fringes of respectable society (and with one foot in the criminal underworld), Döblin sharpens the tools in the traditional realist tool box. He does so by incorporating into his largely realist handiwork new medical, sexological means, as well as psychoanalytic instruments and knowledge. He also modernises the literary tools in the naturalist kit, applying the insights of the medically trained observer of sexual pathologies to real-life murder cases.

It was arguably the case study's emphasis on the individual, and his or her inner life driving social behaviour, especially its extremes such as murder and violence, that was to exert a decisive influence on Döblin's literary production. Moreover, the traditions of medical and criminological case writing were to inform Döblin's approach to literature at a crucial time in his development as a writer, eventually pushing him further in the direction of a forensic type of socially engaged modernism that is epitomised in *Berlin Alexanderplatz*. In Döblin's early historical epics, his focus was more on crowd psychology and behaviour than on the individual.[22] In his futurist work from 1924, *Berge, Giganten und Meere* (*Mountains, Seas and Giants*), we can already see the beginnings of a more pronounced shift towards the individual. More so than this novel, however, it is a much shorter one that seems to hold the key to his aesthetic breakthrough, his true crime novel and medical case study of heterosexual and homosexual relationships, *Die beiden Freundinnen und ihr Giftmord*. A direct line can be traced from this work to Döblin's masterpiece of modernism in *Berlin Alexanderplatz*. Reading Döblin through the prism of the genre of the case study thus makes possible a more nuanced interpretation of his relationship to the two major literary modes of the time, realism and modernism. In addition, it facilitates revision of prevailing conceptions of the relationship between progressive politics and modernism. It can be shown that Döblin's experiments with the case study genre were unthinkable without his expert training in and first-hand knowledge of medicine.

With his mother, Sophie, and four siblings, Döblin had moved to Berlin in 1888, after his womanising and occasionally violent father, Max Döblin, had abandoned the family. As the second youngest sibling, Alfred Döblin was the only member of his immediate family to complete secondary school and enter university; like other writers of his time, such as Gottfried Benn and Arthur Schnitzler, Döblin undertook medical training. From an early age, he harboured literary aspirations while continuing to further his medical training and to establish his career as a medical practitioner and later as a psychiatrist. Döblin's first tentative attempts at writing literature began around 1900, when he was student of medicine in Berlin and Freiburg. His first two novels were written during this time, the second one finding a publisher only much later, in

1919, when it was published under the title *Der schwarze Vorhang* (*The Black Curtain*). After completing his medical training, Döblin worked in various psychiatric clinics, spending a year in Regensburg and two years in Berlin-Buch, and gained further experience in Berlin hospitals, such as the Charité and the municipal Hospital Am Urban, where he met his future wife.

Döblin's friendship with editor, art critic and fellow Jewish writer Herwarth Walden dates from the time of his undergraduate medical studies. When Walden launched the *Der Sturm* (*The Attack*) in 1910, first a monthly periodical and later a gallery that served as a launching pad for expressionism, fauvism, cubism and the futurists, Döblin was one of its ardent supporters. Döblin had yet to publish a full-length novel when the First World War intervened and he was enlisted as a military doctor. In 1916 his first novel, *Die drei Sprünge des Wang-Lun*, appeared while Döblin was still stationed in Saargemünd in Alsace-Lorraine, France. Hailed as a breakthrough in the novel format, the work was a critical success and was even translated into French. However, as he remarked, in the early years there was little or no prospect of making a living from his literature.

Döblin does not appear to have regarded his medical and neurological training as anything more than a means to secure a living, and one independent from his hobby of writing literature. This is not to say that Döblin was not passionate about his medical work and research. He confessed, when reflecting on his life: 'medicine and science had an extraordinary hold on me'.[23] In one autobiographical sketch, he describes spending years of his life, presumably between 1905 and 1911, 'wandering' around mental asylums, evading 'the struggle for so-called existence'.[24] He felt strangely comfortable in the company of the mentally ill, he recalls, and alongside plants, animals and stones claims he tolerated only two types of humans: children and the mad.[25]

Döblin wrote his dissertation on alcohol-induced memory disorders under psychiatrist Alfred Erich Hoche in the years prior to the outbreak of the war. Döblin's lifelong mission to illuminate the causes of mental illness, which was later to drive his forays into literature, stems from his time conducting medical research: 'the darkness that surrounded these sick people was what I wanted to help to illuminate'.[26] According to Döblin, his pre-war years spent in psychiatric clinics eventually led him to turn away from conventional psychiatry and to seek answers in the field of internal medicine. Through the work of Berlin's Institut für Sexualwissenschaft (Institute for Sexual Science) he inevitably became familiar with the latest theories on the 'inner secretions', or hormones. In his words, 'you had to get inside the physiological, not inside brains, but maybe inside the glands, the metabolism'.[27]

After Vienna and Zurich, Berlin was rapidly becoming the third major centre for psychoanalysis.[28] Working in Berlin's large clinics brought Döblin into direct contact with many of the city's sexologists and psychoanalysts, who, under Karl Abraham, were to form the Berlin

Psychoanalytic Institute in 1923.[29] Where Döblin writes that Sigmund Freud's theories were no revelation to him – 'Freud was not a revelation to me personally' – this indifference must be taken with a healthy grain of salt. No doubt representing an underestimation of Freud's impact on himself, Döblin's claim possibly says more about Freud's pre-eminence in the field of psychoanalysis at the time.[30] Psychoanalytic theories that were being formulated and tested in Berlin's hospitals and talked about in the newspapers were even dismissed by some as a 'craze'.[31]

By his own admission, Döblin was anything but indifferent to this craze of psychoanalysis: in 1928 he describes himself possessing a 'great sensitive receptivity, an exceptional capacity for analytical insight namely in the direction of the psychic-unconscious'.[32] When professing in the same sketch to have been more influenced by physiology and neurology than by psychoanalysis, he merely seems to be indicating his preference for physical, somatic and neurological explanatory models of mental illness over purely psychological ones. Like most traditionally trained psychiatrists of the time, he had been schooled in the neurological and physiological determinants of mental illness, but in the post-war years he had increasingly engaged with a whole range of newer psychoanalytic ideas.

Döblin first became interested in psychoanalysis around the time he started working as a doctor in his own practice for social welfare cases. After the First World War and moving his practice to the city's eastside, to 340 Frankfurter Allee in Lichtenberg, he proceeded to train as an analyst in the Berlin Psychoanalytic Institute under the guidance of Ernst Simmel. He went on to join Abraham's reading group and encountered Erich Fromm, Wilhelm Reich and Melanie Klein.[33] Döblin shared the social and political concerns of the Institute and became a member of the Verein Sozialistischer Ärzte (Association of Socialist Doctors), through which he came into contact with the work of Magnus Hirschfeld's Institut für Sexualwissenschaft.

His profound and, as suggested in his memoir, almost uncanny ability to plumb the depths of the psyche's unconscious proved a particular asset in Döblin's first explicit experiment with a medical topic, in *Die beiden Freundinnen und ihr Giftmord*. Because he was trained in many new empirical and clinical disciplines it seemed only natural to Döblin to try to tap into these insights, and to conjoin his two passions in life. His expert medical knowledge could form the basis for experimenting with new forms and styles of writing and allow him to indulge his latest interest.

Like Gottfried Benn, Döblin writes about the split in his life between literature and medicine. In the fashion of the period, he regarded both activities as evidence of the unifying entity of the individual genius, although Döblin never expressed the relationship in these terms.[34] At the heart of Döblin's dualism is, of course, the myth of two cultures – that which C. P. Snow famously called the myth of two opposing cultural spheres.[35] Despite his expertise in both medicine and the arts, Döblin always felt an uneasy tension between his work as a doctor and his endeavours as a writer. In two essays from 1927, 'Der Nervenarzt Döblin über den Dichter Döblin' ('The Nerve Doctor Döblin on the Writer Döblin') and 'Der Dichter Döblin über den Nervenarzt Döblin' ('The Writer Döblin on the Nerve Doctor Döblin'), he writes about the odd relationship between the two different aspects of his life. Not only does Döblin the doctor claim to barely 'know' Döblin the writer, he maintains that his literary works are 'completely foreign to me and I am also completely indifferent to them'.[36] The doctor side of himself does not share the political views or the tastes in literature of his writer self. Döblin the writer, however, appears to have a far better relationship to his namesake in Döblin the doctor, and is at least curious to learn more about the life of a doctor, even to exploit it, if only to find source material for use in his writing. The split between Döblin's two passions in life is presented less in psychological than in sociological terms, and offers a commentary on the increasing specialisation of knowledge in the modern world. The writer is an individualist and a generalist, while the doctor is nothing out of the ordinary, a 'grey soldier in a quiet army', and a specialist.[37] Yet Döblin the writer has an inferiority complex with regard to Döblin the doctor: 'I have defects, probably complexes, and the practised doctor probably sensed something'.[38] Despite the writer's greater fame, he feels defensive towards the doctor, as if intimidated by the knowing gaze of the psychiatrist, whereas the Döblin the doctor is unashamed of his ignorance of literature. From this exchange, it is not hard to adduce the crisis of dominant literary systems of knowledge. Discussing the viability of writing literature in an essay titled 'Ökonomisches aus der Literatur' ('Economic Observations from the Literary Sphere'), Döblin complains bitterly that, despite having published ten books, and selling 6,200 copies, in 1924 he had hardly earned more than 400 Reichsmark per month. He does admit, however, that his 'criminal case' of the two women who tried to poison their husbands sold 3,000 copies and, over the two years 1924 and 1925, earned him a total of 1,200 Reichsmarks.[39]

Criminology and sexology in the literary case study

Döblin wrote his novella *Die beiden Freundinnen und ihr Giftmord* for a new series of crime stories based on real criminal cases. His friend Rudolf Leonhard was keen to commission stories for a new publisher in Berlin, Die Schmiede, and called his series 'Außenseiter der Gesellschaft: Die Verbrechen der Gegenwart' ('Outsiders in Society: The Criminals of Today'). Döblin was to write the first work in what the editor hoped would become a lucrative new series. From Döblin's perspective *Die beiden Freundinnen und ihr Giftmord* combined a number of his professional and personal preoccupations, which he subjected to a new documentary style of treatment. He took a real criminal case as his material, borrowed extensively from journalistic and legal sources and, for embellishment, drew on his medical expertise and his personal experience. Döblin was interested in questions of sadomasochism, madness, sexually motivated violence and female sexuality, and the real criminal case involved all of these themes. From his autobiographical writings it is clear that Döblin also had personal experience of the toll that an abusive marriage could take on women. His sister Meta, who was tragically killed by shrapnel during the attempted November Revolution in Lichtenfelde in 1919, had suffered terribly at the hands of her husband, who, according to Döblin, had married her only for her dowry. 'It was a terrible marriage', he writes.[40]

Döblin's novella centres on a famous legal case from 1923 concerning a woman who poisoned her husband out of love for another woman. Ella Klein and Margarete Nebbe were brought to trial in Berlin for attempting to murder their husbands by poisoning them with arsenic, and their trial touched a raw nerve with readers of the time. Like so many of his contemporaries, Döblin was fascinated and scandalised by the emergence of a new type of female criminal, and the spectre of the 'female poisoner', a phenomenon that Wulffen explored in his popular study *Psychologie des Giftmords* (1917). It reminded him of his sister and the abuse she had suffered, which might easily have escalated into a murder, had she not died during the November Revolution. Döblin recognised the potential of the criminal case for a wider readership, whose fears and anxieties about female sexuality had already been well nurtured by publications such as Richard von Krafft-Ebing's sexological study *Psychopathia Sexualis* (1886), Oskar Panizza's satires and Erich Wulffen's handbooks for lawyers and doctors *Das Weib als Sexualverbrecherin* (1923) and *Psychologie des Verbrechers* (1906, reissued 1908). The Klein–Nebbe case had been sensationalised in the print media in Berlin and the rest of Germany, and taken up by the international press as well. In addition to tackling the issue of the female criminal, it had the added intrigue of female homosexuality, or inversion, along with another modish topic of the day, the 'perversion' of sadomasochism.

Despite having changed the names of the main characters – Ella Klein becomes Elli Link and Margarete Nebbe becomes Margarete (Grete) Bende – Döblin's novella is highly realistic and almost documentary in style. Readers contemporary with Döblin would have been familiar with the real court case from the extensive press coverage, and most would certainly have seen the novella as an exposition of the Klein–Nebbe murder case. Appearances are, however, deceptive, because in the novella the case is carefully crafted, or rather, woven from a bricolage of diverse source material, some medical and psychoanalytic, some journalistic.

On one level, the fictionalised case study composed by Döblin evokes the traditions of legal and medical-forensic case reporting that emerged over the course of the eighteenth century as part of a new 'forensic dispositif' made possible by new testing possibilities, the results of which could be deployed as evidence in trials.[41] Increasingly throughout the nineteenth century, specialist medical knowledge became a topic of interest for a general reading public. In the eighteenth century, the Pitaval tradition of crime writing had already made sensational criminal court cases accessible to a lay reading public, and as middle-class publics expanded over the course of the nineteenth century so did the level of awareness of criminality and pathology, as well as competency in reading such cases. This was partly because in Germany after 1850 legal trials were opened to the public and newspapers were able to report cases of interest with greater fidelity. Moreover, literary writers were – with permission of the court – able to gain access to court materials and ground their own crime narratives in more reliable sources of empirical evidence, such as evidence presented at trials, as well as expert witness statements.[42] With the advent of psychoanalysis, and of sexological theories about 'deviant' sexual behaviour in the twentieth century, the forensic dispositif came to focus on the criminal and her state of mind. By the time of the Klein–Nebbe trial, the courts deployed state-of-the-art medical evidence, often from competing areas within the same discipline, thus from all branches of forensic medicine, neurological psychiatry, sexual medicine and psychology. Of all the schools of psychiatry, however, the newer discipline of psychoanalysis was the least well represented in court cases.[43] This lack of presence during trials can be explained by the fact that institutional acceptance of psychoanalysis developed slowly and with difficulty; this process was shaped by mutual disregard between the practitioners of the court and psychoanalysts, as explored in Chapter 4.

Döblin's literary case writing in *Die beiden Freundinnen und ihr Giftmord* is so faithful to the real case that it is hard to imagine he was not present during the five days of the Klein–Nebbe trial in March 1923. Yet all indications are that he was most likely not present, nor was he an expert witness during the trial, although he knew the doctors who had treated Willi Klein and he had spoken to Ella Klein and Nebbe.[44] Döblin did, however, possess a copy of the *Anklageschrift*, the formal indictment which summarises the court proceedings, and was also familiar with the medical expert witness statements provided by sexologist and psychiatrist Magnus Hirschfeld, and two others, Otto Juliusberger and Friedrich Leppmann. Döblin's other main textual source is the comprehensive newspaper coverage of the trial over those five days; the reports were published in the morning and evening issues of virtually every national and regional newspaper in Germany.

Döblin's literary case study appears to be a good demonstration of the modernist aesthetics of New Objectivity, which aimed to move literature away from conventional psychology and closer to the human and empirical sciences, to be more documentary in style and to be a form of 'factual fantasy' ('Tatsachenphantasie').[45] Read as an elaboration of a criminal case, *Die beiden Freundinnen und ihr Giftmord* actually belongs to a much older tradition of crime writing.[46] With its focus on the criminal, Döblin's story is typical of much of the crime writing that newly emerged from the second half of the nineteenth century onwards.[47] In the vein of a criminal case study, the novella seeks to present a specific example ('Beispiel') of a more general human condition. Yet this instance is not offered as an exemplar, nor as an illustration of a norm or a point of law, nor even of a pathological condition in the usual way of criminal cases.[48] Rather, it might be considered a concretisation of critic André Jolles's simple form of the *Kasus*, the universal form that discusses a criminal event in the context of a deviation from moral or legal norms. In Jolles's schema of 'simple' literary forms, the function of the *Kasus* is to pose questions and weigh up norms of social behaviour.[49] Akin to the riddle, which is a question begging an answer, the *Kasus* poses a moral question via the crime, which often it can only partially answer – frequently by asking further questions. Döblin's story also appears to have much in common with legal and medical case writing, namely in the relationship between the specific instance and the general rule or hypothesis that the case seeks to extrapolate from the example. While the specific modality of this relationship can vary, the general can be inferred from the specific case in inductive forms, or prior to it in deductive forms, or simultaneously when interpretation and representation of the case coincide.[50] The romantic, realist and modernist case of the nineteenth and twentieth centuries gave preference to the inductive method over the deductive.[51]

In writing *Die beiden Freundinnen und ihr Giftmord* Döblin relies heavily on the *Anklageschrift* and the newspaper reports from a host of Berlin newspapers.[52] These sources all reported on the content of the 600 letters exchanged by Klein and Nebbe, and Döblin uses these letters as well. In a rather reductive fashion that was characteristic of newspaper writing of the time, the papers classified the women according to common gender stereotypes of the sadistic, hysterical, unscrupulous woman, and the cold, calculating and inhuman perpetrator.[53] The *Berliner Lokalanzeiger* speaks of two 'dehumanised women ... who wanted to divest themselves of their husbands, who had become a hindrance to them in their abnormal relationship to one another through the unscrupulous, cold and calculating usage of poison'.[54] The demonisation of both women in the press is only slightly mitigated by witnesses who recounted Klein's abusive marriage and Willi Klein's alcoholism. This was a small detail that might have gone unnoticed by most readers, but it struck a chord with Döblin, and was to become the centre-piece of his literary treatment of the trial.

The main change that Döblin makes to extant accounts of the trial is to shift the focus from the inner, psychic realm of the criminal – the principal focus of the newspaper reports – to the space in-between, the intersubjective space between the two women and their conflicts.[55] This innovation enables Döblin to break down the impression that there is a direct, causal link between crime and criminal agent, and perhaps also to deflect attention from the known fact that the actual murder was patently planned. Döblin's other main innovation is to introduce into his novella the concept of the unconscious. This concept had become one of his burning obsessions, and he presents it at the start of his own thinly fictionalised causal chain of events, thereby portraying his characters as figures in a complex game of psychical processes. For *Die beiden Freundinnen und ihr Giftmord* Döblin makes a second shift of emphasis in relation to the case: he intertwines psychological and social causes so as to make each one highly dependent on the other. This sets his account apart from those in the press. He thereby presents the crime as the result of an almost unfathomable confluence of social and psychological factors and conscious and unconscious motives.

Döblin's case writing is deeply experimental, and he seems to have been unsure of how to achieve the desired realistic effect and of how to acknowledge the many baffling aspects of the case. This uncertainty leads him to restate his argument several times within the one work, through the use of slightly different components, published in the original version of *Die beiden Freundinnen und ihr Giftmord*. The story of the murder is supplemented by non-literary and para-literary material, which have largely perplexed critics. At the end of the largely realistic narrative of the case appears a short epilogue with a commentary by the author. Following the epilogue are two one-page, illustrated analyses of the handwriting of each woman, 'Zu Ellis Handschrift' ('On Elli's Handwriting') and 'Zu Margaretes Handschrift' ('On Margarete's Handwriting'). As well, at the close of the volume of the first edition of 1924, and only in this edition, Döblin included an unusual psychiatric addendum, or afterthought to his narrative. Unbound from the text of the novella, and inserted in an envelope glued inside the back cover, the addendum presents a series of psychoanalytic diagrams, printed in colour on ten glossy pages DIN 476 in size. These diagrams represent a further illustration of the case, but in a specialist language and a non-discursive form. Given the title 'Räumliche Darstellung der Seelenveränderung' ('Spatial Representation of the Changes to the Soul'), the addendum comprises seventeen visualisations and two graphs.

Simply by virtue of these heterogeneous components of *Die beiden Freundinnen und ihr Giftmord* as first published, Döblin's literary case study is an anomaly. No doubt it was an indulgence on the part of the publisher, Die Schmiede, and his friend Rudolf Leonhard, who edited the series, to publish it in this form, which is conceivably why the diagrammatic addendum was not included in subsequent editions of the work. The end effect of the first edition is that Döblin rather overstates the intricacies of his interpretation of the Klein–Nebbe murder case; in other words, the impact of the additional, non-literary adjuncts is to overdetermine the myriad causal factors leading to the crime. In the literary narrative Döblin points to various causes of the murder, such as the lesbian relationship between Elli Link and Grete Bende, the violent and loveless marriages, the choice of rat poison, the psychology and pathology of the characters, each playing a role in the eventual crime of murder. Still, Döblin appears to think that his literary account of the case is insufficient, and with the addendum he decides to embellish it in formal, aesthetic terms. By embroidering the literary case study, adding extra-literary elements such as the epilogue and then the addendum, however, Döblin risks staging the case in several discrete acts.[56] In each of these acts, he tries to elucidate the aetiology of the crime, with the help of distinct discursive formations.

In the literary sections Döblin provides his own aetiology of the case, stressing causal factors such as infantilism, homosexuality and the brutality of Elli Link's husband.[57] In the first chapter of the narrative, the story of Elli Link and her abusive relationship with her husband is narrated; the second chapter tells of the lesbian relationship between Elli Link and Grete Bende, and their plot to kill their husbands. Finally, Döblin concludes with a summary of the findings of the trial and the verdict. Yet unlike the court reporters, Döblin is at pains to offer a sympathetic and impartial account, while censoring much of the original evidence produced at the trial. The court transcripts are full of explicit statements taken from the letters. By contrast, Döblin softens his account of Ella Klein/Elli Link's suffering, bringing his story back to this figure as a casualty of marital abuse. An important subtext to Döblin's version is that the husband of Ella Klein/Elli Link belongs to the large army of war-damaged and traumatised veterans from the First World War. He is one of the shell-shocked, unable to live up to ideals of masculinity, and doomed to repeat his wartime trauma in acts of senseless violence directed against his wife.

Döblin's account, however, never imparts the full details of the husband's past and his suffering during the war; instead, Döblin alludes to this in Willi Link's alcoholism and unmotivated violence. Rather, Elli Link is his main focus of attention, as she becomes the victim of a violence that is all-pervasive in society, and that emanates, as sexologists said it would, from damaged returned war veterans, who cannot distinguish between the war front and the home front. Elli Link is more victim than villain in Döblin's account, and the mitigating circumstances Döblin builds into his story point to an important function of his case study. The writer's aim is to humanise the criminal rather than diagnose her or him, and thus to elicit some sympathy and understanding for the plight of Elli Link.

Hence at the level of plot, the narrative is preoccupied with the psychosexual dynamics of Elli Link's marriage – described from the perspectives of both wife and husband – and the plan to murder Elli Link's husband, while the trial and the time in jail are given comparatively little coverage. The language used throughout is literary in the broadest sense, neither strictly medical nor psychoanalytic, although it is replete with allusions to common psychoanalytic terminology of the day. For instance, when referring to the work of the unconscious, Döblin uses the word *unterirdisch* (subterranean). While the behaviour and actions of his characters are clearly viewed through the lens of medical knowledge, Döblin's craft is purely literary.

Döblin's newest passion for psychoanalysis proves to have been the most significant additional influence on *Die beiden Freundinnen und ihr Giftmord*. Ernst Simmel, Döblin's mentor, had experimented in treating war trauma and neuroses – he had been posted in East Prussia during the war as a military doctor. Döblin would have been familiar with Simmel's publications on the topic.[58] Through his other contacts with the Berlin Psychoanalytic Institute, Döblin was exposed to a wide range of psychoanalytic theories and case studies. The main traces of psychoanalysis in *Die beiden Freundinnen und ihr Giftmord* are evident in Döblin's handling of unconscious matter. This can be seen in sections of the novella itself, but also in the schematic addendum, the 'Räumliche Darstellung der Seelenveränderung'. In the literary case study, Döblin alludes in general terms to that which Döblin the doctor, following the lead of Freud, would probably call the unresolved Oedipal complexes of Elli Link and Grete Bende.[59]

In Döblin's story, the 'light-hearted and funloving' Elli naively marries Willi Link because of the man's similarity to her father, and Döblin mentions that Elli's chosen husband even has the same profession as her father.[60] But problems soon start in the marriage, stemming in part from what seems to be Elli's as yet unresolved Oedipal complex. Grete Bende, too, appears to have strong, unresolved Oedipal ties to one parent, her mother: 'Grete had remained unfree due to the close devotedness to her mother'.[61] In keeping with the Oedipal theme, Döblin describes a key turning-point in the Links' marriage in pseudo-psychoanalytic terms as a 'subterranean disappointment' ('unterirdische Enttäuschung').[62] Döblin thus suggests early in his narrative that a 'normal' transference of Elli's desire from her father to the husband becomes impeded. Hence, Elli experiences a 'disappointment' and she regresses to an earlier, apparently pre-sexual stage of development.

Elli's disappointment with her husband, as one of the multiple factors behind the breakdown of the marriage, leads ultimately to the emergence of Elli's homosexuality. To focus on the psychoanalytic addendum at the end of Döblin's case writing is to find this reading reinforced but not enriched in a substantial way. In the addendum, homosexuality is likewise depicted as a complex. It first emerges in Grete Bende, in 'phase 10', and in 'phase 11' in Elli Link. Grete Bende is ascribed a 'normal sexuality' that is 'well developed' and her homosexuality comes to the fore only when she meets Elli Link. The same occurs with Elli Link, whose desire for Bende tapped into dormant tendencies that Döblin identifies in the narrative as 'an old mechanism that was in the past'.[63] The addendum thus suggests that Elli Link's homosexuality is not necessarily congenital or innate, but a response to social or interpersonal circumstances. The emergence of homosexual desire is presented in psychological terms in relation to parental love, as with Freud's Oedipal complex.

Psychoanalysis and literature's answer to life science

The psychiatric addendum included in the 1924 edition of *Die beiden Freundinnen und ihr Giftmord* offers a type of expert commentary on the Klein–Nebbe murder case, in which Döblin reframes the crime and its circumstances in the language of psychology and psychoanalysis. As an additional narrative, the diagrams help to sharpen Döblin's focus on the case, in that they foreground the psychic disposition of the three main characters in relation to one another over the course of a couple of years, taking up the themes of the homosexuality of the two women, all three main characters' sadomasochism and Willi Link's perversion. At the same time, with its specialist, psychiatric discourse, the addendum does little to illuminate the literary account, neither strengthening the coherence of the preceding narrative nor adding greater depth; also, it introduces no additional factors attenuating the crime that are not already apparent in the fictionalised version.

As argued, the addendum serves instead to overdetermine the evidence already in circulation about the Klein–Nebbe murder case. So why did Döblin include it? One answer is that in highlighting the psychological determinants of the case, say, over the social or physiological factors, the pseudo-medical addendum would seem to lend legitimacy to newly emerging psychoanalytic epistemologies about sexuality and perversion. It does so without substantially affecting the literary rendition of the case, which is a rendition capable of much finer analysis. With regard to the genre of the case study, Döblin's creation in the first edition of *Die beiden Freundinnen und ihr Giftmord* is nonetheless significant for what it conveys about the relationship between the literary laboratory and the case study in 1920s Germany. More specifically, *Die beiden Freundinnen und ihr Giftmord* demonstrates the specific contribution that literary cases can make.

By the time of Döblin's experiments with criminology, sexology and psychoanalysis in *Die beiden Freundinnen und ihr Giftmord*, literature had evolved as a medium of communication in unforeseen directions. The demands of realism, empiricism and now modernism all altered the way that writers strived to respond to modern life's many new challenges. Certainly, in Weimar Germany Döblin found a broad, heterogeneous public for his hybrid achievement in the novella. And yet, the experimental nature of Döblin's case writing suggests that while the reading public might have become more capable of embracing greater complexity in literary texts – medical, sexological, legal, psychoanalytic complexity – literature struggled to cope with this complexity.

The remarkable epilogue to *Die beiden Freundinnen und ihr Giftmord* provides a number of clues as to why Döblin overburdened his literary case study.[64] The work began as realistic, documentary-like reportage, but ended as a wild cacophony of discourses and diagrams that do not mesh or meld:

> When I cast my eye over the entire thing, it seems like it was in the story: 'and then the wind came and tore down the tree.' I don't know what type of wind it was and where it came from. The whole is a carpet which consists of many individual bits, of cloth, silk, metal pieces as well as lumps of clay. It is stitched together with straw, wire, yarn. In some places the parts are only loosely connected. Other fragments are connected by glue or glass. And yet it is all seamless and bears the mark of truth. And this is the way it happened: even the actors think so. But it could easily not have happened this way.[65]

In the metaphor of a carpet, woven out of cloth and silk but also metal and clay, Döblin has found a powerful image for his multidisciplinary creation. Unsurprisingly, he is not entirely convinced that the heterogeneity of methods used has created an integrated whole. That some sections of the carpet are woven out of glass, rope, straw and clay – that is, out of material that is normally extraneous to rug weaving – is an admission that he is not happy with the coherence of his work. On inspecting its odd structure, the image of a patchwork proves no exaggeration. Indeed, more than a carpet, the case could be seen to resemble a garment or a coat, even an overcoat; the body woven out of literary fabric, while the rest is made of other disciplinary material. This overcoat could be thought to have, for instance, graphological sleeves from the two analyses of the accused's handwriting included after the epilogue. The same woven overcoat has an added frame or fringe in the epilogue and, at the back, a secret gusset, tucked away out of sight, in the ten unbound leaves containing the psychoanalytic emplotment of the case.

The metaphor of a patchwork carpet or coat aptly captures Döblin's keen sense of the multiple causal factors at play in this intriguing case. Yet he is baffled and bewitched by its complexity. As the patchwork shows, this complexity is unwieldy and irreducible; the coherence of the case is not so much enhanced by the multiple perspectives as undermined by them. Döblin, it seems, balks at the disciplinary richness and determinism of the case – a response all the more perplexing given that he was an expert in most of the specialist discourses included in *Die beiden Freundinnen und ihr Giftmord.*

The contemporary crisis of literature, and the writer's own existential crisis, echo throughout Döblin's epilogue. As a commentary on literature, this aspect of *Die beiden Freundinnen und ihr Giftmord* underscores Döblin's pessimistic perceptions of the limitations of literary case writing. While purporting to offer a commentary on the verdict of the court case, the epilogue ends up negating the value of definitive diagnoses; that is, it undermines the epistemological basis of case writing. Paradoxically, the epilogue serves both to distinguish the difference that literature makes and to negate the ability of the literary case study to make definitive judgements about cases altogether.

The topography of the souls of the three main characters and the seventeen phases of the addendum can be called a curiosity. Undoubtedly it allowed Döblin to display his expert knowledge and his cultural capital – such as his familiarity with Freud's topographical model of the soul, Adler's physiological models and Jung's theories of complexes, as well as his vast knowledge of current psychological and psychoanalytic ideas. As such, the addendum stresses the helplessness of the modernist writer, who cannot turn back the clock to realist and naturalist times, but who cannot solve the challenge of modernity's epistemological complexity and diversity. This complexity of modern life – specifically modern sexual life and the depths of the modern psyche – presented the greatest challenge of all to writers of literature, and in particular to those clinging to New Objectivity. Döblin's compulsion to blur the boundaries between the literary and the psychoanalytic case study in the one publication, and to overburden his literary treatment with additions, points to a severe crisis in aesthetics, one mirrored in the real existential crisis of the 1920s writer, who cannot live solely from literature.

Of course, Döblin was not alone in grappling with the exigencies of modern life through literary forms that no longer seemed fit for purpose. His work therefore reflects much of the multidisciplinarity of the case genre of the period, and the openness of the literary case study to external influences at this historical juncture. Döblin must have been aware that his new type of forensic case study was not designed for the petit-bourgeois readers of 'penny dreadfuls'. He hints at this in the essay about the rift in his life between his literary interests and his professional activities. As a doctor he does not share his namesake's heightened imagination, and does not like to read the sort of literature written by Döblin the writer. He prefers to read factual literature – travelogues, for example. He also prefers books written in a less heavy style: 'it is too heavy for me, you cannot expect worn-out people to work their way through something like that voluntarily'.[66]

Die beiden Freundinnen und ihr Giftmord could be read as a realist case study written in a modernist age. It is a work symptomatic of the inter-war years in Europe, and particularly in Germany, which struggled to overcome the traumas of war neuroses and shell-shock, and found itself faced with a new war on the home front, in domestic violence. Here Döblin attempts to link cause and effect in new ways, to show the impact of war on peacetime – yet, ultimately, the experiment fails, because he locates not one cause or one effect, but multiple factors that all contributed to the violence of the murder. The sheer complexity of modern life in Weimar Germany, of men and women living in the shadow of war and violence, prompted Döblin to take the timeworn form of the case study and give it a twist so violent as to make it virtually unrecognisable. To be sure, he still places a criminal at the centre of his case history, but the female criminal is not presented as a specific instance of a general rule for disciplinary action or prevention. There is no clear moral to her acts or to Döblin's story, no point of law that he makes. Similarly, his findings in the addendum are less than equivocal. Homosexuality is not so much congenital as a response to parental love, and can sometimes be circumstantial. Finally, Döblin's insistence on enriching his account of the murder case with psychoanalysis is less than satisfying. While he claims to have jettisoned psychology entirely, this is not true. Psychoanalysis certainly informs his writing, but the full impact of ideas about the Oedipal complex, sadomasochism and perversions is really felt only in the diagrammatic addendum.

Instead, in the laboratory of literary culture, the exception or deviation from a norm or rule is normalised as a possible modality of the all-too-human. This laboratory functions best, however, when it remains an inexact science. As Bernhard J. Dotzler remarks, all literature transports knowledge but not all knowledge is science.[67] Döblin possibly forgot that literature is not science. Hence the topographical diagrams of the addendum, which were never republished in subsequent editions of *Die beiden Freundinnen und ihr Giftmord*, seem out of place in a literary work. For writers and artists with a commitment to New Objectivity, the solution to the crisis of literature was to reground literary communication about sexuality and female criminals in the empirical life sciences, only to realise, perhaps too late, that literature had a much more sympathetic complement in psychoanalysis. And yet, as contended above, the mere *addition* of psychoanalytic models after the close of the narrative does not necessarily improve readers' understanding of sex crimes. The literary work does not gain from the authentication strategy of the addendum, although to Döblin the literary account must have seemed deficient enough to require further, expert padding. As a result, in this instance, the case study genre became so overdetermined by extra-literary discourses, so overwhelmed by disorder and sheer complexity, that it threatened to separate into its constituent parts altogether. This is indeed what Döblin's patchwork creation did over time, insofar as the hidden gusset of the coat disappeared from public view into the archive. Meanwhile, his literary case survived to the present day, in the public domain, to be republished as part of all subsequent editions of the work.

Döblin's first foray into literary case writing presents an extraordinary case of murder in order to show that extreme behaviours are possible and hence potentially part of the spectrum of the normal. While some kinds of naturalism in literature could be accused of 'inscrib[ing] new normative constraints', overall Döblin's first such treatment of the case study appears to have the opposite effect: by taking deviance as paradigmatic of the normal it disrupts the association of normal sexuality with heterosexuality, and brings the extraordinary or abnormal into the range of possible human behaviours.[68]

This can be seen from the narrative techniques that Döblin uses in *Die beiden Freundinnen und ihr Giftmord*. He combines the neutral focalisation of an objective or heterodiegetic narrator with rapid changes in perspective, switching frequently into free, indirect discourses to present his characters' inner states of mind. The effect is to provide insight into the motivations and psychic dispositions of all his protagonists, and to foster empathy, or at least insight. In addition, such close proximity to the thoughts and emotions of the criminal inevitably humanises her, and furthers a particular type of knowledge about crime. This is a type of knowledge that perhaps only literary genres can foster, though their unique capacity to present what Rita Felski has called a 'social phenomenology'.[69] The distinctiveness of the literary mode is manifest in Döblin's faithfulness to his sources; he quotes directly from the women's letters, while remaining careful to contextualise much of the evidence given at the trial, either through reference to Ella Klein's/Elli Link's terrible inner conflict and pangs of conscience, or through graphic descriptions of her husband's abuse. Döblin seems to have omitted most of the extremely revengeful and hateful parts of the letters, included in the newspapers and court transcripts. Very little of the women's direct coarse language is included in Döblin's story, except for one reference to the husband as a 'bastard'.[70] Döblin's reference to the women's increasing desperation when the rat poison does not take effect is embedded in the broader context of Ella Klein's/Elli Link's husband's continued brutality. This helps to ensure that the reader regards her as the victim of an increasingly perverse, depraved and violent husband, a woman who is driven to murder as a last resort: 'she was affected by her fate like her husband. Her life was in danger'.[71]

Döblin's humanisation of the accused women is assisted by his use of specialist discourse. By choosing not to characterise the women's homosexuality as a perversion, he points to an important function served by the literary case in his time – that of understanding and illuminating from a wide range of perspectives the complexity of female criminality, as distinct from classifying, diagnosing, pathologising or demonising the criminal. Apart from the expert diagrams of the addendum, Döblin uses empathy as his principal means. Empathy, argues Joe Bray, is 'central to developing an understanding of literariness and the value of literature'.[72] Accordingly, Döblin undermines the stereotype of the *Giftmörderin* by complicating the narrative with other circumstances, social, emotional, psychoanalytic, developmental and sexual causes, all of which might have contributed to the act of murder. The hybrid genre of the despecialised and fictionalised case study permits him to achieve all this in one work. The vast scope of this genre can encompass discourses from the empirical human sciences and psychoanalysis; having first distanced them from their conventional professional purpose, Döblin reintegrates them, in a dialectical move typical of the times.[73] The specialist discourses are reframed in terms of literary communication, resynthesised and recoded according to binary categories characteristic of literary work: the categories of the possible and the probable. As the simple form that pits norm against norm – presenting human life as something to be valued and measured against a norm – the case study becomes the ideal method for questioning the certainties of specialist discourse and its truth claims.[74]

The case can thus pose a question without providing an answer, leaving it to the reader to weigh up evidence against other evidence. Döblin's case writing in *Die beiden Freundinnen und ihr Giftmord* emphasises the complexity of murder as the confluence of multiple factors, and hence refuses a monocausal explanation or a clear-cut attribution of guilt; his case delegates this task to the reader. In the laboratory of literature, the deviation is depathologised and reintegrated into the broad spectrum of normality, recoded as a possible modality of the human. The literary case thus manages to resist classifying the murderer as medical and legal discourses do. It defies the dominant forensic dispositif, and ultimately undermines epistemological certainty rather than contributing to it, thus disrupting the knowledge production of the specialist discourses it so deftly borrows from.

Berlin Alexanderplatz: the case study of collective psychopathology

The 'havoc that World War I continues to wreak' on the urban population and relations between the sexes are themes even more pronounced in Döblin's last novel from the 1920s, *Berlin Alexanderplatz: Die Geschichte vom Franz Biberkopf* (*Alexanderplatz Berlin: The Story of Franz Biberkopf*).[75] He first began writing the work late in 1927, possibly inspired by Walter Ruttmann's famous documentary film of the same year, *Berlin – die Symphonie einer Großstadt* (*Berlin: Symphony of a Great City*). *Berlin Alexanderplatz* was first presented to the public in serialised form in the newspaper *Frankfurter Zeitung* in twenty-nine instalments, before being released as a book in October 1929 with a print run of 10,000 copies.[76] It was heralded as the outstanding literary achievement of the year and new editions soon followed. By 1936 it had been translated into nine languages, including English (published in 1931 in New York and London).[77]

Franz Biberkopf, the novel's working-class hero, has served time in Tegel prison for murdering his girlfriend, Ida, and is released into the pulsing metropolis of Berlin at the end of the Weimar Republic and on the eve of the National Socialists' ascent to power. Although determined to lead a 'decent' life, Biberkopf soon falls into disreputable company and loses an arm when his new friend Reinhold thrusts him out of a getaway car. The last section of the novel sees him return to his old ways of living the life of a pimp and a petty criminal with the result that he is almost charged with murder once again when his girlfriend, the devoted Mieze, is murdered by Reinhold. Biberkopf is cleared of any suspicion but is physically and psychologically broken by the experience, falling into a catatonic stupor in Berlin-Buch. He recovers after a close encounter with death and is effectively resurrected as a new man, finally finding a respectable job as a porter in a factory.

Biberkopf's story is told in part as a modern cautionary tale: above all, a tale of extreme, uncontrolled violence, of men pitted against men and, more worryingly, of men against women. As Veronika Fuechtner states: 'in *Berlin Alexanderplatz*, modern life is a war'.[78] While women in this novel are the victims of male violence, the sexes are, as in *Die beiden Freundinnen und ihr Giftmord*, very much at war. Maria Tatar observed that 'Biberkopf hardly ever makes a move that is not in some way coloured by his relationship with the opposite sex ... the women he encounters are habitually presented as the victims of rape or murder and are disempowered or effaced from the written page with a frequency that is nothing short of alarming'.[79]

Berlin Alexanderplatz is regarded as Döblin's greatest contribution to a left-leaning modernism: he abandons many constraints of realism and achieves the much-sought-after synthesis of discourses and knowledge that was lacking in *Die beiden Freundinnen und ihr Giftmord*. The narrative is not strictly linear – instead, Döblin develops a polymodal and polyvocal form of narrative that is similar to but different from the interior monologue characteristic of modernist writers such as Joyce. As Walter Benjamin once remarked:

> The stylistic principle governing [Döblin's] book is that of montage. Petty-bourgeois printed matter, scandalmongering, stories of accidents, the sensational incidents of 1928, folk songs, and advertisements rain down in this text.... Formally, above all the material of the montage is anything but arbitrary. Authentic montage is based on the document. In its fanatical struggle with the work of art, Dadaism used montage to turn daily life into its ally.[80]

The first reviews of the novel immediately compared it to Joyce's masterpiece *Ulysses*, which appeared in English in 1922 and in German translation in 1927. Döblin was quick, however, to deny any direct influence of Joyce, although the comparison no doubt contributed to the international success of the work. Rather than adapting Joyce's technique of stream of consciousness, Döblin's new approach, which he outlined in an essay written around the same time, 'Der Bau des epischen Werks' ('The Construction of the Epic Work'), was to explore the use of the epic mode in combination with even more extensive experimentation with techniques of montage. According to Döblin, the epic is founded on the form of the report, which the author can use for more than merely reporting facts: 'he uses it for his notorious non-facts', and for manipulating reality.[81] The epic draws much of its veracity from the exemplary nature of its characters and action, from its 'powerful fundamental situations, primordial situations of human existence'.[82] Like his contemporary Brecht, Döblin envisaged the epic as a new open form of narrative with no predetermined plot-line, giving the narrator maximum freedom either to intervene or to retreat from his subject matter.[83] The openness of the form allowed him to break down the boundaries between myth and fact, between literary and scientific discourse, the collective and the individual.[84]

In the spirit of this new interest in modernising the epic tradition, Döblin superimposes on the story of Franz Biberkopf a dense layer of mythological, biblical, scientific and popular references, from statistics, descriptions of medical conditions and his own eyewitness reports from a local abattoir, to quotations from the Bible and the story of Job, street ballads, political songs and nursery rhymes. Through further refining the technique of the montage, which he appears to have taken from the new medium of the cinema, Döblin synthesises heterogeneous narrative matter from a wide range of information about the city itself, including short biographical vignettes about its other inhabitants. This time he does not stage his narrative repeatedly through the use of disparate discourses and sources, as seen in *Die beiden Freundinnen und ihr Giftmord*. Instead, he incorporates all his external source material and intertextual allusions directly into his text, often literally with scissors and glue, with inserts marked by letters or symbols or with Dadaistic collages.[85]

By the time Döblin wrote this masterpiece, his literary 'tapestry' was so rich in texture that critics have repeatedly been tempted to say the novel has not one protagonist but many; not the individual criminal but Berlin, the teeming, devouring metropolis, the Whore of Babylon herself. Indeed, the power of external stimuli from the vitalistic life-world of the city is so great that arguably it can no longer be contained by the genre of the individual case study. If Biberkopf's subjective experiences are to be understood as the collective experiences of a new, subjugated urban citizen – and if novelistic character is more an 'anthropomorphic device' than a believable construct with psychological interiority – then Döblin's reinvention of the case study in *Berlin Alexanderplatz* expands the case genre in radical ways, taking it into new territory for the modern novel.[86]

Döblin's novel has been read as both a 'city-epic' and a 'gruesome criminal ballad', which testifies to Döblin's ongoing fascination with the criminal underworld of Berlin.[87] But it is an unconventional crime story, since it picks up the criminal's narrative after his release back into the community and, hence, it is no longer concerned with the threat of crime but with urban criminal life-worlds. The plot is only partially focused on criminal acts, and instead focuses on Biberkopf's rehabilitation and the multiple threats to his successful reintegration into society. Hence Döblin's narrative explodes the boundaries of the criminal case study, not only by virtue of the fact that he seems to regard his main character less and less as a recidivist criminal or a repeat offender and more and more as an everyman – as an individual with allegorical resonances.

Such a perspective on Biberkopf is underscored by Döblin's use throughout the novel of an ironic street-ballad narrator, the narrator of the murder ballad (or *Moritat*), who comments on, interprets and moralises about Biberkopf's fate. This explicit use of an authorial narrator contrasts with the virtual disappearance of the narrator in many of the montage or collage sections, which are stitched together without the aid of commentary. Indeed, the narrative voice is itself 'montage-like': it is 'not a constant preterite presence with a firmly established vantage point, but a compound voice, a series of contrasting attitudes, a prismatically broken point of view in keeping with Döblin's injunction ... to be "decisively lyrical, dramatic, even reflective"'.[88] With multiple masks and personas, including a new-found didacticism that helps him illuminate the case, Döblin's narrator is no longer the objective but the empathetic narrator of the case study, as in *Die beiden Freundinnen und ihr Giftmord*, who had struggled to diagnose or pinpoint the exact causes of the murder. Indeed, the voice of Döblin's narrator summarising the moral of the tale is not taken from the empirical, scientific world of the modern medical case study. Rather, it originates in the disparate sources of the chorus of Greek tragedy and the streets of Berlin:

> We have come to the end of our story. It has proved a long one, but it had to unfold itself, on and on, till it reached its climax, that culminating point which at last illuminates the whole thing.... It was a strange process of revelation. Franz Biberkopf did not walk the street like us. He rushed blindly down this dark street....[89]

Döblin's many departures from the conventions of crime writing in recounting the story of Biberkopf's rise and fall manage to avoid the appeal to theories of racial 'degenerescence' and decline typical of naturalism. As Irene Gammel has observed: 'despite the growing rejection of the heredity-degenerescence model in the twentieth century, the plot of decline remains prominent in twentieth-century social realism'.[90] Despite Biberkopf's best intentions at leading a life of respectability upon his release from jail, he cannot escape from the vicious circle of violence and crime in modern society. This is not because of any innate disposition or hereditary determinism (as associated with alcoholism, for example, in works by Zola and Hauptmann). Ultimately, Biberkopf falls prey to the violence that is endemic to the working-class and criminal milieu in which he moves in Berlin, unable to rise above those underworld circles of pimps and petty criminals or to gain a foothold outside their circles. As such, Biberkopf's fate testifies to the pervasive 'paranoia of proletarianization' that Döblin no doubt himself felt and that affected all middle-class Germans in the midst of the 1929 global stock market crisis.[91]

Döblin's focus on criminality and violence surfaces again towards the conclusion of *Berlin Alexanderplatz*, where Biberkopf's sadistic friend Reinhold Hoffmann lures Mieze, Biberkopf's girlfriend, into a forest and murders her in cold blood. In this powerful scene, Döblin mobilises all the generative possibilities of montage into a highly dramatic finale, simultaneously staging a radically new modernist aesthetic that represents an important innovation in the literary treatment of violent crime. He combines rapid changes of perspective between Hoffmann and Mieze, male to female, villain and victim; he shifts from direct to indirect speech, from authorial commentary to biblical fragments from Ecclesiastes, from a language of emotion to the cold language of the abattoir report. The external influences on Biberkopf, Hoffmann and Mieze are so pervasive – from social and moral pressures to conform, the conflicting drives of envy and jealousy, and the Darwinistic struggles between male rivals – that agency, especially criminal agency, threatens to evaporate altogether.

Although more narrative space is devoted to the female victim's experience of violence, Döblin also allows his male villain to speak. In both *Die beiden Freundinnen und ihr Giftmord* and *Berlin Alexanderplatz*, Döblin deploys various literary devices that allow him to express empathy, in particular, but not only, for his female characters: for the female poisoner in the former and the female victim in the latter. Little narrative space is devoted to the male victim of murder in *Die beiden Freundinnen und ihr Giftmord*, who, it can be safely assumed, deserves his fate. Here Döblin's aesthetics of empathy seek to understand the criminal act from the perspective of the female perpetrator, and are only partially offset by a poetics of shock, designed to evince some horror at least at the circumstances of the murder. Arguably Döblin's densely woven epic montage in *Berlin Alexanderplatz* is far more shocking on many scores. It tells of the murder of Mieze almost at once from all sides, from outside looking in and inside looking out. The plaintive voice of the victim makes it less detached, unleashing more emotional and pathos-laden registers; the insistent repetition of biblical quotes ('there is a time for everything') underscores the terrible inexorability of the young woman's murder.

In the murder scene and elsewhere in the novel, structural violence, or the 'war of daily life', finds its expression in a type of linguistic and narrative violence inflicted upon the literary text.[92] Syntax is disrupted, narrative linearity is fragmented, there is no single subjective perspective, as the point of view shifts back and forth from victim to villain, from outside to inside, from human to animal. Violence and the language of war are all-pervasive, and yet in *Berlin Alexanderplatz* the question of individual guilt and agency is less acute than the problem of the psychopathology of an urban population under siege from multiple quarters.

Overall, Döblin's deep familiarity with medical and psychiatric case writing traditions is less pronounced in *Berlin Alexanderplatz*. His medical training comes to the fore early in the novel in two main passages. The first is in the first chapter (or 'book'), when he inserts a passage from a medical textbook about the causes of sexual impotence: 'Sexual potency depends upon the combined action of (1) the internal secretory system, (2) the nervous system, and (3) the sexual apparatus'.[93] The second occurs immediately after, when the narrator inserts a description of a contemporary treatment: 'Testifortan, authorised patent No. 365695, sexual therapeutic agent approved by Sanitary Councillor Dr Magnus Hirschfeld and Dr Bernhard Schapiro, Institute of Sexual Science, Berlin'.[94] Homosexuality is also not a major concern of the novel, although it does figure in the homoerotic relationship between Mieze and Eva and in the homosexually charged relationship that develops between Reinhold and Franz. The most significant influence from Döblin's medical practice and his long-standing engagement with psychoanalysis, however, can be found in the scene at the end of the novel when Biberkopf, who has become delusional after the murder of Mieze, is admitted to Berlin-Buch. In a scene in which the doctors deliberate over his diagnosis, Döblin manages to parody both Freudian interpretations of psychopathology and his own mentor Hoche's more physiological approach to mental illness in the physicians treating Biberkopf.[95]

More broadly, this accomplished work and his earlier criminal case study in *Die beiden Freundinnen und ihr Giftmord* are aesthetic responses to the enduring impact of the First World War on normative categories of gender and the proletarian classes, and both can be read as attempts to grapple with the legacies of a diseased and traumatised body politic after the First World War.[96] In his first attempt at literary case writing, Döblin sought to integrate the workings, even the discourse, of the unconscious into his representation of violence – with little success. Through experimenting with literary techniques to elicit empathy in his readers, he tried to show how women could be driven to violence. With its disparate components, the first edition of *Die beiden Freundinnen und ihr Giftmord* was an especially fragmented literary case study that reflected in many ways the writer's failure to integrate deep psychology with documentary realism. In the 1920s, Döblin was increasingly involved in the activities of the Berlin Psychoanalytic Institute, which emphasised healing the collective unconscious; consequently, his eyes were opened to the implications of cases of violent crime for the collective psyche of the masses. The Institute was the point of departure for many pioneers of political psychology who strove to incorporate Marxist philosophy and social theory into psychoanalysis.[97] Although he never turned his back on Freudian psychoanalysis, like fellow members of the Berlin Psychoanalytic Institute, by the end of the 1920s Döblin increasingly questioned why Freud was not more concerned with the societal dimensions of his fragile, isolated ego.[98] *Berlin Alexanderplatz* thus reflects many of the new concerns of socially aware Berlin psychoanalysts in Döblin's exploration of the wider socio-political dimensions of violence, its toll on relations between the sexes, and the social cost of war on public health.

Ultimately, however, Döblin was unable to explain the 'how' and 'why' of the specific cases of violent crime that are the focus of his literary treatments. He increasingly preferred narrative chaos or disorder over order, and multiple causal principles over single causes, and he privileged an almost impossibly complex amalgam of historical, social and physiological determinants of violence. Nevertheless, in the later work he found a language capable of convincingly representing the anonymous, impersonal violence that haunted German society in the years of the Weimar Republic, writing a fitting monument to the city of Berlin. *Berlin Alexanderplatz* is thus testament to his vast reservoir of experience 'as a doctor and a writer' acquired from treating patients from criminal and petty bourgeois milieu for an array of different medical, sexological and psychological conditions.

***

Berlin Alexanderplatz cemented Döblin's reputation in Germany as a major novelist and in 1931, shortly after its publication, he was elected into the senate of the literary section of the Prussian Academy.[99] Despite the critical acclaim he achieved through the novel, this was not sufficient for him to be able to give up practising medicine altogether, even though he did close his social welfare practice on the Frankfurter Allee and opened up a private practice in Charlottenburg in 1931. Döblin describes this move away from the poorer districts of Berlin as a 'catastrophic decision' ('katastrophalen Entschluß').[100] It proved to be a crucial turning-point in his life: giving up his licence to work as a social welfare doctor effectively meant he would never practise medicine again.[101] This downturn in his career was, however, soon to pale into insignificance when the National Socialists came to power in 1933 and Döblin found himself blacklisted.

In 1933 Döblin fled to France with six members of his immediate family. After the events of Kristallnacht he wrote: 'everything in Germany had become unbearable, not only politically but intellectually as well'.[102] Initially, he had high hopes that exile would somehow reinvigorate his stagnating career. In France he became close friends with the critic and German scholar Robert Minder, who promoted his work, and Döblin and his family took out French citizenship. In 1940, after his two sons Wolfgang and Klaus were deployed with the French army, Döblin, his wife and youngest son escaped Europe for the USA, joining the community of German exiles in Los Angeles. Without a regular income from his medical practice, and unable to live from his writing, however, Döblin and his family found themselves in dire financial straits. After his contract as a story writer with MGM film studios expired Döblin was almost entirely at the mercy of the generosity of other émigrés, such as Lion Feuchtwanger. Unlike Thomas Mann, who lived a life of relative affluence in exile, Döblin struggled with his loss of relevancy and social status, his precarious financial situation and his grim lack of career prospects. He continued writing on a number of projects, among which was a four-volume epic about revolution, *November 1918*, which he finished in 1941. It was during this time that he converted to Catholicism in a futile attempt to establish himself in America. It was to make little difference, as he was later to write, and he had to 'live like a beggar for years'. He 'was not only condemned to complete silence, disempowered, but even worse than that: degraded, worth less than a native illiterate person who can at least converse with his neighbours'.[103] Those émigrés who were reliant on their language for their livelihood suffered especially, he writes, becoming little more than 'a living corpse'.[104] Oddly, Döblin does not appear to have sought refuge in the émigré psychoanalytic community, for instance in the company of his mentor and fellow Jew and socialist Simmel. Simmel was also living in Hollywood during the war, where he helped to establish psychoanalytic institutes in Los Angeles and San Francisco.[105]

After the war, Döblin returned to Germany with his wife but found the post-war climate singularly unconducive to rebuilding his literary career. He had by now several finished manuscripts but he found it difficult to find a publisher for them. He finished his last novel, *Hamlet oder die lange Nacht nimmt ein Ende* (*Hamlet, or Tales of a Long Night*) in 1947 but he had little success in convincing one of the major publishers, Piper in Munich and Kiepenheuer in Cologne, to publish it. It was only towards the end of his life that, through the stewardship of poet Peter Huchel, he secured an East German publisher for his last work.

These difficulties were compounded by personal problems. At the war's end, Döblin and his wife learned of their son Wolfgang's suicide in 1940, when, as a member of the French armed services, he found himself confronted by German troops. Moreover, Döblin's health problems which had begun during the war continued; in 1949 he was diagnosed with Parkinson's disease, and in 1952 he suffered a further heart attack. Finally, feeling spurned and misunderstood, Döblin decided to leave Germany in 1953 and to resettle in France, where he lived until his death in 1957. He complained in a letter to Huchel in 1954: 'So the reading public does not want to buy anything of mine because I am an emigrant, and in addition to that, someone who served for France'.[106]

When compared with other celebrated modernist writers of the period, such as Franz Kafka, Mann, Joyce and Brecht, Döblin is today far less well known outside the German-speaking world. Even his last work failed to strike a chord with post-war publishers. *Hamlet* took up all the major themes of his earlier novels – the search for self; war; violence; the relationship between the sexes – in an account of an English soldier's peacetime struggles to come to grips with war trauma. In the conservative climate of the post-war period, when international publishers preferred Kafka, Mann and Rilke to more risky and difficult contemporary authors, Döblin, the assimilated Jew who had taken out French citizenship and spent the war in exile, reached an impasse.[107] Cold War politics would also play their part in the lack of interest in Döblin's works: he found more political allies in the German Democratic Republic, but aesthetically he had more in common with West German writers such as Gottfried Benn. Had his health been better, and had he been willing to embrace the socialist experiment in East Germany, Döblin might have obtained a better chance of thriving, by emigrating there.

Döblin's empathetic literary case studies, which combined medical, sexological and social knowledge about human frailty, which he saw epitomised in the acts of criminals, were a masterful synthesis of real-life sources and new forms of expert knowledge. Yet, at least for the time being, the psychoanalytic case study about the low-life criminal failed to appeal as a form that the post-war era was ready to embrace. In West Germany the public was keen to discover new voices and to disavow most continuities with the past. Attention became focused on Gruppe 47, the literary association founded in 1947 that provided a prominent forum for emerging writers to present their experiments with politics and aesthetics. Then again, as one chapter of case writing in literature was closing, a new chapter in the history of the case study was opening: European psychoanalysts fleeing the ravages of German National Socialism and World War Two had exported the genre across the Atlantic Ocean, bringing it to unforeseen discursive contexts and tasks.

Notes

1 Richard Daniel Lehan, *Realism and Naturalism: The Novel in an Age of Transition* (Madison: University of Wisconsin Press, 2005), p. 5.
2 On his own admission, Döblin published 'a handful of publications' on medical topics early in his career. See Alfred Döblin, 'Autobiographische Skizze', in *Schriften zu Leben und Werk*, ed. Erich Kleinschmidt (Olten: Walter-Verlag, 1986), pp. 36–7, p. 36.
3 Andreas Killen, *Berlin Electropolis: Shock, Nerves, and German Modernity* (Berkeley: University of California Press, 2006), pp. 1–2.
4 Killen, *Berlin Electropolis*, p. 2.
5 See Janet Beizer, 'Emma's Daughter: Femininity, Maternity, and "Mothersickness" in *Madame Bovary*', in Suzanne Nash (ed.), *Home and Its Dislocations in Nineteenth-Century France* (Albany: New York Press, 1993), pp. 265–83, p. 266.
6 Roland Dollinger, Wulf Köpke and Heidi Thomann Tewarson (eds), 'Introduction', in *A Companion to the Works of Alfred Döblin* (Rochester: Camden House, 2003), p. 1.
7 See Dollinger, Köpke and Thomann Tewarson, 'Introduction', p. 3.
8 Thomas Mann, 'Letter to Karl Bohm, September 27, 1925', in *Letters of Thomas Mann 1889–1955*, selected and trans. Richard and Clara Winston (Berkeley: University of California Press, 1970), p. 133.
9 See Wulf Köpke, *The Critical Reception of Alfred Döblin's Major Novels* (Rochester: Camden House, 2003), p. 96.
10 See Dollinger, Köpke and Thomann Tewarson, 'Introduction', pp. 5–7.
11 See Döblin's complaint in a letter to Hermann Kesten that none among the émigrés in California 'was laughing', except Stefan Zweig and Thomas Mann. Döblin, 'Letter to Hermann Kesten, 30th January 1942', in *Briefe II*, ed. Helmut F. Pfanner (Dusseldorf: Walter-Verlag, 2001), p. 159.
12 Georg Lukács, *The Historical Novel*, trans. Hannah Mitchell and Stanley Mitchell (London: Merlin, 1978).
13 Döblin, 'Der Geist des naturalistischen Zeitalters', in *Schriften zu Ästhetik, Poetik und Literatur*, ed. Erich Kleinschmidt (Olten: Walter-Verlag, 1989), pp. 168–90, p. 171.
14 Stéphane Michaud, 'L'exception allemande, ou quelques questions au naturalisme européen', *Revue histoire de la littéraire de la France*, 103:3 (2003), pp. 591–6, p. 596.
15 Richard Heinrich, 'Hermann Bahr und der Expressionismus', in Jeanne Benay and Alfred Pfabigan (eds), *Hermann Bahr: Für eine andere Moderne* (Bern: Peter Lang, 2004), pp. 175–88, p. 185. Michaud, 'L'exception allemande', p. 596.
16 Lehan, *Realism and Naturalism*, p. xvi.
17 Lehan, *Realism and Naturalism*, p. 3.
18 Irene Gammel, *Sexualizing Power in Naturalism: Theodor Dreiser and Frederick Philip Grove* (Calgary: University of Calgary Press, 1994), p. 23.
19 See Köpke, *The Critical Reception of Alfred Döblin's Major Novels*, p. 92.
20 The edition used herein is Alfred Döblin, *Die beiden Freundinnen und ihr Giftmord* (Dusseldorf: Artemis & Winkler, 2001).

21 See Russell A. Berman, *The Rise of the Modern German Novel: Crisis and Charisma* (Cambridge: Harvard University Press, 1986).
22 See Dollinger, Köpke and Thomann Tewarson, 'Introduction', p. 6.
23 'Medizin und Wissenschaft fesselten mich außerordentlich.' Döblin, 'Autobiographische Skizze', p. 36.
24 'Dem Kampf um das sogenannte Dasein.' Döblin, 'Autobiographische Skizze', p. 25.
25 Döblin, 'Autobiographische Skizze', p. 25.
26 'Das Dunkle, das um diese Kranken war, wollte ich lichten helfen.' Döblin, 'Autobiographische Skizze', p. 25.
27 'Man mußte hinein in das Leibliche, aber nicht in die Gehirne, vielleicht in die Drüsen, den Stoffwechsel.' Döblin, 'Merkwürdiger Lebenslauf eines Autors', in *Autobiographische Schriften und letzte Aufzeichnungen*, ed. Edgar Pässler (Olten: Walter-Verlag, 1980), pp. 23–9, p. 25.
28 Veronika Fuechtner, *Berlin Psychoanalytic: Psychoanalysis and Culture in Weimar Republic Germany* (Berkeley: University of California Press, 2011), p. 9.
29 Fuechtner, *Berlin Psychoanalytic*, pp. 8–9.
30 '[M]ir persönlich hat Freud nichts Wunderbares gebracht.' Döblin, 'Merkwürdiger Lebenslauf eines Autors', p. 25.
31 See Fuechtner, *Berlin Psychoanalytic*, p. 12.
32 '[G]roße sensible Aufnahmebereitschaft, unerhörte Fähigkeit analytischen Eindringens, namentlich in der Richtung des Seelisch-Unbewußten.' Döblin, 'Erster Rückblick', in *Autobiographische Schriften*, pp. 37–94, p. 62.
33 Veronika Fuechtner, '"Arzt und Dichter": Döblin's Medical, Psychiatric, and Psychoanalytical Work', in Dollinger, Koepke and Thomann Tewarson (eds), *A Companion to the Works of Alfred Döblin*, pp. 111–39, pp. 119–20.
34 See Christoph Hoffmann, 'Literaturforschung. Über medizinische Schriften Gottfried Benns', in Bernhard J. Dotzler and Sigrid Weigel (eds), *'fülle der combination': Literaturforschung und Wissenschaftsgeschichte* (Munich: Wilhelm Fink, 2005), pp. 319–42.
35 Hoffmann, 'Literaturforschung', p. 320.
36 '[I]st mir völlig fremd und auch total gleichgültig.' Quoted in Alfred Döblin, 'Der Nervenarzt Döblin über den Dichter Döblin', in *Autobiographische Schriften*, pp. 33–4, p. 33.
37 Döblin, 'Der Dichter Döblin über den Nervenarzt Döblin', in *Autobiographische Schriften*, pp. 34–5, p. 34.
38 'Ich habe allerlei Defekte, wahrscheinlich Komplexe, und der Routinier da roch wohl so etwas.' Quoted in Döblin, 'Der Dichter Döblin über den Nervenarzt Döblin', p. 34.
39 Döblin, 'Ökonomisches aus der Literatur', in *Schriften zu Leben und Werk*, pp. 77–9, pp. 77–8.
40 'Es war eine schlimme Ehe.' Döblin, 'Erster Rückblick', in *Autobiographische Schriften*, p. 56.
41 Bettina Wahrig, 'Erzählte Vergiftungen: Kriminalitätsdiskurs und Staatsarzneikunde 1750–1850', in Gisela Engel, Susanne Scholz and Johannes Süßmann (eds), *Fallstudien. Geschichte – Theorie – Methode* (Berlin: Trafo, 2007), pp. 97–111, p. 98.
42 Hania Siebenpfeiffer, *'Böse Lust': Gewaltverbrechen in Diskursen der Weimarer Republik* (Cologne: Böhlau, 2005), pp. 73–4.
43 Wolfgang Schäffner, *Die Ordnung des Wahns: Zur Poetologie psychiatrischen Wissens bei Alfred Döblin* (Munich: Wilhelm Fink, 1995), p. 8.
44 See Fuechtner, *Berlin Psychoanalytic*, pp. 188–9.
45 Döblin, 'An Romanautoren und ihre Kritiker?', in *Schriften zu Ästhetik, Poetik und Literatur* (Olten: Walter-Verlag, 1989), p. 123.
46 Joachim Linder, '"Sie müssen das entschuldigen Herr Staatsanwalt, aber es ist

so: Wir trauen Euch nicht…": Strafjustiz, Strafrechtsreform und Justizkritik im *März*, 1907–1911', in Jörg Schönert (ed.), *Erzählte Kriminalität: Zur Typologie und Funktion von narrativen Darstellungen in Strafrechtspflege, Publizistik und Literatur* (Tübingen: Niemeyer, 1991), pp. 533–70, p. 534.

47 Linder, 'Sie müssen das entschuldigen Herr Staatsanwalt, aber es ist so', p. 535.

48 André Jolles, *Einfache Formen. Legende, Sage, Mythe, Rätsel, Spruch, Kasus, Memorabile, Märchen, Witz* (Tübingen: Max Niemeyer, 1968), pp. 178–9.

49 Jolles, *Einfache Formen*, p. 191.

50 Johannes Süßmann, 'Einleitung: Perspektiven der Fallstudienforschung', in Engel, Scholz and Süßmann (eds), *Fallstudien*, pp. 7–27, 20.

51 Medical case writing produced reports that could be used either to illustrate medical theories or to show how medical knowledge should be applied to specific cases. Modern medicine, which has a long tradition of using case reporting of different kinds, has a similar relationship between the specific and the general. See Michael Stolberg, 'Formen und Funktionen medizinischer Fallberichte in der Frühen Neuzeit (1500–1800)', in Engel, Scholz and Süßmann (eds), *Fallstudien*, pp. 81–95.

52 Reports appeared in the morning and evening editions of *Berliner Lokalanzeiger*, *Berliner Tageblatt*, *Deutsche Allgemeine Zeitung*, the liberal *Vossische Zeitung* and the communist-aligned *Vorwärts*.

53 Siebenpfeiffer, *'Böse Lust'*, p. 105.

54 '[E]ntmenschte Frauen … die sich ihrer Männer, die ihnen bei ihrer anormalen Beziehung zueinander unbequem waren … mit Gift skrupellos und kalter Berechnung entledigen wollten.' Quoted in Siebenpfeiffer, *'Böse Lust'*, p. 107.

55 Siebenfeiffer, *'Böse Lust'*, p. 122.

56 My argument here is similar to that advanced by Hania Siebenpfeiffer, who argues that the sections of the work be understood not as a text–para-textual relationship but as individual components of a narrative whole which comment upon and complement one another in their truth claims. Siebenpfeiffer, *'Böse Lust'*, p. 132.

57 Siebenpfeiffer, *'Böse Lust'*, p. 122.

58 Katie Sutton, 'Sexual Pathologies and the Violence of War: Sexological and Psychoanalytic Responses to World War I', *Limbus: Australian Yearbook of German Literary and Cultural Studies*, 7 (2014), pp. 197–218, p. 202.

59 Elli's infantile sexuality and her homosexuality beg to be read in conjunction with a famous psychoanalytic text that also appeared in 1924, namely Sigmund Freud's essay 'The Dissolution of the Oedipus Complex'. See Sigmund Freud, *The Standard Edition of the Complete Psychological Works by Sigmund Freud*, ed. James Strachey, with Anna Freud, Alix Strachey and Alan Tyson, vol. XIX (London: Hogarth Press and Institute for Psychoanalysis, 1961), pp. 173–82.

60 'War leicht und lebenslustig.' Döblin, *Die beiden Freundinnen*, p. 5. (Unless otherwise noted, all translations into English from the novella are by Alison Lewis.)

61 Döblin, *Die beiden Freundinnen*, p. 17.

62 Döblin, *Die beiden Freundinnen*, p. 7.

63 '[E]inen alten Mechanismus, der erledigt war.' Döblin, *Die beiden Freundinnen*, p. 37.

64 Todd Herzog, 'Crime Stories: Criminal, Society, and the Modernist Case History', *Representations*, 80:1 (2002), pp. 34–61, p. 51.

65 'Überblicke ich das Ganze, so ist es wie in der Erzählung: "da kam der wind und riß den Baum um." Ich weiß nicht, was das für ein Wind war und woher er kam. Das Ganze ist ein Teppich, der aus vielen einzelnen Fetzen besteht, aus Tuch, Seide, auch Metallstücke, Lehmmassen dabei. Gestopft ist er aus Stroh, Draht, Zwirn. An manchen Stellen liegen die Teile lose nebeneinander. Manche Bruchstücke sind mit Leim oder Glas verbunden. Dennoch ist alles lückenlos und

trägt den Stempel der Wahrheit. Es hat so sich ereignet; auch die Akteure glauben es. Aber es hat sich auch nicht so ereignet.' Döblin, *Die beiden Freundinnen*, p. 79.

66 'Er ist mir einfach zu schwer, man darf von abgearbeiteten Leuten nicht verlangen, sich durch so etwas freiwillig durchzuarbeiten.' Döblin, 'Der Nervenarzt Döblin über den Dichter Döblin', in *Autobiographische Schriften*, p. 33.

67 Berhard J. Dotzler, 'Wissen in Geschichten. Zur wechselseitigen Erhellung von Literatur, Medien und Wissenschaft', *Berichte zur Wissenschaftsgeschichte*, 32:4 (2009), pp. 319–28, p. 319.

68 Gammel, *Sexualizing Power in Naturalism*, p. 11.

69 Rita Felski, *Uses of Literature* (Malden: Blackwell, 2008), p. 95.

70 Döblin does quote from one letter, in which Ella Klein/Elli Link expresses her exasperation that her husband seems to be resisting the poison: 'Wenn das Schwein doch nur bald krepierte. Das Schwein ist ja so zähe. Heute habe ich ihm Tropfen gegeben, aber ordentlich'. Döblin, *Die beiden Freundinnen*, p. 45.

71 'Sie war von ihrem Schicksal angegriffen wie ihr Mann. Sie war selbst in Lebensgefahr.' Döblin, *Die beiden Freundinnen*, pp. 40–1.

72 Joe Bray, 'The Effects of Free Indirect Discourse: Empathy Revisited', in Marina Lambrou and Peter Stockwell (eds), *Contemporary Stylistics* (New York: Continuum, 2007), pp. 56–67, p. 56.

73 Jürgen Link describes this dialectic between specialisation and reintegration of specialist discourses. Jürgen Link, 'Literaturanalyse als Interdiskursanalyse', in Jürgen Fohrmann and Harro Müller (eds), *Diskurstheorien und Literaturwissenschaft* (Frankfurt am Main: Suhrkamp, 1988), pp. 284–307, p. 285.

74 Ruth Koch, 'Der Kasus und A. Jolles' Theorie von den "Einfachen Formen"', *Fabula*, 14:3 (1973), pp. 194–204, p. 196.

75 Fuechtner, *Berlin Psychoanalytic*, p. 40.

76 See Gabriele Sander, 'Döblin's Berlin: The Story of Franz Biberkopf', in Dollinger, Koepke and Thomann Tewarson (eds), *A Companion to the Works of Alfred Döblin*, pp. 141–60, p. 143.

77 See Sander, 'Döblin's Berlin: The Story of Franz Biberkopf', p. 145.

78 Fuechtner, *Berlin Psychoanalytic*, p. 40.

79 Maria Tatar, *Lustmord: Sexual Murder in Weimar Germany* (Princeton: Princeton University Press, 1995), p. 135.

80 Walter Benjamin, 'The Crisis of the Novel' [1930], in Michael W. Jennings, Howard Eiland and Gary Smith (eds), *Walter Benjamin, Selected Writings, vol. II: 1927–1934* (Cambridge: Belknap Press, 1999), pp. 299–304, 301.

81 '[E]r benutzt sie für seine notorischen Nichtfakta.' Döblin, 'Der Bau des epischen Werkes', in *Aufsätze zur Literatur*, ed. Walter Muschg (Olten: Walter-Verlag, 1963), pp. 103–32, p. 109.

82 'starke Grundsituationen, Elementarsituationen des menschlichen Daseins.' Döblin, 'Der Bau des epischen Werkes', p. 107.

83 Döblin, 'Der Bau des epischen Werkes', p. 114.

84 Devin Fore, 'Döblin's Epic: Sense, Document, and the Verbal World Picture', *New German Critique*, 99 (2006), pp. 171–207, p. 187.

85 See Sander, 'Döblin's Berlin: The Story of Franz Biberkopf', p. 147.

86 Fore, 'Döblin's Epic', pp. 198, 177.

87 Sander, 'Döblin's Berlin: The Story of Franz Biberkopf', p. 143.

88 David B. Dollmayer, *The Berlin Novels of Alfred Döblin* (Berkeley: University of California Press, 1988), p. 71.

89 Alfred Döblin, *Berlin Alexanderplatz: The Story of Franz Biberkopf*, trans. Eugene Jolas (London: Secker & Warburg, 1974), p. 409. 'Wir sind am Ende dieser Geschichte. Sie ist lang geworden, aber sie mußte sich dehnen und immer mehr dehnen, bis sie jenen Höhepunkt erreichte, den Umschlagspunkt, von dem erst Licht auf das Ganze fällt.... Es war ein Enthüllungsprozess besonderer Art. Franz Biberkopf ging nicht die Straße wie wir. Er rannte drauf los, diese

dunkle Straße....' Alfred Döblin, *Berlin Alexanderplatz: Die Geschichte vom Franz Biberkopf* (Munich: DTV, 1965), p. 409.

90 Gammel, *Sexualizing Power in Naturalism*, p. 25.

91 Gammel, *Sexualizing Power in Naturalism*, p. 20.

92 Fuechtner, *Berlin Psychoanalytic*, p. 41.

93 Döblin, *Berlin Alexanderplatz: The Story of Franz Biberkopf*, p. 28. 'Die sexuelle Potenz kommt zustande durch das Zusammenwirken 1. Des innersektorischen Systems, 2. Des Nervensystems und 3. Des Geschlechtsapparates.' Döblin, *Berlin Alexanderplatz: Die Geschichte vom Franz Biberkopf*, p. 27.

94 Döblin, *Berlin Alexanderplatz: The Story of Franz Biberkopf*, pp. 29–30. 'Testifortan, geschütztes Warenzeichen Nr. 365695, Sexualtherapeutikum nach Sanitätsrat Dr. Magnus Hirschfeld und Dr. Bernhard Schapiro, Institut für Sexualwissenschaft, Berlin.' Döblin, *Berlin Alexanderplatz: Die Geschichte vom Franz Biberkopf*, p. 29.

95 See Peter Jelavich, *Berlin Alexanderplatz: Radio, Film, and the Death of Weimar Culture* (Berkeley: University of California Press, 2006), p. 17.

96 Fuechtner, 'Arzt und Dichter', p. 128.

97 See Fuechtner, 'Arzt und Dichter', p. 127.

98 See Fuechtner, 'Arzt und Dichter', p. 127.

99 Döblin, 'Erfolg', in *Schriften zu Leben und Werk*, p. 220.

100 Döblin, 'Erfolg', in *Schriften zu Leben und Werk*, p. 221.

101 Fuechtner, 'Arzt und Dichter', p. 129.

102 '[E]s war alles, nicht nur politisch, auch geistig unerträglich in Deutschland geworden.' Döblin, 'Abschied und Wiederkehr', in *Schriften zu Leben und Werk*, pp. 265–72, p. 267.

103 '[W]ar nicht nur zur völligen Stummheit verurteilt, entmündigt, sondern noch mehr: degradiert, weniger als sein Analphabet des Landes, der sich wenigstens mit seinen Nachbarn unterhalten kann.' Döblin, 'Abschied und Wiederkehr', in *Schriften zu Leben und Werk*, p. 270.

104 Döblin, 'Abschied und Wiederkehr', in *Schriften zu Leben und Werk*, p. 270.

105 See Fuechtner, *Berlin Psychoanalytic*, p. 187.

106 See Döblin, 'Letter to Peter Huchel, 30th September 1954', in *Briefe II*, p. 442.

107 See Döblin, 'Letter to Hermann Kesten, 7th May 1947', in *Briefe II*, pp. 253–4.

6

Viola Bernard and the case study of race in post-war America

Joy Damousi

The writings and political activism of Viola Bernard, a psychoanalyst of German-Jewish background who practised in New York during the twentieth century, provide a further prism through which to consider the genre of the case study, as well as broader questions concerning intersections between culture, politics and the discourses of psychiatry and psychoanalysis. A resilient political and social activist, Bernard was committed to many progressive causes. These included support of trade union activism, black rights, women's rights and civil liberties. Throughout her career she believed that psychiatric and psychoanalytic techniques could be deployed to assist in achieving wider social reforms. She became active in assisting European refugees from German National Socialism, and in 1939 travelled to Europe to examine the plight of refugee children in Britain and France. Merging her commitment to psychoanalysis and psychiatry with social causes, Bernard's study of race – in many of its facets – increasingly took a political form.

Bernard's campaign on the issue of race forms the basis of this chapter. Such a focus deviates from the approach taken in the preceding chapters of this volume. Here the theme is a case study 'in formation' rather than a development or variation in the tradition of the case study genre. The context is the highly charged political environment in the USA from the 1940s to the 1960s. The issue is that of race and the expert field of psychoanalysis: specifically, the development of a profoundly transformative case study narrative about black subjects within this field – and within post-war American politics and society. This chapter demonstrates the difficulties of constructing case studies, or at least advocating them, at certain historic moments that are characterised by political tensions, social unrest, distrust and paranoia. It also highlights the challenges of documenting case histories. When considering the history of case studies in this post-war context, the materials available are necessarily fragmented and disparate. At the time, the discourse of race and psychiatry was emerging in new ways through a range of sources. This chapter draws on a wide variety of sources, including public discussions as these were reflected in the press; specialised talks within the professions of psychiatry and psychoanalysis; and Bernard's personal correspondence. These materials all pertain to an evolving narrative, the writers responding to political and social events as they unfolded.

As the civil rights movement in the USA gained momentum from the 1940s, Bernard was ahead of her time in advocating the urgent need to train more African-Americans for entry into the profession of psychiatry. She believed that African-American people should have access to the best psychiatric assistance available. But for Bernard it was not a matter of merely adding to the field more trained psychiatrists from an African-American background. Her advocacy also involved using her extensive contacts and influence to interrogate the nature of psychiatry and to investigate how the 'problem' of cultural difference was addressed in American psychiatric and psychoanalytic training and practice. Bernard's civil rights campaigning was never simply of academic or theoretical importance. Rather, it took place in political arenas, and involved mobilising fellow advocates as well as expert knowledge on key issues, with the aim of making a profound difference to the lives and rights of black and white Americans.

Bernard's activism points to the ways in which her exploration of the 'case' of the 'Negro' – as African-Americans were then termed – became framed by cultural and political considerations.[1] This was especially notable in the position she took concerning the civil liberties of African-Americans, and in her attempts to promote them inside the medical profession, in psychiatry and in the wider society, such that she became a leading supporter of black civil rights in post-war America.

Although this chapter is centred on the emerging case study of race and its intersection with medicine during the post-war period, Bernard's work on cases of 'sexual deviance' links her practice and ethos as a psychoanalyst to earlier chapters in this volume. Many of Bernard's patients were middle-class women who struggled with their sexual identity and subjectivity when they deviated from the 'norm' of heterosexuality. Bernard offered psychoanalytic treatments that resisted labelling these women as deviant. As such, Bernard was progressive for her era insofar as she was reluctant to label and dismiss homosexual and bisexual behaviours, at a time when sexual behaviours other than heterosexual were considered abnormal, and were, indeed, often illegal.[2] This defiance of contemporary practices and assumptions also emerged in Bernard's advocacy of black rights at a volatile period of social upheaval in American history.

Viola Bernard: medicine, McCarthyism and black rights

Viola Bernard was the child of a German-Jewish couple Jacob Wertheim and his second wife, Emma Stern. Wertheim was the owner of the United Cigar Company and among the founders of the Federation of Jewish

Philanthropies. His death in 1920 left his family in comfortable circumstances.[3] Born in 1907 in New York City, Bernard undertook her undergraduate studies at Smith College, Barnard College, Johns Hopkins University and New York University. In 1936 she was one of only four women to receive her medical degree at Cornell University. Bernard completed her postgraduate work in psychoanalysis at the New York Psychoanalytic Society and Institute, from where she graduated in 1942. In 1945 she received her certification from the American Psychoanalytic Association. In the same year, she assisted Sandor Rado in establishing the Columbia University Center for Psychoanalytic Training and Research – the first university-based training programme in the world.

Bernard's own case notes were less in the literary style of some analysts and more flavoured by her medical background. Case notes on black patients she may have analysed have yet to be located. Most of her cases were not written up for publication, but those accessible in her archived papers are illuminating for their discussion of sexuality: atypically for the time, she approached homosexuality neither as a pathology nor as a medical condition. When compared with European psychoanalysis, psychoanalysis in the USA was conspicuously medicalised as a profession.[4] Despite this context for her practice, and although her training was firmly in medicine, Bernard did not always frame her examination of case histories in terms of medicalisation.[5]

A long-term social and political activist, during the 1930s, Bernard was a financial supporter of the People's Press, a trade unionist news service which was later attacked as a communist front organisation. She was active in civil liberties causes and during the 1950s was unofficially blacklisted as a person deemed unsuitable for US government employment. One of her key interests was the role that she believed psychiatry could play in empowering African-Americans. In the hostile ideological climate of the Cold War she encountered severe opposition to this idea, which propelled her into the political limelight.

In 1952 Bernard was at the pinnacle of her influence as a prominent New York psychiatrist, supporter of civil and liberal causes and a leading philanthropist. Also in 1952 she testified before the House Un-American Activities Committee (HUAC). Formed in 1938 to monitor German National Socialist activity, this committee of the US House of Representatives became best known for the interrogation of alleged communists. Promoted by Cold War warrior Joseph McCarthy, HUAC reached the peak of its influence during the 1940s and 1950s, when artists such as film directors and actors came under its scrutiny. Investigations resulted controversially in the blacklisting of the 'Hollywood Ten', driving those in the film industry underground, or forcing them to leave the USA altogether.[6] Under J. Edgar Hoover as leader of the Federal Bureau of Investigation, psychoanalysts were subject to the closest scrutiny. Inevitably the focus fell on foreign-born analysts, but even those not foreign-born, like Bernard, did not escape surveillance. As Elizabeth Danto has argued, psychoanalysts often showed traits that were anathema to the 'Americanism' of the day, namely a 'history of left-wing affiliations, an openness to sexuality, [they were] frequently atheists, and often Jewish'. Bernard displayed all of these traits, which collectively represented a catalogue of 'moral weakness'.[7]

When asked about her affiliations, Bernard was direct and forthright in her testimony to HUAC. 'Politically', Bernard informed those judging her, 'I have always considered myself a liberal. I oppose totalitarianism of the left or right. I believe in the freedom and dignity of the individual and am convinced that these are best preserved and protected in a democratic society'. She believed her medical specialisations – in child welfare and mental health – to be a means of contributing to a 'better and healthier America'. Her exemplary record of public service, she argued, 'must prove that I am thoroughly loyal to my country and its institutions'.[8] In this climate of surveillance and interrogation, Bernard's activity in a range of political causes was interpreted as mildly subversive at best and destructive at worst. Her testimony also coincided with the fervour and rapid rise of the civil rights movement, before it burst upon the political scene and developed into an unstoppable wave that engulfed American society.[9]

The recriminations that followed Bernard's testimony to HUAC were severe. Two years later, in 1954, Bernard was delisted as a consultant for the US Department of Health, Education and Welfare on the grounds of pro-communist activity. Such an attack upon a senior and influential member of the medical profession was unusual. It was based on Bernard's membership of several organisations: the American Committee for Protection of Foreign Born, and a number of other groups, including American Women for Peace, as well as her part ownership and financial support of a corporation that was community initiated and controlled – the People's Press. Bernard staunchly defended these connections as nothing more than loose affiliations, and asserted that her association with such initiatives did not reflect disloyalty. Bernard was also a member of the Physicians Forum Conference for Health Care Without Discrimination; she was a candidate for election to the board. The accusations of subversive activity become so pronounced that she resigned as a consultant to the US Public Health Service, and as a member of the Training Committee of the National Advisory Mental Health Council. The pressure became too much to bear:

> there is no basis for questioning my loyalty to the US[.] I am submitting my resignation lest my continued association reflect adversely in the slightest degree on the National Mental Health Program. I value the importance of this Program so highly that I prefer resigning to the faintest risk of incurring even the most minimal handicap to this vital service for the mentally ill.[10]

Bernard believed that the 'misuse of security measures' would increasingly exclude from service to the USA 'loyal and devoted professional individuals' who, in her view, had attempted to 'help solve social problems of vital importance to our democratic way of life'.[11] Despite the manifest hostility towards her political standing, she remained steadfast in her determination to assist minority groups. This was especially apparent in her support for African-Americans in pursuit of careers in psychiatry. For example, in 1945 Bernard wrote to her colleague Dr Frederick Weil, thanking him for seeing twenty-year-old student Archie Parsons in order to administer a Rorschach test, the popular test used, especially in the post-war period, to observe personality and emotional states. This appointment was important to Bernard. Parsons was an African-American student at the University of Michigan; he had sought advice from Bernard regarding the possibility of a career in psychiatry and she was keen to promote the option to him. In her letter to Weil, Bernard suggested that Weil charge his usual fee, but send the bill to her, which she paid from a fund used to support African-American students. The tests raised no concerns, and Bernard wrote to Parsons encouraging him to call on her if there was anything with which she could assist.[12] Other African-Americans wrote to Bernard in deepest appreciation of her efforts to encourage them into psychiatry, even though they decided not to take that career path themselves.[13] Bernard was a staunch supporter and provided strong letters of reference for African-American psychiatrists. The first African-American medical resident accepted into the Department of Psychiatry at Bellevue Hospital, Dr Charles Brown, received a glowing reference from Bernard.[14]

Yet, in the profession of psychiatry, the question of race was not unproblematic. Through the twentieth century, psychiatry had long been perceived as the enemy of minority groups. As such, in what ways did Bernard envisage that psychiatry would indeed provide a framework for liberation during the immediate post-war period? How did the Cold War thwart her progressive stance on the rights of African-Americans to enter into areas of medical practice such as psychiatry?

'Mental hygiene' and minority groups

In his comprehensive history of psychoanalysis in America, Nathan Hale has described 1945–65 as the period of the rapid rise of psychoanalytic psychiatry. In the American context, psychoanalysis – the practice based in Freudian principles and theories – emerged from the ashes and traumas of the First World War. The traditional methods of psychiatry, which involved an examination of mental disorders based on hereditary and neurological models, were increasingly challenged after the First World War by methods advocated by Freud and his followers. They favoured psychodynamic approaches that emphasised social and cultural factors. By the mid-twentieth century, psychoanalysis was becoming increasingly popular in America, and many psychiatrists with medical backgrounds began to train in this approach and to apply its methods. Bernard was one such medically trained psychiatrist who practised as a psychoanalyst. While psychiatry is medically based and psychoanalysis considers socio-cultural circumstances, both rely on individual case histories as a methodology and practice.[15]

Hale cites astonishing statistics concerning the importance of psychoanalysis after the Second World War. He notes that 78 per cent of those who took up psychiatry after graduating from the US army's neuropsychic training programme were psychoanalysed 'or planned to be psychoanalysed'.[16] Private practice was on the increase. Hale estimates that, in 1947, more than half of all American psychiatrists were in private practice, or worked in outpatient clinics, a 20–30 per cent increase since 1940. By 1958, only 16 per cent of members of the American Psychiatric Association worked full-time in mental hospitals, reflecting a trend away from mental hospital services to those within a community setting. From 1948 to 1976, the numbers of qualified psychiatrists also increased, six-fold. This generation of younger psychiatrists emerged in the USA in the late 1950s, and dominated until the mid-1960s; each saw 'about seven patients a day for 45 or 50 minutes each, an average of three times a week for about 18 months'.[17] Analysts from the preceding generation had prescribed drugs and shock treatments, and their treatments had differed. However, psychoanalysts held most of the teaching positions and dominated the psychiatric profession. Hale notes that the 'new generation of analysts was a talented group, and by the 1960s they had assumed leadership of the American psychoanalytic movement and partially dominated American psychiatry'.[18] Hale characterises the period between 1945 and 1965 as one of widespread popularity for psychoanalytic psychiatry in America. Psychoanalytic writings found expression in the popular arena through films, literature and magazines, and, over this period, ideas from Sigmund Freud found expression in a wide range of cultural forms.[19]

While acknowledging the shifting parameters of progressive psychiatry in post-war America, Hale's history does not, however, take into account the politics of race in psychoanalysis. A focus on race as a challenge to the discourse of psychiatry illuminates an unknown history that fundamentally reconceptualises our understanding of the importance of the civil rights movement for the development of modern psychiatry – and thus for the development of the psychiatric case study capable of acknowledging racial as well as sexual difference.

The issue of 'mental hygiene' had preoccupied black activist groups for decades. The year 1939 saw the formation of the Committee for the Development of Mental Hygiene Resources for Negroes in Raleigh, North Carolina. Rosa Kittrell initiated the movement. Kittrell was training to be a social worker when she experienced 'the onset of mental illness'.[20] Through this experience she was moved to work for 'better psychiatric care for her people'. She wished to see created and to help create a 'hospital of high standards for the care of mentally ill Negro patients and for the training of professional workers in psychiatry and mental hygiene'. Towards this end, she organised the White Plains Mental Hygiene Group, which eventually became the Committee for Mental Hygiene for Negroes. The aim was to establish several regional groups. By 1941, there were three in existence – in the cities of White Plains and New York, and in Alabama state.[21] The Committee's constitution stipulated that its key purpose was to 'develop a movement to secure better Psychiatric and Mental Hygiene Recourses [*sic*] for Negroes ... [these] would appear to be best embodied in a Psychiatric Institute or Hospital incorporated in or attached to a Medical School'.[22] The work of the Committee was regularly reported in the *Journal of the National Medical Association*. In 1943, when Bernard was part of the Harlem Clinic of the Board of Education Bureau of Child Guidance, the journal noted that she staunchly 'advocated the admission of Negro physicians to existing facilities in psychiatry. Dr Bernard pointed out that excellent training opportunities are open to Negroes in Social Work and Psychology but are very limited in psychiatry'.[23]

In Bernard's view, the crucial issue was provision of resources and opportunities for training more psychiatrists from within the African-American community. Her campaign on this matter simultaneously addressed a wider issue that held importance for her: that of the therapeutic treatment of 'difference'. She considered it problematic that those identified with minority groups should be treated by those in majority groups. She asked how psychiatry handled the difference.

> Inherent in psychiatric practice is an interpersonal relationship, charged with feeling. Inevitably inter-racial relationships are especially filled with emotion. The situation may become therapeutically impossible when patients of minority groups have emotional disturbances making them seek help, can only be treated by physicians of the majority group. The resultant tensions may well preclude the type of confidence in the doctor that is an essential part of good practice. This is not to say that Negro patients should necessarily go to Negro psychiatrists. There should, however, be available for all patients a varied range of therapists to meet different needs.... To have only white psychiatrists available creates a wall at the outset.[24]

The benefit of such a varied range of therapists would also flow to the psychiatric community. Bernard observed that severe limitations and 'theoretical misconceptions' would follow if conclusions were 'too often based on data from a middle-class white group, interpreted by investigators of the same social group. The psychiatric body of knowledge needs the contributions of colleagues who represent the whole community, including its Negro members'.[25] Several clinics had opened in the Harlem area – the Harlem Hospital Clinic, the Northside Center for Child Development and the Bureau of Child Guidance – and 'all are struggling with overwhelming case loads', Bernard stated. Equally, she argued, leadership should come 'from the Negro community'.

The barriers to leadership faced by African-Americans were deeply embedded within existing restrictions to education, since admission into medical colleges was strictly limited. Bernard believed that the twin evils of exclusion and segregation 'have placed a formidable barrier in the way of medical education for Negroes'; prejudice further barred the way to training in the specialties, including psychiatry. Nonetheless, she remained confident that social change could be ushered into the medical system. 'If upheaval is the forerunner of progress', she boldly proclaimed in 1948, 'then we are on the threshold of major gains in the field of mental hygiene'.[26]

What was the upheaval Bernard had identified? The war years, she believed, had created a major shift 'on the whole question of psychiatry'. She argued that there had developed 'a widespread acceptance of the fact that psychiatric guidance is needed by millions of children and adults who are not actually or potentially insane'. Mental illness, she declared, had been recognised as an illness, not a scandal. Recent discoveries and developments in psychiatry had suggested progress in the field: drug therapy combined with psychotherapy; shock treatment; group therapy. These 'advances have served to diminish greatly the sense of hopelessness which has long permeated the whole area of mental illness. An equally significant development has been the use of clinical teams of psychiatrists, psychologists and social workers'.[27]

A major deficiency that Bernard identified was in the area of training the 'Negro' psychiatrists, whom she considered vital to the assistance of black communities. The wider politics of race loomed large in her promotion of the training of such psychiatrists. The onus was on white, middle-class psychiatrists, who needed to move beyond their racialised conceptions and recognise the inner life of all, not just white, communities:

> As psychiatrists in the United States in 1947, we need to understand intimately the inner mental life and meaning of behavior of the total population with its many social, economic and racial groups. Some of our theoretical misconceptions are doubtless traceable to the fact that conclusions are too often based on data from a middle-class white group, interpreted by investigators of the same social group. The psychiatric body of knowledge needs the contributions of colleagues who represent the whole community, including its Negro members. Many errors of theoretic concepts, based on incomplete sampling, could be corrected by teamwork between investigators of different ethnic and social deviation.

The 'Negro' needing psychiatric care could be accommodated only in state-run mental institutions – 'private inter-racial sanatoria are practically non-existent'.[28] The few psychiatric facilities in the Harlem district, for instance, had employed very few specialists – 'virtually the only private care the patient can seek is at the hands of a non-specialist'. Therefore, Bernard claimed, 'Negro' patients who could afford and would prefer to be treated in 'private inter-racial sanitoria' were nonetheless committed to state hospitals. The way to improve this situation would be to increase the number of 'Negro' psychiatrists and interracial services. Bernard believed that the solution to the overall problem largely depended upon the 'Negro' community taking some leadership itself.[29] Towards this end, Bernard tackled the discrimination inherent in the medical schools and colleges. There were very few medical colleges who admitted 'Negro' students, and the few 'Negro' admissions to those institutions represented no more 'than a token'. The medical profession more generally had tried to draw attention to the plight of 'Negroes'; National Health Negro Week took place in 1944 to highlight the poor health of African-Americans.[30]

The psychoanalyst, too, Bernard believed, needed to take account of 'his own cultural position and social attitudes', conscious and unconscious, 'with particular reference to prejudice'. This belief informed her larger platform of training analysts from a wider range of ethnic, religious and social backgrounds. For Bernard the need for sociologically inclusive training constituted a major issue, with notable implications for countertransference. She held that the 'respective subcultural groups to which patient and analyst belong can be regarded as constituting a special dynamic factor of the analytic situation and as such can be provocative of countertransference'.[31]

Bernard examined the different aspects of the patient–analyst dynamic, but the issue of prejudice was one in which she was most interested to explore the implications of the background of patient and analyst. 'We know that the personal training provided the major safeguard against countertransference hazards, but often the unconscious foundations and psychodynamics of prejudice have not been worked with and worked through in the analyst's own analysis'.[32] As such, Bernard believed the 'personal training' of psychoanalysts to be inadequate. If an analyst has insufficiently analysed 'his own unconscious material' pertaining

> to his own group memberships and those of others, he and his patients may be insufficiently protected from the transference of a variety of positive and negative countertransference reactions stimulated by the ethnic, religious and racial elements that are present in the analytic situation, the patient's personality, and in the specific content of the patient's material.[33]

Bernard was acutely aware of the black–white divide informing these discussions. 'Although', she observed, the white analyst 'may be a member of a minority group, such as Jewish, he is also a member of the dominant white majority, vis-à-vis the Negro patient'.[34] How is this often negotiated? It needs to be done carefully and delicately, but denial is the typical response. On the other hand, the analyst must avoid becoming caught up 'in exaggerating his response to the patient as a Negro rather than as an individual whose total being and specific life experience, including that of being colored, is the analyst's natural field of interest'.[35] To Bernard, it appeared that, while some white analysts 'seem compelled to overemphasize the effects of being Negro on their patient's personality difficulties, others have an apparent need to deny and sidestep any such effects altogether'.[36] Either of these options seemed 'fallacious' to her, as they reflected 'a preconceived bias on the part of the analysts who should, instead, themselves be guided by what the material reveals'.[37]

In Bernard's view, there was a real danger that a 'Negro' stereotype would emerge, 'the psychoanalytic stereotype – whose frustrations will always come back to race'. While urging analysts to examine their own cultural experience, she did not wish to begin constructing the 'white analyst' in a stereotyped manner. She argued strongly for closer 'cultural matching', because, according to her understanding, 'the negative emotional experience still overwhelmingly exceeds the positive experience between white and Negroes'.[38] Bernard suggested that analysts recognise more and more 'the need for informing themselves as fully as possible about social and cultural processes and patterning'.[39] Ahead of her time, then, she saw an imperative to undertake transcultural analyses, 'whereby the analyst's understanding of social and cultural meaning is extended and deepened'.[40] Bernard advised analysts to scrutinise their 'motivations, attitudes and expectations' when embarking on psychoanalysing members of the African-American community. This was necessary at least until 'prejudice and discrimination are significantly reduced in the general social setting'.[41]

Psychoanalytic ideas

In advocating for analysts from a wide background to be admitted into training programmes, Bernard also argued for a more transcultural analysis to be incorporated into psychoanalytic discourse in America. In doing so she was giving voice to ideas that were widely in circulation; others had already discussed racial issues in terms of transference, countertransference and race.[42] Indeed, during the 1950s and 1960s, transference and countertransference in interracial analyses had become a major preoccupation among some analysts. In their discussion of this topic, published in 1968 in the *Journal of the American Psychoanalytic Association*, analysts Judith Schachter and Hugh Butts found it necessary to be cognisant of the 'current social revolution' and its impacts on the analytic relationship.

> Many patients are involved in the interracial tensions which permeate our society. The major efforts being made to upset the structured patterns of discrimination are an important factor in the patient's awareness of choice and increase the possibilities of interracial analysis. We do not discuss, although we recognise, that on the conscious level, Negro–white relationships are directly related to the values, ethics, group norms, and sociopolitical philosophy of participants, and this fact plays a part in the material both patient and analyst choose to work with as well as in the nonverbal cues the patient receives.[43]

The authors drew the conclusion that, while racial differences between analyst and patient involve 'issues of unconscious meaning at various levels analogous to differences in sex between analyst and patient', only 'rarely do they create an either unanalysable barrier or a serious obstacle to treatment'. In their consideration of several cases, Schachter and Butts believed that while interracial analysis indicates 'the difficulties to be anticipated', 'these are apparently no greater than the obstacles encountered in analyses in which race is not an issue'. Such sentiments were not confined to professional exchanges between analysts, but influenced the wider population.

In the following decades Bernard's activism in support of permitting more 'Negroes' to enter medical school remained a key aspect of her personal and public discussions regarding the question of race and psychoanalysis. The year 1976 found her continuing her campaign. In correspondence with John Rhoads, then Professor of Psychiatry at Duke University, she revealed the way in which this issue had remained a preoccupation for her. 'The medical school has a reasonable proportion of blacks', observed Rhoads, 'but none seem to be interested in going into psychiatry. In fact, in the last several years, we recruited the only one who was interested. I'm not sure what the reason for this is, but it certainly is a matter of concern'. He also shared another concern with Bernard – that of the 'problem of middle-class therapists in dealing with patients from different cultural backgrounds'.[44] Discussions on the same issue had been continuing in various medical journals. In 1970 Maynard Calnek published an article titled 'Racial Factors in the Countertransference: The Black Therapist and the Black Client' in the *American Journal of Orthopsychiatry*, arguing that the 'American racial situation' had created difficulties in 'working successfully with black clients'. He maintained that 'racial factors must be acknowledged and dealt with by the therapist', and that the black community and black therapist 'should be the reference points for diagnosis and therapy with any black person'.[45]

During the 1970s race was hotly debated as a case study topical for the practice of psychiatry, and of more general, public importance. For example, in 1970 the Psychiatric Society of Westchester County's Committee on Social Issues presented a 'position paper' on 'white racism'. The Committee was chaired by Norbert Bromberg, who noted that the paper was not a 'scientific' paper, but was meant to

> contribute to the public's understanding of those aspects of an issue in which the organization issuing the statement has some expertise. Unlike the scientific paper, it does not attempt to add to the scientific knowledge of the specialist, nor even to be an exhaustive and complete study of the subject, although such a study should be undertaken by the authors of the statement.

The organisation undertook to examine this subject because there were 'psychological factors beyond those of other group prejudices that are important for psychiatrists and the public to understand'.[46]

This position paper is especially compelling, since, in directly linking racism with psychiatry, it offers a key context for understanding the milieu in which Bernard's activism took place, and within which psychiatry and psychoanalysis were endowed with a political purpose. The paper expounds how racism 'is rooted' in the 'conscious' and the 'unconscious', the authors believing it 'hardly possible for any white man in the United States to be completely free of at least unconscious racism, so pervasive is it in our culture'. From this prevalence it follows that, 'in times of stress, even the most liberal and enlightened may regress to racist stereotypes and preconceptions'. The psychological and psychiatric assessment was easily made. Racism was to be found in 'residuals of a very early phase of development in which images of others and self-images are regarded as "all good" or "all bad"'.

> [The] more completely this split persists, the less subject it is to rational modification. The blatant racist preserves an essentially 'all good' image of himself, which he protects from contamination by projecting the 'all bad' onto the black man. The Black, consequently, may be seen as indolent, suspicious, deceitful, violent, dirty, or salacious, i.e., possessing whatever traits the white man would find objectionable in himself.

Even when 'whites' have a 'better' conception of this characterisation, 'the Black's position in our society makes him an available object for the projection of unacceptable impulses and also for direct discharge of sadistic drives. Slavery, after all, was rationalized by the fiction that black people were subhuman'.[47] On a clinical level, the authors observed that the 'degrading' conditions in which black people were living constituted 'a severe hazard to personality development': 'early and repeatedly the black child is made aware that black men live in a child-like, passive, feminine, and inferior position vis-à-vis white men'.

The response of the white man, too, is described as complex: 'racist cultural values offer ... infantile solutions to psychic conflicts over love and hate'. The expression of this is set forth as a 'sense of entitlement, self-aggrandizement and denigration of others. The same is true of any Black extremist who develops his own racism. In the White racist, in place of identification with Blacks as fellow humans, there is sadism which reinforces infantile elements in his personality'. The report concluded that an 'understanding of these irrational forces and factors in the psychological structure of racism is indispensible to its elimination'.[48]

The paper's proposed 'solutions' and actions for psychiatrists and psychologists are telling. They include distinctive recommendations for action by the Psychiatric Society of Westchester County. 'Most psychiatrists are of white middle-class background'; it was the responsibility of the individual to 'remove one's blind spots'. In clinical practice the psychiatrists' responsibilities included paying 'more attention ... to racist attitudes in the course of therapy with White patients'. Significantly, however, the paper stipulated that 'psychiatrists should be in the forefront of those interpreting racism to the community' – by promoting leadership positions to members of all races, which would further cooperation between the races and help to combat racism as a cultural value. The critical assessment of some members of the profession in relation to racism remains striking. 'Some psychiatrists view the black struggle with condescension and subtle defensiveness, eventually sacrificing human understanding to rhetoric which defends the status quo'.[49]

Black activists themselves were not always convinced of the productive use of psychoanalysis or psychiatric case studies for the black population. Moreover, the question of whether 'a white psychiatrist can actually psychoanalyse a Negro under pressure of racial conflict' drew vitriolic and sharp responses from black activists, such as the outspoken and strident black journalist James Hicks. Hicks was a pioneering correspondent who edited the *New York Amsterdam News* from 1955 to 1966 and again from 1972 to 1977. During this time, the *Amsterdam News* became one of America's most widely circulated and most influential weekly newspapers on black rights. During the civil rights movement of the 1950s and 1960s, Hicks reported the incidents of violence throughout the country for the *Amsterdam News*.[50] On the issue of psychoanalysis he was especially vocal. He noted that a group of psychiatrists

> say that it is almost impossible for a white psychiatrist to psychoanalyze a Negro who is under the pressure of racial conflict (and what Negro is not under pressure) because since the white psychiatrist represents the image of the cause of the Negro's conflict, by tradition and force of habit will not permit the white psychiatrists to really look into his inner mind and see the turmoil within. It goes without saying that if the white man can't find what's wrong with the Negro he can't offer him any cure.[51]

In the same article Hicks stated emphatically, 'I'd like to make it plain that I agree with [this] group of psychiatrists – I know that NO white man could ever psychoanalyze me because I couldn't bring myself to tell a white man ALL my innermost thoughts, even if he took me on a ride to Paradise on Cloud 17'.[52] He persisted in this vein, arguing that 'if ALL Negroes would tell white people what they really think of them many white people would commit suicide'. Furthermore, 'since I'm not going to tell him what he wants to know when I'm not under pressure – I KNOW I'm not going to tell him all the things that are on my mind when I'm under pressure'.[53]

The New York City government announced in 1961 that it planned to spend $90,000 'to pay a "psychiatric patrol" from the Jewish Board of Guardians to float around Harlem to "watch" or "study" juvenile delinquents with a view toward snatching them off the streets and forcing them on some white psychiatrist's couch'.[54] The proposal focused on gang leaders in Harlem. Even the idea that the Youth Board of the City of New York would commit to such an initiative was 'insulting'. Hicks expressed his outrage at this 'idiotic' suggestion:

> Good, bad or indifferent, the children of Harlem belong to the parents of Harlem, and these parents are not going to sit idly by and let a group of people from the Jewish Board of Guardians, the Polish Board of Guardians, the Chinese Board of Guardians or any other 'board of guardians' experiment without permission on the minds of their children as if they were white mice or guinea pigs.... For the benefit of these ill-informed social scientists downtown, we would inform them that Harlem is not yet a 'compound' or 'reservation' set aside for Negroes where white scholars may conduct scientific experiments on the minds of Negroes. And the people of Harlem will never allow this area to become such a reservation.[55]

Hicks declared: 'let[']s curb juvenile delinquency this summer. But first, let['] s curb the delinquent adults on our Your Board!'[56] If the very concept of a 'study' of black children by white experts disgusted Hicks, he found especially affronting any efforts to study them psychoanalytically. To Hicks, these efforts resonated with earlier 'scientific' experimentation by whites, when blacks were treated like 'guinea pigs'. Hicks was adamant that the political agenda intrinsic to studies of blacks by whites – whatever form the studies took – was highly offensive.

Bernard and the role of psychology in challenging racial segregation

Bernard assisted those working for racial equality beyond the medical sphere. In August 1959, prominent left-wing activist and rights agitator Carl Braden was charged with contempt of Congress and sentenced to a year's imprisonment 'for refusing to answer certain questions of him by a subcommittee of the House Un-American Committee in Atlanta Ga., in July, 1958. He challenged the committee's right to ask the questions.' Bernard paid his bail of $1,000. As a celebrated activist for racial equality, Braden was the target of attacks by white supremacists and was barred from employment in Kentucky. He worked for the Southern Conference Educational Fund (SCEF) and developed its civil rights cause through the *Southern Patriot*, the organisation's monthly newspaper.[57]

Bernard took an exceptionally active role on the issue of segregation. In 1952 she was a signatory to a submission to the US Supreme Court that outlined the effects of the segregation of racial and ethnic groups.[58] The *Southern Patriot* discussed this issue at length in 1956, and particularly the psychiatric benefits of integration. Pro-segregationists were claiming that 'mixing children in public schools would have harmful emotional effect on both races'.[59] A survey conducted by the New Orleans Medical Association and the Medical Advisory Committee of the SCEF asked the following question: 'From a professional point of view, how would you characterize the psychiatric effect of racially integrated schools on white and Negro children?' The results revealed a greater openness to desegregation than might have been expected. Eighteen doctors thought that 'integration would either be beneficial or would have little effect'; eleven 'declared it beneficial'; of the seven anticipating it to have little effect, three qualified their answers with 'in the long run'. Four 'considered there were harmful possibilities in the ending of segregation'. Two 'thought both races would suffer; one believed that whites would be harmed while Negroes would benefit'.[60]

Bernard's view on this question was clear. The notion of desegregation was not perfect, but it was the better option and any difficulties that might arise from it could be treated.

> With desegregation some Negro children will probably feel discrimination in more personally-directed and immediately painful forums than in their all-Negro schools. But at least this form of trauma is more accessible therapeutically than the chronic indirect hurt to personality of legally sanctioned exclusion and restriction.[61]

Of the two conditions, then, desegregation was the lesser of evils.

> As the choice of the lesser evil it seems preferable, from the mental-health standpoint, for some Negro children to suffer the transitional and current psychological hardships of desegregation which are relatively more recognisable and correctable, than to experience the more insidious and less treatable life-long psychic damage from segregation.[62]

Other psychiatrists agreed. One 'young, Louisiana-born doctor' commented in the following way on segregation in schools:

> There can be little question of the detrimental effect on the psychic development of any discriminated-against group, by a system which teaches them that they are inferior, but which requires them to compete for the necessities and niceties of life on an equal economic level. The results, in decreased contentment, undeveloped potential, and the fostering of resentments and hostility likely to be acted out against the frustrating community, should be obvious.[63]

Ideas about the impact of racial and ethnic integration on the white population were the source of some contention. It was a 'complex subject', noted the same young doctor, 'but since there are no demonstrable biological differences between races on any significant level, there can be no advantage for a group to grow up with the belief, totally false, that they are significantly better, and thus entitled to greater privilege and more of the world's goods. This does not produce mature people'.[64] Another medical doctor commented on the 'emotional transition' that segregation would entail:

> Initially there is likely to be some reserve and suspiciousness on the part of both races. Especially in the upper grades the children will at first try to remain separate and associate only with their own color. Some, inflamed by their elders, may become involved in fighting.

It was predicted that, over time, however, children would cease to see only colour differences and would gradually

> come to accept the individuals of the other race according to each one's worth as a student and a human being. The ultimate effect will be a lessening of irrational prejudice generally.... The Negro children will live with less fear, envy and suppressed hostility towards whites. In turn the white children will have less irrational fear of Negroes and less guilt feelings towards them.[65]

Others believed in the necessity of a gradual adaptation to desegregation. 'I favor a gradual integration beginning first with kindergarten and in 13 years integration will be complete. A sudden, cataclysmic change can only lead to disaster!' Dr Martial Boudreaux wrote with a strident voice:

> The fears that any mixture of the races will lead to increases of disease, significant lowering of intelligence, or psychiatric difficulties in either race, to my view are unfounded.... These methods of rationalization are common in history. They, in one form or another, have been used to give a pseudo-logical or scientific front for action that has motivations other than the stated ones. Hitler used them effectively in Germany, except the prejudice was primarily against the Jew rather than the American Negro. Perhaps it is forgotten that one of the reasons we fought so hard in World War II was to assert that racial intolerances were not compatible with freedom and democracy.[66]

The matter of public health in general was much debated in the *Southern Patriot*. One paediatrician in the 'integrated city' of St Louis commented:

> child health, particularly in the South, where so much domestic work is done by Negroes, cannot be segregated.... With regard to school contacts, whether with teachers or pupils, if the school hygiene program of observation and examination of children is well and conscientiously conducted ... integration should have no appreciable effect upon the children's health. So far, it certainly has not.[67]

Alfred Yankauer, another medical doctor, dismissed segregationists because their views were not 'based upon logic and therefore not answerable by logic. In fact, there are harmful effects of inferior housing, dense populations and inadequate facilities'.[68]

Bernard was perhaps most directly involved in the cause of public health and its relation to segregation through her support of the court cases litigated by the National Association for the Advancement of Colored People (NAACP) and its Legal and Educational Fund against state laws 'which required segregated schools [and] violated the equal protection clause of the Fourteenth Amendment of the United States Constitution'. The NAACP has a long history in the civil rights movement. Founded in 1909, its guiding principle was to fight for equal citizenship rights for

African-Americans. When the Association was formed, open violation of civil rights and lynching of blacks continued, despite the Thirteenth, Fourteenth and Fifteenth Amendments to the US Constitution which had been adopted between 1865 and 1870, and which explicitly enshrined equal political rights for all, as well as the illegality of denying the right to vote on the grounds of 'race, color, or previous condition of servitude'.[69]

The NAACP fought for full desegregation. Since the late 1940s, psychologist Kenneth Clark had been collecting material on the damage that segregation caused to children. Clark's work was not confined to schools. He and his researchers had been charting the effects of segregation in housing, employment and health, and on the learning capacities of white and 'Negro' children. With this research in hand, the NAACP took the next step in its campaign against segregation.[70] At a meeting in 1950, all members of the NAACP, including its branch and state conferences, decided to tackle the question of educational segregation in a bold move; the psychical and psychological harm of segregation was immediate and devastating in its impact on 'Negro' children, and action needed to be swift and direct.[71] As part of this strategy, Robert L. Carter, a lawyer in the NAACP, decided to draw on the wider expertise and knowledge of a range of specialists, including psychiatrists, psychologists and social scientists such as sociologists and anthropologists, to produce material explaining the detrimental impact of segregation on 'Negro' children.[72] Bernard was one such specialist who became involved in the enterprise of writing up and publicising the relevant studies.

In a landmark decision of May 1954, *Brown v. Board of Education*, the US Supreme Court found segregation in schools to be unconstitutional. Bernard assisted with the preparation of this case, especially in terms of the medical and psychological impact of desegregation. In developing material for the court case, Carter, the Assistant Counsel, wrote to Bernard in October 1952, to express appreciation of her efforts. Carter was fulsome in his praise of the work she had done and the material she had provided:

> It is difficult to express in words our gratitude and elation for your support and generous cooperation. Certainly, we realize that if we succeed in destroying the legal foundation upon which segregation is based in these or in subsequent cases, most of the credit must go, not to us lawyers, but to those social scientists who have made it possible to demonstrate the injurious and hurtful consequences of segregation as a pattern of American life.[73]

In June 1954, shortly after the historic ruling in *Brown v. Board of Education*, Carter wrote to Bernard in ecstasy over their success. In a moving letter he again expressed his thanks for her assistance:

> You are undoubtedly as overjoyed as we with the May 17th decisions of the United States Supreme Court in the school segregation cases. It now

> seems certain that the basic objectives of the NAACP's legal program – elimination of legally enforced segregation and discrimination in all aspects of American life – will be realized much sooner than any of us had dared hope. While the staff here feels justly proud in being on the winning side of such a great issue, all of us realize that we did not and could not have done this job alone.[74]

In the context of this victory, Carter wrote in powerful terms of Bernard's indispensable role:

> You were one of those who greatly aided in the successful preparation, development and presentation of the theory which won the vote for the Court. I wish to express to you on behalf ... [of] our entire staff, our deep and sincere appreciation for the part you played in what may well be one of the greatest victories for democracy in our generation.[75]

The NAACP looked to the future for further support from Bernard:

> Much remains to be done. Having contributed so much, we feel confident that we can include you among those to whom we can turn for help in the planning and implementation of a sound program designed to give effect to the May 17th ruling at the community level and in extending that ruling to other areas. While the task ahead is formidable indeed, all of us, I believe, feel we can now approach that difficult job with high optimistic hope.[76]

Bernard's involvement in the pursuit of desegregation in schools across the USA continued. In July 1954, a conference of social scientists for the legal division of the NAACP convened to consider several issues associated with segregation. Discussion focused on the key question of the pace of desegregation: there were forms of 'gradual' transition and there were forms of 'immediate' desegregation. Central to these considerations were the 'doubts and anxieties concerning the readiness, the procedure by which and the rate at which the general public can accept changes in race relations.... It is assumed that the period of preparation and education will reduce resistance or opposition to desegregation or other changes in racial practices'.[77] The pace of change was a major concern for Bernard, and she stressed the importance of highlighting the shift in public opinion on this issue. She wrote to Clark,

> Doesn't the evidence show in employment, housing, and military desegregation, that reform for integration grew out of changed and growing public feeling for integration sufficient to create the necessary pressure for the reform – and that then the legally enforced and sanctioned policy of desegregation induced the necessary social behavior.[78]

Shifts had already taken place in public opinion, 'as evidenced by the steps towards – the fact of – the reactions to – the Supreme Court Decision'. According to Bernard, the best move forward was to ensure that the legal sanctions had been implemented. 'The unequivocal decree of the court, and the setting up thereby [*sic*] of the strongest legal sanctions and enforcement would offer the best means of creating the further attitudinal climate for smooth and effective implementation'.[79]

The September 1952 submission to the US Supreme Court titled 'The Effects of Segregation and Consequences of Desegregation: A Social Science Statement' articulated the psychological thinking of progressives of the time, like Bernard. The concept of the 'inferiority complex' was central to a discussion of self-worth and conflict. One finding stated:

> as minority group children learn the inferiority status to which they are assigned – as they observe the fact that they are almost always segregated and kept apart from others who are treated with more respect by the society as a whole – they often react with feelings of inferiority and a sense of personal humiliation. Many of them become confused about their own personal worth.[80]

Indeed, personal dignity, self-respect and conflict were themes that emerged from the statement to the Supreme Court:

> On the one hand, like all other human beings they require a sense of personal dignity; on the other hand, almost nowhere in the larger society do they find their own dignity as human beings respected by others. Under these conditions, the minority group child is thrown into a conflict with regard to his feelings about himself and his group. He wonders whether his group and he himself are worthy of no more respect than they receive. This conflict and confusion leads to self-hatred and rejection of his own group.[81]

To consider why segregation produces this impact, it was necessary to bring to bear on the issue insights from psychological and sociological knowledge. Such insights included 'the role of various environmental influences in producing feelings of inferiority, confusions in personal roles, various types of basic personality structures and the various forms of personal and social disorganization'. The emphasis here was on 'feelings of inferiority and doubts about personal worth', which involved an awareness of 'social status difference'. Enforced segregation produced flow-on effects, such as defeatism and a low level of aspiration among children in segregated schools. Moreover, minority group children displayed a hypersensitivity and anxiety about their relations with the larger society.[82] Segregation had the potential to be detrimental to all children, although for children in the majority group, the effects were comparatively obscure. These children learn 'the prejudices of society' and are taught 'to gain personal status in an unrealistic and non-adaptive way'. The culture then condones 'hostility and aggression against whole groups of people' believed to be weaker than the majority group.[83] Those subject to segregation often 'develop patterns of guilt feelings, rationalizations and other mechanisms which they must use in an attempt to protect themselves from recognizing the essential injustice of their unrealistic fears and hatreds of minority groups'.[84]

The problem of violence was mentioned as a significant source of ongoing concern. The submission document included the observation that studies of 'urban riots ... found that race riots occurred in segregated neighborhoods', while there was 'no violence in sections of the city where the two races lived, worked and attended school together'.[85] An important message of the argument set forth in the Social Science Statement related to intelligence, and the supposed inferior intelligence of minority groups. It declared that 'fears based on the assumption of innate racial differences in intelligence are not well founded'.[86] Submitted in September 1952 as the appendix to the appellant's brief in *Brown v. Board of Education*, the Statement was published eight months later in the *Minnesota Law Review*; it was at the forefront of promoting civil rights, by drawing on studies undertaken within the discipline of psychology. Bernard's role in generating the expert submission was central, and she provided much insight and energy to this enterprise.

The wave of resistance to the Supreme Court decision of May 1954 was immediate and sustained. Bernard's consideration of public opinion was germane. As white resistance heightened, the court ruling and the NAACP's belief in judicial rulings were to be severely challenged. For instance, the activities of the NAACP were effectively barred inside the boundaries of the State of Alabama, limiting its operations.[87] The campaign for desegregation continued during the 1950s. In 1955, NAACP members Rosa Parks and Edgar ('E. D.') Nixon helped to spearhead the bus boycott in Alabama's capital city of Montgomery. The protest aimed to end racial segregation on the city's public transportation system.[88] Eventually, the tactics of 'nonviolent mass protest, targeted litigation, and deft political lobbying had helped shatter the southern caste system. The Civil Rights Act of 1964 and the Voting Rights Act of 1965 dismantled the legal framework for segregation'.[89]

Related to the issue of racial segregation was that of child delinquency. Bernard worked closely with the public school system to attempt to address this. In 1959, the Department of Public Welfare made publicly available statistics and information about the increasing rise of delinquency among poor children and white and 'non-white' children.[90]

The Jewish community

Viola Bernard's interests in cultural change and psychiatry extended to other kinds of advocacy, such as writing and speaking out against anti-Semitism. In 1945, Max Horkheimer from the American Jewish Committee had written to Bernard when the committee was searching for expertise on 'the nature and extent of anti-Semitism, particularly as it relates to psycho-dynamic motivations'. Horkheimer went on to note that they 'should like ... to discuss this project with a group of leaders in the field and for that purpose are calling an initial meeting'.[91]

The Jewish community's concern to understand support for German National Socialism continued into the 1960s, and the American Jewish Committee sought Bernard's advice, also assisting her with research into young people and their series of 'Swastika daubings'.[92] The Committee's support for such research was not due to 'morbid curiosity', but to a wish for a fuller understanding of psychological and psychiatric issues behind such behaviours. Aggressive, public displays of anti-Semitic behaviour became an ongoing cause of concern across the USA. In 1960, Bernard was involved in discussions about increasing anti-Semitism and the links between these and 'crazes and fads of less destructive nature'.[93] Her public comments drew the supportive attention of other doctors, such as Anthony Votos, who wrote to her: 'I couldn't help but write after reading your comments in today's *Times*. There is much more destructive hatred in today's anti-Semitic outbursts than even seemingly astute clinicians are willing to admit'.[94]

Of additional interest to Bernard was the question of Jewish identity, and several organisations and institutions sought her view on ways in which Jewish identity and the self might be addressed psychoanalytically. She conferred with her colleagues. In correspondence about the nature of anti-Semitism, others contacted Bernard regarding their psychoanalytic patients. In 1946, Bluma Swerdloff from the Department of Scientific Research contacted Bernard, raising questions about cultural shifts within Jewish families, and the impact of such shifts on family functioning. In relation to one particular patient of Bernard's, several questions were asked about responses to cultural change:

> We learned in the background history that there were a number of inter-marriages in the maternal family. We were wondering what the mother's attitude was to her sister who married a non-Jew. There seemed to be much feeling about the brother who married a Gentile girl but little was said about the sister.[95]

The patient's attitude to 'Jewishness' became central to the discussion:

> Did the parent have any reactions to the dependence of his parents on their relatives? We are interested in this because we feel that it might throw further light as to the parents' own attitude towards their Jewishness. It was our feeling, for instance, that the mother's ambivalent attitude to her own Jewishness is a reflection of her ambivalence to her mother. We are also concerned as to how the mother's attitude to Jewishness and her father's reflect themselves in the patient's attitude towards being a Jew. The fact of being Jewish seems to have different meaning for the father and the mother. The father seems to have a more ethical approach and the mother seems to accept some of the ritual without ideological understanding.[96]

Circumcision also becomes the focus of discussion, Bernard's correspondent noting that the patient's 'feeling about his own penis seems significant. Did he make any comments about circumcision? How does this patient compare how own penis [*sic*] with that of others, for example, his cousin Robert's?'[97]

***

In dedicating her activism to black and also Jewish causes, Bernard was part of an activist movement with a long-standing history in America.[98] Her empathy for historically marginalised groups emerged from her own commitment to justice and equality – causes that she believed were vital for psychoanalysts to pursue. An examination of Bernard's efforts, both within and beyond the disciplinary sphere of psychiatry, to develop case materials in support of minority groups, especially in relation to the African-American community, is illuminating. Bernard's key contribution lies in her efforts to use the case study in psychiatry to explore issues of race in ways which she perceived were empowering to those from the African-American community. Furthermore, as a professional case writer, Bernard aimed to create a space for African-American psychiatrists themselves to become case writers, in ways which addressed issues of power, civil rights and self-determination at a time when these questions were at the forefront of American society.

This chapter also points to ways in which case studies can be overtly political – in terms of theorisation, at a professional level, and also with regard to wider movements for change in the broader society. It suggests, too, the difficulties of developing case narratives capable of convincing the public at large during particular historic moments, and within highly charged political environments. The 1940s and 1950s were characterised by rigid racial segregation and denial of human rights for America's black community. The immediate post-war period saw the dramatic rise of the civil rights movement. These issues and concerns placed Bernard at the progressive end of the racial politics of the day; none was a theoretical abstraction for Bernard. She was a key activist in establishing organisations and lobby groups for African-American rights, and in doing so provided expert knowledge to those agitating for reform.

Bernard's role as a medical expert in the campaign to end racial segregation in schools resonates strongly with Erich Wulffen's influence as a legal expert in the first decades of the twentieth century. As with Wulffen's career in the law, Bernard's career highlights the rise of the 'expert' in medicine. Although separated by time and place, the influence exerted by Wulffen and by Bernard was considerable, due in good part to recognition of their expertise; both shaped and were shaped by the political and legal culture of their respective eras. The case-based common law (or case law) of the USA enabled Bernard to change US regulations to the benefit of her cause, since by definition in a common law system a single case ruling has binding powers. In Wilhelmine and Weimar Germany,

Wulffen experienced frustrations occasioned by the fact that German civil law responded extremely slowly to change. Yet the comparatively lesser importance of legal cases in his context also enabled him to reinvent the case study genre more radically, and target a range of readerships for promoting his ideas. Such differences point to two themes of the present volume: the historical contingency of all case study modalities, and hence ways in which they illuminate cultural and political developments of the day.

Notes

1 The use of the term 'Negro' in the present chapter reflects usage characteristic of the time and place under discussion.

2 See Joy Damousi, 'Viola Bernard and the Analysis of "Alice Conrad": A Case Study in the History of Intimacy', *Journal of the History of Sexuality*, 22:3 (2013), pp. 474–500; Joy Damousi, 'Sexuality and the Public Case Study in the United States, 1940–1965', in Joy Damousi, Birgit Lang and Katie Sutton (eds), *Case Studies and the Dissemination of Knowledge* (New York: Routledge, 2015), pp. 133–51.

3 A. C. Long Health Sciences Library, Columbia University, New York City, Archives and Special Collections (hereafter CU), Viola Wertheim Bernard Papers, 1918–2000, 'Historical/Biographical Note', given at http://library-archives.cumc.columbia.edu/finding-aid/viola-wertheim-bernard-papers-1918-2000, accessed 29 June 2015.

4 Nathan G. Hale, *The Rise and Crisis of Psychoanalysis in the United States: Freud and the Americans 1917–1985* (New York: Oxford University Press, 1995), pp. 3–9.

5 Damousi, 'Viola Bernard and the Analysis of "Alice Conrad"', p. 481.

6 John Joseph Gladchuk, *Hollywood and Anticommunism: HUAC and the Evolution of the Red Menace, 1935–1950* (New York: Routledge, 2006).

7 Elizabeth Ann Danto, '"Have you no Shame" – American Redbaiting of Europe's Psychoanalysis', in Joy Damousi and Mariano Ben Plotkin (eds), *Psychoanalysis and Politics: Histories of Psychoanalysis under Conditions of Restricted Political Freedom* (New York: Oxford University Press, 2012), pp. 213–32, p. 222. For Bernard's examination of sexuality, see Damousi, 'Viola Bernard and the Analysis of "Alice Conrad"'.

8 CU, Viola Wertheim Bernard Papers, 1918–2000, Box 311, Folder 3, 'Answers to Interrogatories'.

9 Robert Cook, *Sweet Land of Liberty? The African-American Struggle for Civil Rights in the Twentieth Century* (London: Longman, 1998), p. 112.

10 CU, Viola Wertheim Bernard Papers, 1918–2000, Box 311, Folder 2, Viola Bernard to Dr R. H. Felix, June 1954.

11 CU, Viola Wertheim Bernard Papers, 1918–2000, Box 311, Folder 2, Viola Bernard to Dr R. H. Felix, June 1954.

12 CU, Viola Wertheim Bernard Papers, 1918–2000, Box 341, Folder 9, Viola W. Bernard to Frederick S. Weil, 23 October 1945; Box 341, Folder 9, Viola Bernard to Archie Parsons, 4 December 1945.

13 CU, Viola Wertheim Bernard Papers, 1918–2000, Box 341, Folder 9, Garnet T. Ice to Viola Bernard, 12 April 1946; 15 February 1947.

14 CU, Viola Wertheim Bernard Papers, 1918–2000, Box 341, Folder 9, Viola Bernard to Dr B. E. Boothe, 4 June 1947.

15 Hale, *The Rise and Crisis of Psychoanalysis*, p. 246.

16 Hale, *The Rise and Crisis of Psychoanalysis*, p. 246.
17 Hale, *The Rise and Crisis of Psychoanalysis*, p. 247.
18 Hale, *The Rise and Crisis of Psychoanalysis*, p. 247.
19 Hale, *The Rise and Crisis of Psychoanalysis*, pp. 276–99.
20 CU, Viola Wertheim Bernard Papers, 1918–2000, Box 338, Folder 4.2, Records Documenting 'A Committee for Mental Hygiene for Negroes'.
21 CU, Viola Wertheim Bernard Papers, 1918–2000, Box 338, Folder 4.2, Records Documenting 'A Committee for Mental Hygiene for Negroes'.
22 CU, Viola Wertheim Bernard Papers, 1918–2000, Box 338, Folder 4.1, 'The Committee for the Development of Mental Hygiene Resources for Negroes: Constitution and By-Laws'.
23 *Journal of the National Medical Association*, 35:4 (July 1943), p. 146.
24 CU, Viola Wertheim Bernard Papers, 1918–2000, Box 384, Folder 11, Viola Bernard, 'Mental Hygiene and the Negro Community', unpublished article, 1948, pp. 1–7, p. 5.
25 Bernard, 'Mental Hygiene and the Negro Community', unpublished article, 1948, p. 5
26 Bernard, 'Mental Hygiene and the Negro Community', unpublished article, 1948, p. 7.
27 Bernard, 'Mental Hygiene and the Negro Community', unpublished article, 1948, p. 1.
28 Bernard, 'Mental Hygiene and the Negro Community', unpublished article, 1948, p. 5.
29 Bernard, 'Mental Hygiene and the Negro Community', unpublished article, 1948, p. 6.
30 Documented in the *Journal of the National Medical Association*, 36:4 (1944), p. 118; also 36:6 (1944), p. 202.
31 *Journal of the National Medical Association*, 36:4 (1944), p. 118; also 36:6 (1944), p. 202.
32 Viola Bernard, 'Psychoanalysis and Members of Minority Groups', *Journal of the American Psychoanalytic Association*, 1:2 (1953), pp. 255–68, p. 258.
33 Bernard, 'Psychoanalysis and Members of Minority Groups', p. 259.
34 Bernard, 'Psychoanalysis and Members of Minority Groups', p. 259.
35 Bernard, 'Psychoanalysis and Members of Minority Groups', p. 261.
36 Bernard, 'Psychoanalysis and Members of Minority Groups', p. 262.
37 Bernard, 'Psychoanalysis and Members of Minority Groups', p. 262.
38 Bernard, 'Psychoanalysis and Members of Minority Groups', p. 265.
39 Bernard, 'Psychoanalysis and Members of Minority Groups', p. 266.
40 Bernard, 'Psychoanalysis and Members of Minority Groups', p. 266.
41 Bernard, 'Psychoanalysis and Members of Minority Groups', p. 263.
42 Judith S. Schachter and Hugh F. Butts, 'Transference and Countertransference in Interracial Analyses', *Journal of the American Psychoanalytic Association*, 16:4 (1968), pp. 792–808.
43 Schachter and Butts, 'Transference and Countertransference in Interracial Analyses', pp. 792–3.
44 CU, Viola Wertheim Bernard Papers, 1918–2000, Box 335, Folder 2.1, John M. Rhoads to Viola Bernard, 27 May 1976.
45 Maynard Calnek, 'Racial Factors in the Countertransference: The Black Therapist and the Black Client', *American Journal of Orthopsychiatry*, 40:1 (1970), pp. 39–46, p. 45.
46 CU, Viola Wertheim Bernard Papers, 1918–2000, Box 340, Folder 4.5, Norbert Bromberg to Alexander Carlen, 23 July 1970.
47 'Report of Ad Hoc Committee on Social Issues. Position Paper: White Racism', Presented by the Psychiatric Society of Westchester County's Committee on Social Issues, 1970, p. 1, sourced at CU, Viola Wertheim Bernard Papers,

1918–2000, Box 340, Folder 4.5. Note that all relevant quotations herein reproduce the inconsistent capitalisation found in this source.
48 'Report of Ad Hoc Committee on Social Issues: Position Paper: White Racism', p. 1.
49 'Report of Ad Hoc Committee on Social Issues: Position Paper: White Racism', p. 1.
50 Wolfgang Saxon, 'James Hicks, 70, Journalist, Ex-*Amsterdam News* Editor' (Obituary), *New York Times*, 22 January 1986, www.nytimes.com/1986/01/22/obituaries/james-hicks-70-journalist-ex-amsterdam-news-editor.html, accessed 4 May 2015.
51 James L. Hicks, 'Tired Guinea Pigs', *New York Amsterdam News*, 20 May 1961, n.p., news clipping sourced at CU, Viola Wertheim Bernard Papers, 1918–2000, Box 341, Folder 13.2.
52 Hicks, 'Tired Guinea Pigs'.
53 Hicks, 'Tired Guinea Pigs'.
54 Hicks, 'Tired Guinea Pigs'.
55 James L. Hicks, 'Who's Delinquent?', *New York Amsterdam News*, 20 May 1961, n.p., news clipping sourced at CU, Viola Wertheim Bernard Papers, 1918–2000, Box 342, Folder 1.2.
56 Hicks, 'Who's Delinquent?'
57 CU, Viola Wertheim Bernard Papers, 1918–2000, Box 338, Folder 10.2, 'News from Southern Conference Educational Fund'; Box 338, Folder 10.1, Jim Dombrowski, Executive Director, Southern Conference Educational Fund, to Dr Bernard, 5 February 1959; Box 338, Folder 10.5, Records Documenting *Carl Braden v. US* (1961); Box 338, Folder 10.1, *Pittsburgh Courier* and *New York Courier*, 22 April 1961, news clippings.
58 CU, Viola Wertheim Bernard Papers, 1918–2000, Box 343, Folder 3.13, 'The Effects of Segregation and the Consequences of Desegregation: A Social Science Statement', Supreme Court of the United States, 1952.
59 *Southern Patriot*, 14:5 (1956), p. 1.
60 *Southern Patriot*, 14:5 (1956), p. 1.
61 *Southern Patriot*, 14:5 (1956), p. 1.
62 *Southern Patriot*, 14:5 (1956), p. 1.
63 *Southern Patriot*, 14:5 (1956), p. 1.
64 *Southern Patriot*, 14:5 (1956), p. 1.
65 *Southern Patriot*, 14:5 (1956), p. 1.
66 *Southern Patriot*, 14:5 (1956), p. 1.
67 Alfred Yankauer, *Southern Patriot*, 14:5 (1956), p. 4.
68 Yankauer, *Southern Patriot* (1956), p. 4.
69 Adam Fairclough, 'Foreword', in Kevern Verney and Lee Sartain (eds), *Long Is the Way and Hard: One Hundred Years of the National Association for the Advancement of Colored People (NAACP)* (Fayetteville: University of Arkansas Press, 2009), p. vii.
70 Gilbert Jonas, *Freedom's Sword: The NAACP and the Struggle Against Racism in America, 1909–1969* (New York: Routledge, 2005), pp. 55–6.
71 Jonas, *Freedom's Sword*, p. 58.
72 Jonas, *Freedom's Sword*, p. 58.
73 CU, Viola Wertheim Bernard Papers, 1918–2000, Box 343, Folder 3.1, Robert L. Carter to Viola Bernard, 6 October 1952.
74 CU, Viola Wertheim Bernard Papers, 1918–2000, Box 342, Folder 3.1, Robert L. Carter to Viola Bernard, 23 June 1954.
75 CU, Viola Wertheim Bernard Papers, 1918–2000, Box 342, Folder 3.1, Robert L. Carter to Viola Bernard, 23 June 1954.
76 CU, Viola Wertheim Bernard Papers, 1918–2000, Box 342, Folder 3.1, Robert L. Carter to Viola Bernard, 23 June 1954.

77 CU, Viola Wertheim Bernard Papers, 1918–2000, Box 343, Folder 3.12, 'Summary and Integration of Discussion and Conclusions of the 23 July 1954 Conference of Social Scientists'.

78 CU, Viola Wertheim Bernard Papers, 1918–2000, Box 343, Folder 3.5, Viola Bernard to Ken (Kenneth Clark), 14 August 1954.

79 CU, Viola Wertheim Bernard Papers, 1918–2000, box 343, folder 3.5, Viola Bernard to Ken (Kenneth Clark), 14 August 1954.

80 Kenneth B. Clark, Isidor Chein and Stuart W. Cook, 'The Effects of Segregation and the Consequences of Desegregation: A Social Science Statement', Brief Filed with the US Supreme Court on 22 September 1952, p. 4, sourced at CU, Viola Wertheim Bernard Papers, 1918–2000, Box 343, Folder 3.13. The brief appeared under the same title in the *Minnesota Law Review*, 37 (May 1953), pp. 427–38.

81 Clark, Chein and Cook, 'The Effects of Segregation and the Consequences of Desegregation', p. 4.

82 Clark, Chein and Cook, 'The Effects of Segregation and the Consequences of Desegregation', p. 9.

83 Clark, Chein and Cook, 'The Effects of Segregation and the Consequences of Desegregation', p. 6.

84 Clark, Chein and Cook, 'The Effects of Segregation and the Consequences of Desegregation', p. 6.

85 Clark, Chein and Cook, 'The Effects of Segregation and the Consequences of Desegregation', p. 15.

86 Clark, Chein and Cook, 'The Effects of Segregation and the Consequences of Desegregation', p. 12.

87 Yvonne Ryan, 'Leading from the Back: Roy Wilkins's Leadership of the NAACP', in Verney and Sartain (eds), *Long Is the Way and Hard*, pp. 43–58, p. 47.

88 For a detailed examination of the Montgomery bus boycott, see Taylor Branch, *Parting the Waters: America in the King Years, 1954–63* (New York: Simon & Schuster, 1988), pp. 143–205.

89 Simon Hall, 'The NAACP and the Challenges of 1960s Radicalism', in Verney and Sartain (eds), *Long Is the Way and Hard*, pp. 75–85, p. 79.

90 CU, Viola Wertheim Bernard Papers, 1918–2000, Box 342, Folder 5.5, Carl F. Hansen to Viola Bernard, 8 April 1959.

91 CU, Viola Wertheim Bernard Papers, 1918–2000, Box 338, Folder 7.2, Max Horkheimer to Dr Bernard, 7 April 1945.

92 CU, Viola Wertheim Bernard Papers, 1918–2000, Box 338, Folder 8.2, Edwin J. Luckas to Dr Viola Bernard, 28 July 1960.

93 CU, Viola Wertheim Bernard Papers, 1918–2000: Box 338, Folder 17.1, *New York Times*, 11 January 1960, news clipping; also Box 338, Folder 17.1, Viola Bernard to Dr Anthony Votos, 15 September 1960.

94 CU, Viola Wertheim Bernard Papers, 1918–2000, Box 338, Folder 17.1, Dr Anthony Votos to Dr Bernard, 11 January 1960.

95 CU, Viola Wertheim Bernard Papers, 1918–2000, Box 342, Folder 1.2, Bluma Swerdloff to Viola Bernard, 13 June 1946.

96 CU, Viola Wertheim Bernard Papers, 1918–2000, Box 342, Folder 1.2, Bluma Swerdloff to Viola Bernard, 13 June 1946.

97 CU, Viola Wertheim Bernard Papers, 1918–2000, Box 342, Folder 1.2, Bluma Swerdloff to Viola Bernard, 13 June 1946.

98 Cheryl Lynn Greenberg, *Troubling the Waters: Black–Jewish Relations in the American Century* (Princeton: Princeton University Press, 2006), pp. 163, 169, 197, 203.

Conclusion

Birgit Lang, Joy Damousi and Alison Lewis

This volume delineates the changing forms of the case study across disciplines and decades, mapping circuits of knowledge through which the sexed and gendered human subject became a persistently urgent topic of enquiry in the Western world. *A History of the Case Study* presents an analysis of case writing about the human subject from a critical juncture in its formation in the second half of the nineteenth century, when, as claimed by Michel Foucault, sexuality came to be regarded as a conceptual part of human nature. According to Foucault's famous dictum, notions of sexuality 'organized sex as a "fictitious unity"' of distinct parts and functions, feelings and behaviours; new categories for describing and policing sex produced a new object of enquiry.[1]

The case study became the genre *par excellence* for discussing human sexuality across the humanities and the life sciences. Through the first sixty years of the twentieth century, sexologists, psychoanalysts, lawyers, medical practitioners and literary writers continued to avail themselves of the highly malleable and flexible parameters of the case study, and to repurpose it for their own ends. As demonstrated in the foregoing chapters, notions of the modern sexed subject have thus become inseparable from the emergence and development of the case study genre itself: in the newer fields of psychoanalysis and sexology, in literature, in the law and in areas of legal and social reform, practitioners and theorists gravitated towards astoundingly similar modes of narration, each modifying the case study genre for their own disciplinary purposes. Our history of the case study has focused on key moments in the genre's past, occasions when and where its conventions were contested from within particular disciplines. Such contestation has often involved reconceptualising the case study's epistemological foundations. This volume has taken the reader on a transcontinental journey from the imperial world of fin-de-siècle Central Europe and the Austro-Hungarian Empire to the inter-war metropolises of Weimar Germany, and to the USA in the post-war years. At all of these moments, and in all of these contexts, the case study has been evolving; fostering transformation; migrating across cultures and the globe; instrumental in asking and prompting questions about the human subject – the sexed subject, the criminal subject, the segregated black subject and so on.

Today, the case study remains a nomadic genre, one that stubbornly refuses to find a definite home in a discrete discipline. In medicine and the social sciences, the past forty years have witnessed a turn away from the case study as a scientific method of enquiry: case writing is now situated at the opposite end of 'best evidence' randomised control trials.[2] The demotion of the medical case study to a method used mainly in clinical practice is a direct result of the scientific turn in these fields, which prioritises large sample sizes and serialisation. Evidence-based research methods have replaced the more discursive, even searching style of case histories or case studies. Still, in medical practice, for complex cases, recent years have seen a renewed interest in organising specialist meetings of the various medical experts involved in patient treatment. Such gatherings of experts return the patient to the centre of attention in clinical practice. Nonetheless, as Warwick Anderson argues, in the clinic the mechanism of creating an individual case file and adding to an archive is more significant than the contents of the repository.[3]

In psychoanalysis, a traditional stronghold of the case study genre, case writings continue to play a pivotal role in academic discourse; they remain part of the psychoanalytic training regime, and journal writing about patients is still a relatively common practice, even if such cases are not necessarily published. Characteristic of the fin de siècle, and focused on the presentation of new psychological phenomena, the long case study format has been superseded. This acknowledged, Peter Wegner has pointed to the fresh qualities of the modern psychoanalytic case study; its ability to encapsulate in a unique way the history of interaction between patient and analyst.[4]

The literary case study as an empirically based form of writing about criminologically or sexologically interesting cases was to suffer a fate similar to the medical case study. The realism of New Objectivity in Weimar Germany soon ceded ground to disparate strains of literary modernism: fascist modernism as found in the works of Ernst Jünger; the socialist-inflected modernism of Bertolt Brecht; and Thomas Mann's more stylistically conservative modernism. Alfred Döblin's brand of left-liberal modernism did not fare well in the post-war era and his literary case studies of the working classes did not capture the tastes of post-war readers. Instead, the works of Mann – his novels about the bourgeoisie – proved more popular with critics and publishers. Interestingly, as the more readable of the German writers, Mann maintained aspects of the tradition of the literary criminal case study elaborated by Erich Wulffen, and by Döblin in his unfinished novel from 1954, *Bekenntnisse des Hochstaplers Felix Krull. Der Memoiren, erster Teil* (translated into English in 1955 as *Confessions of Felix Krull, Confidence Man: The Early Years*). Like one of Wulffen's expert case studies, and Wulffen's several case stories about imposture, Mann's unfinished novel was also inspired by Romanian con man Georges Manolescu.

The post-war European writer who owes perhaps the largest debt to Döblin is Günter Grass, winner of the 1999 Nobel Prize in Literature. In interviews, Grass repeatedly invoked Döblin as a forebear. However, Grass's literary works are less influenced by Döblin's experiments with empirical case writing and psychoanalysis than by his realism and irony. Instead, the literary case study derived from the courts and legal settings continues to find its more conventional home in contemporary crime fiction and the detective novel. Both have become transnational genres that occupy middlebrow and popular segments of the literary market. In the English-speaking world, the bestselling works of Lisa Scottoline, a litigation expert, currently exemplify popular writing in the case study tradition outlined in this book. In Germany, the works of Bernhard Schlink comprise the leading contemporary example of crime fiction developed from the author's first-hand legal experience. As a professor of law, and a judge of the Constitutional Court, Schlink wrote his crime novels under a pseudonym, until in 1995 he published *Der Vorleser* (*The Reader*) about a Holocaust war criminal, which became an international bestseller. *Der Vorleser* is in many ways a fitting heir to the European literary case study of the early 1920s. At its core is a narrative about a codependent, sadomasochistic relationship between a young man and a strong, older woman. Like Döblin's *Die beiden Freundinnen und ihr Giftmord* (*Two Girlfriends Commit Murder by Poison*) of 1924, Schlink's novel also has a crime at its centre. However, in *Der Vorleser* 'the crime' takes the plural form of Nazi war crimes committed in occupied Poland.

Ferdinand von Schirach is another contemporary writer who has continued in Döblin's tradition of the literary crime novel. Also a trained lawyer, Schirach shot to fame in 2009 with the publication of a collection of realistic short stories taken from his legal practice titled *Verbrechen* (*Crime*). Written in a detached, minimalist style reminiscent of Döblin's *Die beiden Freundinnen und ihr Giftmord*, Schirach's riveting combination of ghastly real-life cases and terse prose affirms the lasting appeal of the case study genre in the realm of crime fiction. Different from Döblin, however, Schirach's latest explorations of the German justice system in the realm of fiction such as *Der Fall Collini* (*The Collini Case*) and *Tabu* (*Taboo*) have not found favour with literary critics, despite referencing the case study genre.

The medical case study in literary or fictional guise is proving to be a similarly long-lived case modality. The heirs to this strand of case writing are too numerous and dispersed to discuss here. Suffice it to say that ailing or troubled states of mind – or psychopathology, to use a psychiatric term – remain a staple theme in contemporary literature around the world. Traces of the case study genre are especially discernible in the writing about sickness and disability that takes the form of self-help books targeted at a popular audience, reflecting a trend that began to flourish during the 1960s. Pathography and autopathography are new forms of popular, empirically based writing (termed 'life-writing') about sickness, often written from the perspective of the affected victim or sufferer.[5] Today, these first-person case studies fill row upon row of bookshop shelves, meeting a strong public desire – a desire not that far removed from those of readers in Wulffen's and Döblin's day – to communicate strange or miraculous cases taken from real life.

In broad terms, popular pathography has allowed the case study genre to maintain its prominence in the humanities and to retain its importance as a means of conveying topical, expert knowledge. The widely translated collections of case histories penned by recently deceased English neurologist Oliver Sacks are good illustrations of this trend; his works *Awakenings* (1973), *The Man Who Mistook His Wife for a Hat and Other Clinical Tales* (1985) and *Musicophilia* (2007) are all based on Sacks's own medical practice, and present unusual neurological disorders. Self-help books, in turn, popularise expert knowledge from the patient's perspective: the popularity of life-writing about illness reflects the much higher levels of knowledge about medicine in the wider population today. The same popularity is, of course, also a product of far greater levels of tolerance with regard to the spectrum of possible and acceptable sexual behaviours by comparison with 1900, when the writers of the first pathographies struggled to communicate expert medical perspectives to a lay readership.

While early sexologists and psychoanalysts resorted to illustrating their insights about sexuality through reference to 'great men' and individuals considered creative geniuses, today's case studies about non-heteronormative sexuality and gender are often written in the first instance by journalists for the print media and by lay writers for social media. In mainstream media, recent years have seen a growing interest in personal stories about gender reassignment, which have been packaged as stories about transgender personalities and celebrities such as Olympian Bruce/Caitlyn Jenner. The case of Conchita Wurst, born Tom Neuwirth, the bearded gay transvestite who won the Eurovision Song Contest in 2014, captured the imaginations of LGBTI and music communities around the globe. Attesting to the enduring power of case studies that confound expectations of gender and sexual identity, Wurst's story has been told through various case modalities – media reports, interviews, YouTube blogs and now in the conventional autobiography, *Ich Conchita, Meine Geschichte. We are Unstoppable* (2015). Sales of this memoir quickly prompted a second print run. Such success demonstrates that the case study as set forth by the patient or subject herself (rather than by the treating doctor, presiding judge or defending lawyer) has become the dominant form through which the lives of modern transgendered, transsexual and intersex subjects are narrated.

Another legacy of the art and science of case writing outlined in this volume can be observed in scholarly writing, whether in the disciplines of cultural history or of social sciences such as ethnography, linguistics and anthropology. The case study of an endangered indigenous language in Australia and the case study of foreign language pedagogy in the university classroom are just two of the varied types of case studies that have become staple forms of academic writing today. In tertiary teaching, the case study method has retained importance in psychology and psychiatry, as in medicine. Other fields, such as law and commerce, have moved on from the more traditional approaches to teaching through cases; those approaches tended to use case studies that presented dilemmas after the dilemmas had been resolved. The new 'immersive' case method teaching aims to train students to use the case study genre to imitate realistic situations as they unfold, in an attempt – according to the Harvard Law School – to promote students' 'legal imagination'.[6]

The academic disciplines of biography and autobiography have become especially privileged forms of case writing, and even when they subvert their own conventions the results are not that dissimilar to the modernist experiments that took place during the first few decades of the twentieth century. Moreover, some of Australia's most prominent contemporary writers have built their reputations on case studies. Helen Garner's *The First Stone: Some Questions About Sex and Power* (1995) dealt sympathetically with the controversial real case of a college master at the University of Melbourne who was charged with indecent assault. Subsequent books, *Joe Cinque's Consolation* (2004), which explored the murder trial of a young law student, and her latest work, *This House of Grief: The Story of a Murder Trial* (2014), likewise based on a trial attended by Garner, all follow on in the case writing traditions established during the first half of the twentieth century.

Outside of the realms of scholarship and the media, case writing is today regularly undertaken for the purposes of public advocacy. Whether in case histories presented to official commissions investigating sexual abuse in the Church, or materials submitted to government enquiries into the effects of racism on black youths, the case study of the human subject and its relationship to institutional power is an enduring form for communicating the stories of individuals and groups; for making the stories public, as part of seeking significant change. Indeed, at present, the case study is perhaps most fittingly 'at home' in the spheres of public advocacy and popular media. Uniquely suited to conveying the singularity of individual lives and identity, the case study is a modern genre that has not yet outgrown its original purpose – that of placing sexuality, gender and certain extremes of behaviour such as violent crime directly under the spotlight. If it has been superseded by other scientific methods in medicine, the case study genre undoubtedly continues to offer writers, both lay and expert, a means for fathoming the riddle that is the human self.

Notes

1 Michel Foucault, *The History of Sexuality, vol. I: An Introduction*, trans. Robert Hurley (New York: Vintage Books, 1990), p. 154.
2 Teresa Paslawski, 'Case Study Research in Medicine', in Albert J. Mills, Gabrielle Durepos and Elden Wiebe (eds), *Encyclopedia of Case Study Research* (London: Sage, 2010), pp. 107–9.
3 Warwick Anderson, 'The Case of the Archive', in Joy Damousi, Birgit Lang and Katie Sutton (eds), *Case Studies and the Dissemination of Knowledge* (New York: Routledge, 2015), pp. 15–30, p. 24.
4 Peter Wegner, 'Die Fallgeschichte als Instrument psychoanalytischer Forschung', in Gerd Kimmerle (ed.), *Zur Theorie der psychoanalytischen Fallgeschichte* (Tübingen: Diskort, 1988), pp. 9–44, p. 36.
5 See Anne Hunsaker Hawkins, *Reconstructing Illness: Studies in Pathography*, 2nd edition (West Lafayette: Purdue University Press, 1999).
6 Todd D. Rakoff and Martha Minow, 'A Case for Another Case Method', *Vanderbilt Law Review*, 60:2 (2007), pp. 597–607, p. 602.

Select bibliography

Published primary material

Abraham, Karl, 'Die Geschichte eines Hochstaplers im Lichte psychoanalytischer Erkenntnis', *Imago. Zeitschrift für Anwendung der Psychoanalyse auf die Geisteswissenschaften*, 9:4 (1925), pp. 355–70

Abraham, Karl, 'The History of an Impostor in the Light of Psychoanalytical Knowledge', *Psychoanalytic Quarterly*, 4 (1935), pp. 570–87

Arndt, Rudolf, *Lehrbuch der Psychiatrie für Ärzte und Studirende* (Vienna: Urban & Schwarzenberg, 1883)

Bernard, Viola, 'Psychoanalysis and Members of Minority Groups', *Journal of the American Psychoanalytic Association*, 1:2 (1953), pp. 255–68

Cadivec, Edith, *Bekenntnisse und Erlebnisse*, ed. Michael Farin (Munich: Belleville, 2008)

Clark, Kenneth B., Isidor Chein and Stuart W. Cook, 'The Effects of Segregation and the Consequences of Desegregation: A Social Science Statement', brief filed with the US Supreme Court on 22 September 1952, published under the same title in the *Minnesota Law Review*, 37 (May 1953), pp. 427–38

Döblin, Alfred, *Aufsätze Zur Literatur*, ed. Walter Muschg (Olten: Walter-Verlag, 1963)

Döblin, Alfred, *Autobiographische Schriften und letzte Aufzeichnungen*, ed. Edgar Pässler (Olten: Walter-Verlag, 1980)

Döblin, Alfred, *Berlin Alexanderplatz: Die Geschichte vom Franz Biberkopf* (Munich: DTV, 1965)

Döblin, Alfred, *Berlin Alexanderplatz: The Story of Franz Biborkopf, trans. Eugene Jolas (London: Secker & Warburg, 1974)*

Döblin, Alfred, *Briefe II*, ed. Helmut F. Pfanner (Dusseldorf: Walter-Verlag, 2001)

Döblin, Alfred, *Die beiden Freundinnen und ihr Giftmord* (Dusseldorf: Artemis und Winkler, 2001)

Döblin, Alfred, *Schriften zu* Ästhetik, *Poetik und Literatur*, ed. Erich Kleinschmidt (Olten: Walter-Verlag, 1989)

Döblin, Alfred, *Schriften zu Leben und Werk*, ed. Erich Kleinschmidt (Olten: Walter-Verlag, 1986)

Freud, Sigmund, *Gesammelte Werke, chronologisch geordnet*, vols I–XVIII, ed. Anna Freud, in collaboration with M. Bonaparte, E. Bibring, W. Hoffer, E. Kris and O. Isakower (London: Imago, 1940–68)

Freud, Sigmund, *The Standard Edition of the Complete Psychological Works of Sigmund Freud*, vols I–XXIV, ed. James Strachey, with Anna Freud, Alix Strachey and Alan Tyson (London: Hogarth Press and Institute for Psychoanalysis, 1950–74)

Jung, Carl Gustav, 'Besprechung von Erich Wulffen "Der Sexualverbrecher"', *Jahrbuch für psychoanalytische und psychopathologische Forschungen*, 2:2 (1910), p. 747

Krafft-Ebing, Richard von, *Neuere Forschungen auf dem Gebiet der Psychopathia Sexualis*, 1st edition (Stuttgart: Enke, 1890)

Krafft-Ebing, Richard von, *Psychopathia Sexualis. Eine klinisch-forensische Studie*, 1st edition (Stuttgart: Enke, 1886)

Lombroso, Cesare, *Der geniale Mensch* (Hamburg: Richter, 1890)

Lombroso, Cesare, *The Man of Genius*, trans. H. Havelock Ellis (London: Scott, 1891)

Mann, Thomas, *Letters of Thomas Mann 1889–1955*, selected and trans. Richard and Clara Winston (Berkeley: University of California Press, 1970)

Manolescu, Georges, *Ein Fürst der Diebe. Memoiren* (Groß-Lichterfelde Ost: Paul Langenscheidt, 1905)

Manolescu, Georges, *Gescheitert. Aus dem Seelenleben eines Verbrechers* (Groß-Lichterfelde Ost: Paul Langenscheidt, 1907)

Mill, John Stuart, 'On Liberty', *Essays on Politics and Society. Collected Works of John Stuart Mill*, vol. XVIII (Toronto: University of Toronto Press, 1977), pp. 213–310

Möbius, Paul Julius, *Goethe* (Leipzig: Barth, 1903)

Möbius, Paul Julius, *J.-J. Rousseaus Krankheitsgeschichte* (Leipzig: Vogel, 1889)

Möbius, Paul Julius, *Über das Pathologische bei Goethe* (Leipzig: Barth, 1898)

Möbius, Paul Julius, *Über den physiologischen Schwachsinn des Weibes*, 5th edition (Halle a.S.: Marhold, 1903)

Möbius, Paul Julius, *Über Kunst und Künstler* (Leipzig: Barth, 1901)

Möbius, Paul Julius, *Über Schopenhauer* (Leipzig: Barth, 1903)

Nunberg, Hermann and Ernst Federn (eds), *Protokolle der Wiener Psychoanalytischen Vereinigung*, vols I–IV (Gießen: Psychosozial-Verlag, 2008)

Panizza, Oskar, *Abschied von München. Ein Handschlag* (Zurich: Schabelitz, 1897)

Panizza, Oskar, *Das Rothe Haus. Lesebuch zu Religion, Sexus und Wahn*, ed. Michael Bauer (Munich: Allitera, 2003)

Panizza, Oskar, 'Genie und Wahnsinn, Vortrag', *Münchner Flugschriften*, 1:4/5 (1891), reprinted in Oskar Panizza, *Die kriminelle Psychose, genannt Psichopatia criminalis* (Munich: Matthes & Seitz, 1978), pp. 85–117

Panizza, Oskar, *Meine Verteidigung in Sachen 'Das Liebeskonzil': nebst dem Sachverständigen-Gutachten des Dr. M. G. Conrad und dem Urteil des k. Landgerichts München I* (Zurich: Schabelitz, 1895)

Panizza, Oskar, *Psichopatia criminalis: Anleitung um die vom Gericht für notwendig erkanten Geisteskrankheiten psichjatrisch zu eruiren und wissenschaftlich festzustellen; für Ärzte, Laien, Juristen, Vormünder, Verwaltungsbeamte, Minister etc.* (Zurich: Zürcher Diskußionen, 1898)

Rahmer, Sigismund, *August Strindberg. Eine pathologische Studie* (Munich: Reinhardt, 1907)

Rahmer, Sigismund, *Heinrich von Kleist als Mensch und Dichter. Nach neuen Quellenforschungen* (Berlin: Reimer, 1909)

Rousseau, Jean-Jacques, *Confessions*, trans. Angela Scholar (Oxford: Oxford University Press, 2000)

Sacher-Masoch, Leopold von, *Das Vermächtnis Kains. Novellen. Erster Theil. Die Liebe. Erster Band* (Stuttgart: Cotta, 1870) (*Love*, part 1)

Sacher-Masoch, Leopold von, *Das Vermächtnis Kains. Novellen. Erster Theil. Die Liebe. Zweiter Band* (Stuttgart: Cotta, 1870) (*Love*, part 2)

Sacher-Masoch, Leopold von, 'Eine Autobiographie', *Deutsche Monatsblätter. Centralorgan für das literarische Leben der Gegenwart*, 2:3 (1879), pp. 259–69

Sacher-Masoch, Leopold von, *Ueber den Werth der Kritik. Erfahrungen und Bemerkungen* (Leipzig: Ernst Julius Günther, 1873)

Sacher-Masoch, Leopold von, 'Venus in Furs', in Gilles Deleuze and Leopold von Sacher-Masoch, *Masochism: Coldness and Cruelty, and Venus in Furs*, trans. Jean McNeil (New York: Zone Books, 1991), pp. 143–271

Sacher-Masoch, Wanda von, *Lebensbeichte. Meine Lebensbeichte. Memoiren (1905) sowie Masochismus und Masochisten. Nachtrag zur Lebensbeichte (1908). Mit einem Dossier*, ed. Lisbeth Exner and Michael Farin (Munich: Belleville, 2003)

Sadger, Isidor, *Heinrich von Kleist. Eine pathographisch-psychologische Studie* (Wiesbaden: Bergmann, 1909)

Sadger, Isidor, 'Kranke Dichter und Krankendichtung', *Deutsche Revue*, 22:4 (1897), pp. 36–44
Sadger, Isidor, *Recollecting Freud*, ed. Alan Dundes (Madison: University of Wisconsin Press, 2005)
Schlichtegroll, Carl Felix von, *Sacher-Masoch: enthaltend Sacher-Masoch und der Masochismus sowie 'Wanda' ohne Maske und Pelz nebst einem Dossier*, ed. Lisbeth Exner and Michael Farin (Munich: Belleville, 2003)
Stekel, Wilhelm, *Die Träume der Dichter. Eine vergleichende Untersuchung der unbewussten Triebkräfte bei Dichtern, Neurotikern und Verbrechern (Bausteine zur Psychologie des Künstlers und des Kunstwerks)* (Wiesbaden: Bergmann, 1912)
Tucholsky, Kurt, 'Old Bäumerhand, der Schrecken der Demokratie', in *Gesammelte Werke in zehn Bänden*, ed. Mary Gerold-Tucholsky and Fritz J. Raddatz, vol. IV (Reinbek bei Hamburg: Rowohlt Verlag, 1975), pp. 556–9
Turgenev, Ivan Sergeevich, 'The Superfluous Man', in *The Essential Turgenev*, ed. and intro. Elizabeth Cheresh Allen (Evanston: Northwestern University Press, 1994), pp. 104–51
Wulffen, Erich, *Das Weib als Sexualverbrecherin. Ein Handbuch für Juristen, Polizei- und Strafvollzugsbeamte*, Ärzte *und Laienrichter* (Berlin: Paul Langenscheidt, 1923)
Wulffen, Erich, *Der Mann mit den sieben Masken. Roman* (Dresden: Reißner, 1917)
Wulffen, Erich, *Der Sexualverbrecher. Ein Handbuch für Juristen, Verwaltungsbeamte und* Ärzte (Groß-Lichterfelde Ost: Paul Langenscheidt, 1910)
Wulffen, Erich, 'Ein kriminalpsychologisches Experiment', *Monatsschrift für Kriminalpsychologie und Strafreform*, 2 (1905), pp. 734–38
Wulffen, Erich, *Frau Justitias Walpurgisnacht. Roman* (Berlin: Duncker, 1913)
Wulffen, Erich, *Irrwege des Eros. Mit einer Einleitung Mütter und Töchter* (Hellerau bei Dresden: Avalun, 1928)
Wulffen, Erich, *Kriminalpsychologie. Psychologie des Täters. Ein Handbuch für Juristen, Justiz-, Verwaltungs- und Polizeibeamte*, Ärzte, *Pädagogen und Gebildete aller Stände* (Berlin: Paul Langenscheidt, 1926)
Wulffen, Erich, *Manolescu und seine Memoiren. Kriminalpsychologische Studie* (Groß-Lichterfelde Ost: Paul Langenscheidt, 1907)
Wulffen, Erich, *Psychologie des Verbrechers. Ein Handbuch für Juristen*, Ärzte, *Pädagogen und Gebildete aller Stände* (Groß-Lichterfelde Ost: Paul Langenscheidt, 1908)

Secondary material

Aust, Hugo, *Novelle* (Stuttgart: Metzler, 1990)
Bakhtin, Mikhail M., *Speech Genres and Other Late Essays*, trans. Vern W. McGee, eds Caryl Emerson and Michael Holquist (Austin: University of Texas Press, 1986)
Barbin, Herculine, *Herculine Barbin dite Alexina B., présenté par Michel Foucault* (Paris: Gallimard, 1978)
Barbin, Herculine and Michel Foucault, *Herculine Barbin: Being the Recently Discovered Memoirs of a Nineteenth-Century French Hermaphrodite* (New York: Pantheon Books, 1980)
Bauer, Heike, *English Literary Sexology: Translations of Inversion, 1860–1930* (Basingstoke: Palgrave Macmillan, 2009)
Bauer, Michael, *Oskar Panizza. Ein literarisches Portrait* (Munich: Hanser, 1984)
Bauer, Michael, 'Panizza, Leopold Hermann Oskar', *Neue Deutsche Biographie*, 20 (2001), pp. 30–2
Beachy, Robert, 'The German Invention of Homosexuality', *Journal of Modern History*, 82:4 (2010), pp. 801–38
Becker, Peter, *Verderbnis und Entartung. Eine Geschichte der Kriminologie des 19. Jahrhunderts als Diskurs und Praxis* (Göttingen: Vandenhoeck & Ruprecht, 2002)

Becker, Peter, 'Weak Bodies? Prostitutes and the Role of Gender in the Criminological Writings of 19th-Century German Detectives and Magistrates', *Crime, History and Societies*, 3:1 (1999), pp. 45–70

Beizer, Janet, 'Emma's Daughter: Femininity, Maternity, and "Mothersickness" in Madame Bovary', in Suzanne Nash (ed.), *Home and Its Dislocations in Nineteenth-Century France* (Albany: New York Press, 1993), pp. 265–83

Berkenkotter, Carol, *Patient Tales: Case Histories and the Uses of Narrative in Psychiatry* (Columbia: University of South Carolina Press, 2008)

Berlant, Lauren, 'On the Case', *Critical Inquiry*, 33:4 (2007), pp. 663–72

Berlant, Lauren and Michael Warner, 'Sex in Public', *Critical Inquiry*, 24:2 (1998), pp. 547–66

Berman, Russell A., *The Rise of the Modern German Novel: Crisis and Charisma* (Cambridge: Harvard University Press, 1986)

Boeser, Knut, 'Panizza und Rushdie. Vom gefährlichen Leben der Schriftsteller in moralischen Zeiten', in Knut Boeser (ed.), *Der Fall Oskar Panizza: ein deutscher Dichter im Gefängnis; eine Dokumentation* (Berlin: Hentrich, 1989), pp. 220–9

Bourdieu, Pierre, *The Field of Cultural Production: Essays on Art and Literature*, ed. Randal Johnson (New York: Columbia University Press, 1993)

Bourdieu, Pierre, *The Rules of Art: Genesis and Structure of the Literary Field*, trans. Susan Emanual (Stanford: Stanford University Press, 1996)

Brady, Seán, *John Addington Symonds (1840–1893) and Homosexuality: A Critical Edition of Sources* (New York: Palgrave Macmillan, 2012)

Brown, Peter D. G., *Oskar Panizza: His Life and Works* (New York: Peter Lang, 1983)

Brown, Peter D. G., 'The Continuing Trials of Oskar Panizza: A Century of Artistic Censorship in Germany, Austria, and Beyond', *German Studies Review*, 24:3 (2001), pp. 533–56

Calnek, Maynard, 'Racial Factors in the Countertransference: The Black Therapist and the Black Client', *American Journal of Orthopsychiatry*, 40:1 (1970), pp. 39–46

Charles, Marilyn, *Psychoanalysis and Literature: The Stories We Live* (Lanham: Rowman & Littlefield, 2015)

Cleary, Joe, 'Realism after Modernism and the Literary World-System', *Modern Language Quarterly*, 73:3 (2012), pp. 255–68

Crapanzano, Vincent, 'The Postmodern Crisis: Discourse, Parody, Memory', in Amy Mandelker (ed.), *Bakthin in Contexts: Across the Disciplines* (Evanston: Northwestern University Press, 1995), pp. 137–50

Crouthamel, Jason, 'Male Sexuality and Psychological Trauma: Soldiers and Sexual Disorder in World War I and Weimar Germany', *Journal of the History of Sexuality*, 17:1 (2008), pp. 60–84

Crozier, Ivan, 'Philosophy in the English Boudoir: Havelock Ellis, Love and Pain, and Sexological Discourses on Algophilia', *Journal of the History of Sexuality*, 13:3 (2004), pp. 275–305

Crozier, Ivan, 'Pillow Talk: Credibility, Trust and the Sexological Case History', *History of Science*, 46:4 (2008), pp. 375–404

Damousi, Joy, 'Viola Bernard and the Analysis of "Alice Conrad": A Case Study in the History of Intimacy', *Journal of the History of Sexuality*, 22:3 (2013), pp. 474–500

Damousi, Joy, Birgit Lang and Katie Sutton (eds), *Case Studies and the Dissemination of Knowledge* (New York: Routledge, 2015)

Damousi, Joy and Mariano Ben Plotkin (eds), *Psychoanalysis and Politics: Histories of Psychoanalysis Under Conditions of Restricted Political Freedom* (New York: Oxford University Press, 2012)

Davidson, Arnold I., 'Sex and the Emergence of Sexuality', *Critical Inquiry*, 14:1 (1987), pp. 16–48

Deutsch, Helene, 'The Impostor: Contribution to Ego Psychology of a Type of Psychopath [Reprint from 1955]', *Psychoanalytic Quarterly*, 80:4 (2011), pp. 1005–24

Dingeldey, Hugo, 'Erich Wulffen', in Alexander Baumgarten and Hugo Dingeldey (eds), *Erich Wulffen. Festschrift zu seinem siebzigsten Geburtstag* (Berlin: HRW, 1932), pp. 12–40

Doan, Laura, *Disturbing Practices: History, Sexuality, and Women's Experience of Modern War* (Chicago: University of Chicago Press, 2013)

Dollinger, Roland, Wulf Köpke and Heidi Thomann Tewarson (eds), *A Companion to the Works of Alfred Döblin* (Rochester: Camden House, 2003)

Dotzler, Bernhard J., 'Wissen in Geschichten: Zur wechselseitigen Erhellung von Literatur, Medien und Wissenschaft', *Berichte zur Wissenschaftsgeschichte*, 32:4 (2009), pp. 319–28

Dotzler, Bernhard J. and Sigrid Weigel (eds), *'Fülle der combination': Literaturforschung und Wissenschaftsgeschichte* (Munich: Wilhelm Fink, 2005)

Düsterberg, Rolf, *'Die gedrukte Freiheit'. Oskar Panizza und die Zürcher Diskussionen* (Frankfurt: Peter Lang, 1984)

Eco, Umberto, *The Open Work* (Cambridge: Harvard University Press, 1989)

Elder, Sace, *Murder Scenes: Normality, Deviance, and Criminal Violence in Weimar Berlin* (Ann Arbor: University of Michigan Press, 2010)

Elms, Alan C., 'Sigmund Freud, Psychohistorian', *Annual of Psychoanalysis*, 31 (2003), pp. 65–78

Engel, Gisela, Susanne Scholz and Johannes Süßmann (eds), *Fallstudien. Geschichte – Theorie – Methode* (Berlin: Trafo, 2007)

Englisch, Paul, *Geschichte der erotischen Literatur* (Stuttgart: Julius Püttmann, 1927)

Ette, Ottmar (ed.), *Wissensformen und Wissensnormen des ZusammenLebens: Literatur – Kultur – Geschichte – Medien* (Berlin: de Gruyter, 2012)

Eulenburg, Albert, *Sadismus und Masochismus* (Wiesbaden: Bergmann, 1902)

Exner, Lisbeth, *Leopold von Sacher-Masoch* (Reinbeck bei Hamburg: Rowohlt, 2003)

Farin, Michael (ed.), *Leopold von Sacher-Masoch. Materialien zu Leben und Werk* (Bonn: Bouvier, 1987)

Felman, Shoshana, *Literature and Psychoanalysis: The Question of Reading, Otherwise* (Baltimore: Johns Hopkins University Press, 1982)

Felski, Rita, *Uses of Literature* (Oxford: Blackwell, 2008)

Fleck, Ludwik, 'Some Specific Features of the Medical Way of Thinking (1927)', in Robert S. Cohen and Thomas Schnelle (eds), *Cognition and Fact: Materials on Ludwik Fleck* (Dordrecht: Springer, 1986), pp. 39–46

Ford, James M., *Patriarchy and Incest from Shakespeare to Joyce* (Gainesville: University Press of Florida, 1998)

Forrester, John, 'If p, Then What? Thinking in Cases', *History of the Human Sciences*, 9:3 (1996), pp. 1–25

Foucault, Michel, *Herculine Barbin: Being the Recently Discovered Memoirs of a Nineteenth-Century French Hermaphrodite*, trans. Richard McDougall (Brighton: Harvester Press, 1980)

Foucault, Michel, *The History of Sexuality, vol. I: An Introduction*, trans. Robert Hurley (New York: Vintage Books, 1990)

Frommel, Monika, 'Internationale Reformbewegung zwischen 1880 und 1920', in Jörg Schönert (ed.), *Erzählte Kriminalität. Zur Typologie und Funktion von narrativen Darstellungen in Strafrechtspflege, Publizistik und Literatur zwischen 1770 und 1920* (Tübingen: Niemeyer, 1991), pp. 447–96

Frow, John, *Genre* (New York: Routledge, 2006)

Fuchs, Thomas, 'Temporality and Psychopathology', *Phenomenology and the Cognitive Sciences*, 12:1 (2013), pp. 75–104

Fuechtner, Veronika, *Berlin Psychoanalytic: Psychoanalysis and Culture in Weimar Republic Germany* (Berkeley: University of California Press, 2011)

Furst, Lilian R., *Just Talk: Narratives of Psychoanalysis* (Lexington: University Press of Kentucky, 1999)

Galassi, Silviana, *Kriminologie im Deutschen Kaiserreich. Geschichte einer gebrochenen Verwissenschaftlichung* (Stuttgart: Franz Steiner, 2004)

Gammel, Irene, *Sexualizing Power in Naturalism: Theodor Dreiser and Frederick Philip Grove* (Calgary: University of Calgary Press, 1994)

Giddens, Anthony, *The Transformation of Intimacy: Sexuality, Love and Eroticism in Modern Societies* (Stanford: Stanford University Press, 1992)

Gliboff, Sander, *H. G. Bronn, Ernst Hackel, and the Origins of German Darwinism: A Study in Translation and Transformation* (Cambridge: MIT Press, 2008)

Gratzke, Michael, *Liebesschmerz und Textlust. Figuren der Liebe und des Masochismus in der Literatur* (Würzburg: Könighausen & Neumann, 1997)

Greenacre, Phyllis, 'The Impostor', *Psychoanalytic Quarterly*, 27 (1958), pp. 359–82

Greenberg, Udi E., 'Criminalization. Carl Schmitt and Walter Benjamin's Concept of Criminal Politics', *Journal of European Studies*, 39:3 (2009), pp. 305–19

Greve, Ylva, *Verbrechen und Krankheit: die Entdeckung der 'Criminalpsychologie' im 19. Jahrhundert* (Cologne: Böhlau, 2004)

Grundmann, Reiner and Nico Stehr, *Experts: The Knowledge and Power of Expertise* (New York: Routledge, 2011)

Guenther, Katja, *Localization and Its Discontents: A Genealogy of Psychoanalysis and the Neuro Disciplines* (Chicago: University of Chicago Press, 2015)

Gundlach, Horst, 'Germany', in David B. Baker, *The Oxford Handbook of the History of Psychology: Global Perspectives* (Oxford: Oxford University Press, 2012), pp. 255–88

Habermas, Jürgen, *The Structural Transformation of the Public Sphere: An Inquiry into Category of Bourgeois Society*, trans. Thomas Burger (Cambridge: MIT Press, 1989)

Habermas, Jürgen, 'What Is Universal Pragmatics?', in Thomas McCarthy (ed.), *Communication and the Evolution of Society* (London: Heinemann, 1979), pp. 1–68

Habermas, Rebekka, *Frauen und Männer des Bürgertums. Eine Familiengeschichte (1750–1850)* (Göttingen: Vandenhoeck & Ruprecht, 2000)

Hacking, Ian, 'Between Michel Foucault and Erving Goffman: Between Discourse in the Abstract and Face-to-Face Interaction', *Economy and Society*, 33:3 (2004), pp. 277–302.

Hacking, Ian, 'Language, Truth, and Reason', in *Historical Ontology* (Cambridge: Harvard University Press, 2002), pp. 159–77

Hale, Nathan G., *The Rise and Crisis of Psychoanalysis in the United States: Freud and the Americans, 1917–1985* (Oxford: Oxford University Press, 1995)

Hauser, Renate, 'Einleitung', in Richard von Krafft-Ebing, *Eine Studienreise durch Südeuropa 1869/70*, ed. Renate Hauser (Graz: Leykam, 2000), pp. 10–19

Hawkins, Anne Hunsaker, *Reconstructing Illness: Studies in Pathography*, 2nd edition (West Lafayette: Purdue University Press, 1999)

Herzog, Todd, 'Crime Stories: Criminal, Society, and the Modernist Case History', *Representations*, 80 (2002), pp. 34–61

Herzog, Todd, *Crime Stories: Criminalistic Fantasy and the Culture of Crisis in Weimar Germany* (New York: Berghahn, 2009)

Hett, Benjamin Carter, *Death in the Tiergarten: Murder and Criminal Justice in the Kaiser's Berlin* (Cambridge: Harvard University Press, 2004)

Hilken, Susanne, Matthias Bormuth and Michael Schmidt-Degenhard, 'Psychiatrische Anfänge der Pathographie', in Matthias Bormuth, Klaus Podoll and Carsten Spitzer (eds), *Kunst und Krankheit. Studien zur Pathographie* (Göttingen: Wallstein, 2007), pp. 11–26

Hilliard, Russell B. and Robert L. Spitzer, 'Letter to the Editor: Change in Criterion of Paraphilias in DSM-IV-TR', *American Journal of Psychiatry*, 157:7 (2002), p. 1249, http://ajp.psychiatryonline.org/article.aspx?Volume=159&page=1249&journal ID =13, accessed 31 August 2012

Hoff, Paul, *Emil Kraepelin und die Psychiatrie als klinische Wissenschaft* (Berlin: Springer, 1994)

Houlbrook, Matt, 'Commodifying the Self Within: Ghosts, Libels, and the Crook Life Story in Interwar Britain', *Journal of Modern History*, 85:2 (2013), pp. 321–63

Hunter, Kathryn Montgomery, *Doctors' Stories: The Narrative Structure of Medical Knowledge* (Princeton: Princeton University Press, 1991)

Hutcheon, Linda, *A Theory of Parody: The Teachings of Twentieth-Century Art Forms* (New York: Methuen, 1985)

Jacobs, Joela, '*Verbrechen wider die Natur.* Oskar Panizza's First Encounter with Censorship', in Godela Weiss-Sussex and Charlotte Woodford (eds), *Protest and Reform in German Literature and Visual Culture, 1871–1918* (Munich: Iudicium, 2015), pp. 125–38

Jolles, André, *Einfache Formen. Legende, Sage, Mythe, Rätsel, Spruch, Kasus, Memorabile, Märchen, Witz* (Tübingen: Max Niemeyer, 1930)

Jonas, Gilbert, *Freedom's Sword: The NAACP and the Struggle Against Racism in America, 1909–1969* (New York: Routledge, 2005)

Jones, Ernest, *Sigmund Freud Life and Work, vol. 2: Years of Maturity 1901–1919* (London: Hogarth Press, 1955)

Kelly, Alfred, *The Descent of Darwin: The Popularization of Darwinism in Germany, 1860–1914* (Chapel Hill: University of North Carolina Press, 1981)

Killen, Andreas, *Berlin Electropolis: Shock, Nerves, and German Modernity* (Berkeley: University of California Press, 2006)

Kimmerle, Gerd (ed.), *Zur Theorie der psychoanalytischen Fallgeschichte* (Tübingen: Diskort, 1988)

Koch, Ruth, 'Der Kasus und A. Jolles' Theorie von den "Einfachen Formen"', *Fabula*, 14:3 (1973), pp. 194–204

Könemann, Sophia, 'Von "Menschen-Bälgen", "kostbaren Rassen" und "Canarienvögeln": Fetischismus in Oskar Panizzas Erzählung "Der Corsetten-Fritz"', in Sophia Könemann and Anne Stähr (eds), *Das Geschlecht der Anderen. Figuren der Alterität: Kriminologie, Psychiatrie, Ethnologie und Zoologie* (Bielefeld: Transcript, 2011), pp. 171–86

Köpke, Wulf, *The Critical Reception of Alfred Döblin's Major Novels* (Rochester: Camden House, 2003)

Kraepelin, Emil, *Psychiatrie: ein Lehrbuch für Studirende und Aerzte*, 6th edition (Leipzig: Barth, 1899)

Lang, Birgit, 'Translation as Transposition. Leopold von Sacher-Masoch, Darwinian Thought, and the Concept of Love in German Sexual Modernity', in Heike Bauer (ed.), *Sexology and Translation: Cultural and Scientific Encounters* (Philadelphia: Temple University Press, 2015), pp. 19–35.

Lang, Birgit and Katie Sutton, 'The Aesthetics of Sexual Ethics: *Geschlecht und Gesellschaft* and Middle-Class Sexual Modernity in *Fin-de-siècle* Germany', *Oxford German Studies*, 44:2 (2015), pp. 177–98

Lees, Andrew, *Cities, Sin, and Social Reform in Imperial Germany* (Ann Arbor: University of Michigan Press, 2002)

Lehan, Richard Daniel, *Realism and Naturalism: The Novel in an Age of Transition* (Madison: University of Wisconsin Press, 2005)

Leitner, Marina, *Ein gut gehütetes Geheimnis. Die Geschichte der psychoanalytischen Behandlungs-Technik von den Anfängen in Wien bis zur Gründung der Berliner Poliklinik im Jahr 1920* (Gießen: Psychosozial-Verlag, 2001), pp. 13–19

Leitner, Marina, *Freud, Rank und die Folgen. Ein Schlüsselbegriff für die Psychoanalyse* (Vienna: Turia und Kant, 1998)

Lensing, Leo, '"Freud and the Child Woman" or "The Kraus Affair"? Textual "Reconstruction" of Fritz Wittels's Psychoanalytic Autobiography', *The German Quarterly*, 69 (1996), pp. 322–32

Lieberman, E. James, *Acts of Will: The Life and Work of Otto Rank* (New York: Free Press, 1985)

Linder, Joachim, '"Sie müssen das entschuldigen Herr Staatsanwalt, aber es ist so: Wir trauen Euch nicht…": Strafjustiz, Strafrechtsreform und Justizkritik im März, 1907–1911', in Jörg Schönert (ed.), *Erzählte Kriminalität: Zur Typologie und Funktion von narrativen Darstellungen in Strafrechtspflege, Publizistik und Literatur* (Tübingen: Niemeyer, 1991), pp. 533–70

Lothane, Henry Zvi, 'Romancing Psychiatry: Paul Schreber, Otto Gross, Oskar

Panizza – Personal, Social and Forensic Aspects', in Werber Felber, Albrecht Götz von Olenhusen, Gottfried Maria Heuer and Bernd Nitzschke (eds), *Psychoanalyse und Expressionismus. 7. Internationaler Otto-Gross-Kongress, Dresden* (Marburg: LiteraturWissenschaft.de, 2010), pp. 461–93

Lukács, Georg, *The Historical Novel*, trans. Hannah Mitchell and Stanley Mitchell (London: Merlin, 1978)

Lukács, Georg, 'The Playful Style,' in *Essays on Thomas Mann*, trans. Stanley Mitchell (New York: Howard Fertig, 1978), pp. 98–134

Lynn, David J. and George E. Vaillant, 'Anonymity, Neutrality, and Confidentiality in the Actual Methods of Sigmund Freud: A Review of 43 Cases, 1907–1939', *American Journal of Psychiatry*, 155:2 (1998), pp. 163–71

Madea, Burkhard, 'Case Histories in Forensic Medicine', *Forensic Science International*, 165 (2007), pp. 111–14

Madsen, Ole Jacob, '"I am a philosopher of the particular case": An Interview with the 2009 Holberg Prizewinner Ian Hacking', *History of the Human Sciences*, 26:3 (2013), pp. 32–51

Mak, Geertje, *Doubting Sex: Inscriptions, Bodies and Selves in Nineteenth-Century Hermaphrodite Case Histories* (Manchester: Manchester University Press, 2012)

May, Ulrike, 'Ein Traum (1897) und ein Brief (1902): Zur frühen Beziehung zwischen Freud und Isidor Sadger', *Luzifer-Amor. Zeitschrift zur Geschichte der Psychoanalyse*, 12:24 (1999), pp. 25–48

May-Tolzmann, Ulrike, 'Zu den Anfängen des Narzißmus: Ellis – Näcke – Sadger – Freud', *Luzifer-Amor. Zeitschrift zur Geschichte der Psychoanalyse*, 4:8 (1991), pp. 50–88

McGuire, William (ed.), *The Freud/Jung Letters: The Correspondence Between Sigmund Freud and C. G. Jung* (Princeton: Princeton University Press, 1974)

Michaud, Stéphane, 'L'exception allemande, ou quelques questions au naturalisme européen', *Revue histoire de la littéraire de la France*, 103:3 (2003), pp. 591–6

Michler, Werner, *Darwinismus und Literatur. Naturwissenschaftliche und literarische Intelligenz in* Österreich, *1859–1914* (Vienna: Böhlau, 1999)

Mitscherlich-Nielsen, Margarete, 'Sittlichkeit und Kriminalität. Psychoanalytische Bemerkungen zu Karl Kraus', *Psyche*, 29:2 (1975), pp. 131–53

Mosse, George L., *Nationalism and Sexuality: Respectability and Abnormal Sexuality in Europe* (New York: Fertig, 1985)

Müller, Jürgen, *Der Pazjent als Psychiater: Oskar Panizzas Weg vom Irrenarzt zum Insassen* (Bonn: Narrenschiff, 1999)

Müller, Jürgen, 'Oskar Panizza: Psychiatrist, Antipsychiatrist, Patient. The Man Behind Emil Kräpelin's Case Report on "Paraphrenias"', *International Journal of Psychiatry in Clinical Practice*, 4:4 (2000), pp. 335–8

Müller, Klaus, *Aber in meinem Herzen sprach eine Stimme so laut: homosexuelle Autobiographien und medizinische Pathographien im neunzehnten Jahrhundert* (Berlin: Rosa Winkel, 1991)

Nitzschke, Bernd, *Die Psychoanalyse Sigmund Freuds: Konzepte und Begriffe* (Wiesbaden: VS Verlag, 2011)

Noll, Richard, *American Madness: The Rise and Fall of Dementia Praecox* (Cambridge: Harvard University Press, 2011)

Noyes, John K., *The Mastery of Submission: Inventions of Masochism* (Ithaca: Cornell University Press, 1997)

Oosterhuis, Harry, 'Sexual Modernity in the Works of Richard von Krafft-Ebing and Albert Moll', *Medical History*, 56:2 (2012), pp. 133–55

Oosterhuis, Harry, *Stepchildren of Nature: Krafft-Ebing, Psychiatry, and the Making of Sexual Identity* (Chicago: University of Chicago Press, 2000)

Paslawski, Teresa, 'Case Study Research in Medicine', in Albert J. Mills, Gabrielle Durepos and Elden Wiebe (eds), *Encyclopedia of Case Study Research* (London: Sage, 2010), pp. 107–9

Person, Jutta, *Der pathographische Blick. Physiognomik, Atavismustheorien und Kulturkritik* (Würzburg: Königshausen & Neumann, 2005)

Peukert, Detlev, *Weimar Germany* (New York: Hill & Wang, 1992)

Phiddian, Robert, 'Satire and the Limits of Literary Theory', *Critical Theory*, 55:3 (2013), pp. 44–58

Polubojarinowa, Larissa, 'Österreichischer Realismus als ein Problem der Literaturgeschichte (Leopold von Sacher-Masoch, Maria von Ebner-Eschenbach)', in Werner Wiesinger (ed.), *Akten des X. Internationalen Germanistenkongresses Wien 2000. Epochenbegriffe. Grenzen und Möglichkeiten* (Bern: Lang, 2002), pp. 477–82

Pope, Rob, *Creativity. Theory, History, Practice* (New York: Routledge, 2005)

Rakoff, Todd D. and Martha Minow, 'A Case for Another Case Method', *Vanderbilt Law Review*, 60:2 (2007), pp. 597–607

Rimmon-Kennan, Shlomith, *Discourse in Psychoanalysis and Literature* (Routledge Revivals) (Hoboken: Taylor & Francis, 2014)

Ringer, Fritz, *The Decline of the German Mandarins: The German Academic Community, 1890–1933* (Hanover: University Press of New England, 1969)

Robertson, Stephen, 'What's Law Got To Do With It? Legal Records and Sexual Histories', *Journal of the History of Sexuality*, 14:1/2 (2005), pp. 161–85

Rohrwasser, Michael, *Freuds Lektüren. Von Arthur Conan Doyle bis zu Arthur Schnitzler* (Gießen: Psychosozial-Verlag, 2005)

Rosario, Vernon A., *The Erotic Imagination: French Histories of Perversity* (New York: Oxford University Press, 1997)

Rose, Louis, *The Freudian Calling: Early Viennese Psychoanalysis and the Pursuit of Cultural Science* (Detroit: Wayne State University Press, 1998)

Rudnytsky, Peter, *Reading Psychoanalysis: Freud, Rank, Ferenczi, Groddeck* (Ithaca: Cornell University Press, 2002)

Rudnytsky, Peter, *The Psychoanalytic Vocation: The Legacy of Otto Rank and Donald Winnicott* (New Haven: Yale University Press, 1991)

Sauerteig, Lutz D. H., 'Loss of Innocence: Albert Moll, Sigmund Freud and the Invention of Childhood Sexuality Around 1900', *Medical History*, 56:2 (2012), pp. 156–83

Savoia, Paolo, 'Sexual Science and Self-narrative: Epistemology and Narrative Technologies of the Self Between Krafft-Ebing and Freud', *History of the Human Sciences*, 23:5 (2010), pp. 17–41

Schachter, Judith S., and Hugh F. Butts, 'Transference and Countertransference in Interracial Analyses', *Journal of the American Psychoanalytic Association*, 16:4 (1968), pp. 792–808

Schaffner, Anna Katharina, *Modernism and Perversion: Sexual Deviance in Sexology and Literature, 1850–1930* (Basingstoke: Palgrave Macmillan, 2012)

Schäffner, Wolfgang, *Die Ordnung des Wahns: Zur Poetologie psychiatrischen Wissens bei Alfred Döblin* (Munich: Wilhelm Fink, 1995)

Schauz, Desiree and Sabine Freitag (eds), *Verbrecher im Visier der Experten: Kriminalpolitik zwischen Wissenschaft und Praxis im 19. und frühen 20. Jahrhundert* (Stuttgart: Steiner, 2007)

Sealey, Anne, 'The Strange Case of the Freudian Case History. The Role of Long Case Histories in the Development of Psychoanalysis', *History of the Human Sciences*, 24:1 (2011), pp. 36–50

Shaklan, Steven Brett, '"So Many Foreign and Useless Words!" Ivan Turgenev's Poetics of Negation', in Robert Reid and Joe Andrew (eds), *Turgenev: Art, Ideology and Legacy* (Amsterdam: Rodopi, 2010), pp. 41–60

Siebenpfeiffer, Hania, *'Böse Lust': Gewaltverbrechen in Diskursen der Weimarer Republik* (Cologne: Böhlau, 2005)

Siemens, Daniel, 'Explaining Crime. Berlin Newspapers and the Construction of the Criminal in Weimar Germany', *Journal of European Studies*, 39:3 (2009), pp. 336–52

Sigusch, Volkmar, 'Erich Wulffen', in Volkmar Sigusch and Günter Grau (eds), *Personenlexikon der Sexualforschung* (Frankfurt: Campus, 2009), pp. 783–8

Simpson, Paul, *On the Discourse of Satire: Towards a Stylistic Model of Satirical Humour* (Amsterdam: John Benjamins, 2003)

Sprengel, Peter, *Darwin in der Poesie. Spuren der Evolutionslehre in der deutschsprachigen Literatur des 19. und 20. Jahrhunderts* (Würzburg: Könighausen und Neumann, 1998)

Springman, Luke, 'Poisoned Hearts, Diseased Minds, and American Pimps: The Language of Censorship in the *Schund und Schmutz* Debates', *German Quarterly*, 68:4 (1995), pp. 408–29

Stark, Gary D., 'Trials and Tribulations: Authors' Responses to Censorship in Imperial Germany, 1885–1914', *German Studies Review*, 12:3 (1989), pp. 447–68

Steinberg, Holger, *'Als ob ich zu einer steinernen Wand spräche'. Der Nervenarzt Paul Julius Möbius. Eine Werkbiografie* (Bern: Huber, 2005)

Steinberg, Holger, *Kraepelin in Leipzig. Eine Begegnung von Psychiatrie und Psychologie* (Bonn: Narrenschiff, 2001)

Strozier, Charles B. and Daniel Offer, 'Freud and His Followers', in Charles B. Strozier and Oliger Abdyli (eds), *The Leader: Psychological Essays* (New York: Springer, 2011), pp. 13–30

Sulloway, Frank J., 'Reassessing Freud's Case Histories. The Social Construction of Psychoanalysis', *Isis*, 82 (1991), pp. 245–75

Sutton, Katie, 'Sexual Pathologies and the Violence of War: Sexological and Psychoanalytic Responses to World War I', *Limbus: Australian Yearbook of German Literary and Cultural Studies*, 7 (2014), pp. 197–218

Tatar, Maria, *Lustmord: Sexual Murder in Weimar Germany* (Princeton: Princeton University Press, 1995)

Timms, Edward (ed.), *Freud and the Child Woman: The Memoirs of Fritz Wittels* (New Haven: Yale University Press, 1995)

Timms, Edward, *Karl Kraus, Apocalyptic Satirist. Culture and Catastrophe in Habsburg Vienna* (New Haven: Yale University Press, 1986)

Timms, Edward, 'The "Child-Woman": Kraus, Freud, Wittels, and Irma Karczewska in Fin-de-Siécle Vienna', in Edward Timms and Ritchie Robertson (eds), *Vienna 1900: From Altenberg to Wittgenstein* (Edinburgh: Edinburgh University Press, 1990), pp. 87–107

Üding, Gert and Bernd Steinbrink, *Grundriss der Rhetorik. Geschichte – Technik – Methode* (Stuttgart: Metzler, 2011)

Uhl, Karsten, *Das 'verbrecherische Weib'. Geschlecht, Verbrechen und Strafen im kriminologischen Diskurs 1800–1945* (Münster: LIT, 2003)

Vanheule, Stijn, *Subject of Psychosis: A Lacanian Perspective* (Basingstoke: Palgrave Macmillan, 2011)

Verney, Kevern and Lee Sartain (eds), *Long Is the Way and Hard: One Hundred Years of the National Association for the Advancement of Colored People (NAACP)* (Fayetteville: University of Arkansas Press, 2009)

Warner, Michael, 'Publics and Counterpublics', *Public Culture*, 14:1 (2002), pp. 49–90

Weikart, Richard, *From Darwin to Hitler: Evolutionary Ethics, Eugenics, and Racism in Germany* (Basingstoke: Palgrave Macmillan, 2009)

Weindling, Paul, 'Bourgeois Values, Doctors and the State', in David Blackbourn and Richard J. Evans (eds), *The German Bourgeoisie* (New York: Routledge, 1991), pp. 198–223

Wetzell, Richard F., *Inventing the Criminal: A History of German Criminology, 1880–1945* (Chapel Hill: University of North Carolina Press, 2000)

Wetzell, Richard F., 'Psychiatry and Criminal Justice in Modern Germany, 1880–1933', *Journal of European Studies*, 39 (2009), pp. 270–89

Whitney, Davis, *Queer Beauty: Sexuality and Aesthetics from Winckelmann to Freud and Beyond* (New York: Columbia University Press, 2010)

Williams, Linda Ruth, *Critical Desire: Psychoanalysis and the Literary Subject* (London: Edward Arnold, 1995)

Zimmermann, Christian von, *Biographische Anthropologie. Menschenbilder in lebensgeschichtlicher Darstellung (1830–1940)* (Berlin: de Gruyter, 2006)

Index